Ciro Esposito · Philippe Montupet · Steven Rothenberg (Eds.

Gastroesophageal Reflux in Infants and Children

Diagnosis, Medical Therapy, Surgical Management

Springer-Verlag Berlin Heidelberg GmbH

Ciro Esposito · Philippe Montupet · Steven Rothenberg (Eds.)

Gastroesophageal Reflux in Infants and Children

Diagnosis, Medical Therapy, Surgical Management

With 78 Figures, 35 in Color and 23 Tables

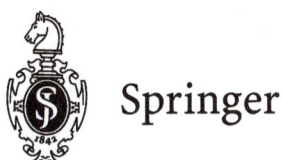

Springer

Ciro Esposito
Chair of Pediatric Surgery
Department of Clinical and Experimental Medicine
Magna Graecia University of Catanzaro
Via Tommaso Campanella 115
88100 Catanzaro, Italy

Philippe Montupet
University Paris XI
7 Rue du Laos
70015 Paris, France

Steven Rothenberg
Mother and Child Hospital at Presbyterian/
St Lukes Medical Center
Denver, Colorado, USA

Additional material to this book can be downloaded from http:// extras.springer.com.

ISBN 978-3-642-62349-3   ISBN 978-3-642-18906-7 (eBook)
DOI 10.1007/978-3-642-18906-7

Library of Congress Cataloging-in-Publication Data

Bibliographic information published by Die Deutsche Bibliothek
Die Deutsche Bibliothek lists this publication in the Deutsche Nationalbibliografie;
detailed bibliographic data is available in the Internet at http://dnb.ddb.de

Springer-Verlag is a part of Springer Science+Business Media

springeronline.com

© Springer-Verlag Berlin Heidelberg 2004
Originally published by Springer-Verlag Berlin Heidelberg New York 2004

Editor: Gabriele M. Schröder, Heidelberg, Germany
Desk Editor: Stephanie Benko, Heidelberg, Germany
Production: ProEdit GmbH, 69126 Heidelberg, Germany
Cover: Frido Steinen-Broo, EStudio Calamar, Spain
Typesetting: K. Detzner, 67346 Speyer, Germany

Printed on acid-free paper   21/3150 ML   5 4 3 2 1 0

It was a pleasure reading the excellent articles of the many distinguished experts who contributed to this excellent volume on *The Gastroesophageal Reflux in Infants and Children* edited by Professors Ciro Esposito, Philippe Montupet, and Steven Rothenberg.

Knowledge in the biomedical and surgical sciences changes at an ever increasing rate. In the specific field of gastroesophageal reflux in children, the newly developed knowledge is impressive in terms of both results – recovery from reflux – and acceptance by patients and families and their pediatricians.

With the explosive development of modern biomedical science, medical and surgical practices become more and more specialized, thus increasing the need for focusing, in the recent literature, on specific issues. At the same time specialized issues require multidisciplinary interactions: pediatric surgeons, pediatricians, radiologists, pediatric gastroenterologists and others must cooperate as a team. For this reason, this volume is targeted not only at pediatric surgeons and pediatricians, but also at several other types of specialists.

As pediatricians, our main concern is child care, but we also have been and will be involved in teaching as required by the modern interactive methods of teaching/learning. At the same time we should not lose sight of the fact that these are not distinct areas of activity and that they must go hand-in-hand with a research-oriented environment. The quality of each of the three – child care, education, research – is improved through interaction. Obviously, this is not to say that every single pediatrician or pediatric surgeon will be involved in all three types of activity; it is only meant as a plea for the maintenance of free communication and integration among these three systems and types of activity in the pediatric field. We all need to work on maintaining strong links among research, teaching, and health care.

This work by Ciro Esposito, Philippe Montupet and Steven Rothenberg is a nice example of how production of new scientific knowledge, transmission of newly produced knowledge and application of newly developed principles, methods and techniques to practice may find an excellent synthesis for the common benefit of the researchers, educators, and practicing specialists engaged in the field.

Armido Rubino
Department of Pediatrics,
School of Medicine
University of Naples Federico II

The idea to write this book had its initial spark in May 2002 after the IPEG Meeting in Genoa.

The editors' aim was to create a book focused on gastroesophageal reflux disease (GERD) in pediatric patients in which there was a collaboration between pediatricians, pediatric surgeons, pediatric gastroenterologists and other specialists involved in the care of children affected by this pathology.

Over the past 10 years, a revolution has taken place in the management of infants and children affected by GERD. With the development of new medical treatments (proton pump inhibitors) as well as significant advancements in the field of pediatric surgery with advanced laparoscopic techniques, the management of GERD has changed dramatically.

The purpose of this book is to inform pediatricians and pediatric surgeons about commonly used diagnostic, medical and surgical procedures now adopted in children with GERD. We believe that this book meets the needs of all the physicians who wish to deepen their understanding and get "up to date" with GERD in infants and children.

All the authors who have participated in this project are considered leading world experts in the management of children with GERD, and we are extremely grateful to them for their participation and for devoting the time required to produce such outstanding reviews.

We think that it is important that pediatric surgeons continue to collaborate closely with pediatric gastroenterologists for the best treatment of the children and infants affected by GERD. Only a combined approach with thorough evaluation, sound clinical judgement and meticulous surgical care can help us improve this part of child care with good functional results and without complications.

Ciro Esposito, Philippe Montupet, Steven Rothenberg

Contents

List of Contributors

Peter Ahrens
Darmstädter Kinderkliniken Prinzessin Margaret
Dieburgerstr. 31
64876 Darmstadt
Germany

Craig T. Albanese
Department Of Surgery
HSW 1601513 Parnassus Ave.
San Francisco
CA 94143–0570
USA

Hossein Allal
Pediatric Surgery Unit
CHU Montpellier
Montpellier
France

Giuseppe Amici
Pediatric Surgery
Unversity of Ancona
Via Corridoni 11
60123 Ancona
Italy

Giuseppe Ascione
Pediatric Surgery
"Federico II" University
Via Pansini 5
80131 Naples
Italy

Renata Auricchio
Department of Pediatrics
"Federico II" University
Via Pansini 5
80131 Naples
Italy

Nicolas M. A. Bax
Wilhelmina Children's Hospital
University Medical Center Utrecht
Utrecht
The Netherlands

Francois Becmeur
Service de Chirurgie Infantile
CHU Hautepierre
Avenue Moliere
67098 Strasbourg
France

Fares Benmiloud
La Timone Children's Hospital
Rue Saint-Pierre, 264
13385 Marseille cedex 5
France

Adrian Bianchi
The Royal Manchester Children's Hospital
Pendlebury M27 4HA
UK

Gabriella Boccia
Department of Pediatrics
"Federico II" University
Via Pansini 5
80131 Naples
Italy

Patrick Bontems
Department of Gastroenterology-Hepatology
Queen Fabiola Children's Hospital
Free University of Brussels
Brussels
Belgium

Osvaldo Borrelli
Department of Pediatrics
Division of Pediatric Gastroenterology
University of Rome "La Sapienza"
Viale Regina Elena 324
00161 Rome
Italy

Jesus Broto
Valle de Hebrón Hospital
Autonomous University
Barcelona
Spain

Samy Cadranel
Department of Gastroenterology-Hepatology
Queen Fabiola Children's Hospital
Free University of Brussels
Brussels
Belgium

Francesco S. Camoglio
·Pediatric Surgery
University of Verona
Verona
Italy

Guillaume A. Cargill
Centre d'Explorations Fonctionnelles Digestives
77 rue Vergniaud
F 75013 Paris
France

Marco Castagnetti
La Timone Children's Hospital
Rue Saint-Pierre, 264
13385 Marseille cedex 5
France

Moti M. Chowdhury
Department of Paediatric Surgery
Institute of Child Health
30, Guilford Street
London WC1N 1EH
UK

Ray E. Clouse
Division of Gastroenterology
Washington University School of Medicine
St Louis
Missouri
USA

Salvatore Cucchiara
Department of Pediatrics
Division of Pediatric Gastroenterology
University of Rome "La Sapienza"
Viale Regina Elena 324
00161 Rome
Italy

Marcello Dòmini
Department of Pediatric Surgery
University of Bologna
S.Orsola-Malpighi Hospital
Via Massarenti 11
40138 Bologna
Italy

Ciro Esposito
Chair of Pediatric Surgery
Department of Clinical and Experimental Medicine
Magna Graecia University of Catanzaro
Via Tommaso Campanella 115
88100 Catanzaro
Italy

Giovanni Esposito
Pediatric Surgery
"Federico II" University
Via Pansini 5
80131 Naples
Italy

José Estevão-Costa
Division of Pediatric Surgery
Faculty of Medicine of Porto
Hospital S. João
4200–319 Porto
Portugal

Luca Giacomello
Pediatric Surgery
University of Verona
Verona
Italy

Jean-Michel Guys
La Timone Children's Hospital
Rue Saint-Pierre, 264
13385 Marseille cedex 5
France

Nigel Hall
Department of Paediatric Surgery
Institute of Child Health
30, Guilford Street
London WC1N 1EH
UK

Bruno Hauser
AZ Kinderen-Vrije Universiteit Brussel
Laarbeeklaan 101
1090 Brussels
Belgium

Paul Hyman
Pediatric Gastroenterology
Kansas University Medical Center
Children's Center
3901 Rainbow Blvd.
Kansas City, KS 66160
USA

Vincenzo Jasonni
Department of Surgery
School of Paediatric Surgery
Giannina Gaslini Research Institute for Children
University of Genoa
Genoa
Italy

Tarun Kumar
University of Tennessee, Memphis
777 Washington Avenue, P220
Memphis, TN 38105
USA

Jacob C. Langer
Hospital for Sick Children
5555 University Ave
Toronto, ON M5G 1X8
Canada

Antonio Leggio
Pediatric Surgery
University of Bari
Bari
Italy

Mario Lima
Department of Pediatric Surgery
University of Bologna
S.Orsola-Malpighi Hospital
Via Massarenti 11
40138 Bologna
Italy

Thom E. Lobe
University of Tennessee at Memphis
777 Washington Avenue, Suite P220
Memphis, TN 38105
USA

Carlo Di Lorenzo
Children's Hospital of Pittsburgh
Department of Pediatric Gastroenterology
3705 Fifth Avenue at De Soto Street
Pittsburgh, PA 15213
USA

Girolamo Mattioli
Department of Surgery
School of Paediatric Surgery
Giannina Gaslini Research Institute for Children
University of Genoa
Genoa
Italy

Peter J. Milla
Gastroenterology Unit
Institute of Child Health
University College
London
United Kingdom

Stephen Miller
Department of Radiology
Hospital for Sick Children
Toronto, Ontario
Canada

Philippe Montupet
University Paris XI
7 Rue du Laos
70015 Paris
France

Azad Najmaldin
Pediatric Surgery
St. James University Hospital
Leeds, LS2 9JT
UK

Emanuele Nicolai
SDN – Napoli
Via Gianturco 113
80131 Naples
Italy

Jose Boix Ochoa
Valle de Hebrón Hospital
Autonomous University
Barcelona
Spain

Pedro Olivares
Hospital Infantil La Paz
Madrid
Spain

Susan R. Orenstein
Pediatric Gastroenterology
Children's Hospital of Pittsburgh
One Children's Place
Pittsburgh, PA 15213-2583
USA

Alberto Ottolenghi
Pediatric Surgery
University of Verona
Verona
Italy

Anna Pasquini
Pediatric Surgery
University of Verona
Verona
Italy

Gabriella Pelusi
Department of Pediatric Surgery
University of Bologna
S.Orsola-Malpighi Hospital
Via Massarenti 11
40138 Bologna
Italy

Agostino Pierro
Department of Paediatric Surgery
Institute of Child Health
30, Guilford Street
London WC1N 1EH
UK

Ashwin Pimpalwar
Department of Pediatric Surgery
The Leeds Teaching Hospitals NHS Trust
Leeds
UK

Carmelo Romeo
Unit of Neonatal Surgery
Department of Medical and Surgical Pediatric Sciences
University of Messina
Messina
Italy

Steven Rothenberg
Mother and Child Hospital at Presbyterian/
St Lukes Medical Center
Denver
Colorado
USA

Giovanni Ruggeri
Department of Pediatric Surgery
University of Bologna
S.Orsola-Malpighi Hospital
Via Massarenti 11
40138 Bologna
Italy

Mahmoud Sabri
Children's Hospital of Pittsburgh
Department of Pediatric Gastroenterology
3705 Fifth Avenue at De Soto Street
Pittsburgh, PA 15213
USA

Marco Salvatore
Department of Biomorphological Sciences
Faculty of Medicine
University of Naples Federico II
Naples
Italy

Silvia Salvatore
AZ Kinderen-Vrije Universiteit Brussel
Laarbeeklaan 101
1090 Brussels
Belgium

Michèle Scaillon
Department of Gastroenterology-Hepatology
Queen Fabiola Children's Hospital
Free University of Brussels
Brussels
Belgium

Jurgen Schleef
Clinic of Pedriatic Surgery,
Graz University Medical School
Auenbruggerplatz 34,
Graz 8010
Austria

Alessandro Settimi
Pediatric Surgery
"Federico II" University
Via Pansini 5
80131 Naples
Italy

Andrea Soricelli
Diagnostic Imaging
Faculty of Sciences of Movement
University of Naples Parthenope
Naples
Italy

Annamaria Staiano
Department of Pediatrics
University of Naples "Federico II"
Naples
Italy

Isabelle Talon
Service de Chirurgie Infantile
CHU Hautpierre
Avenue Moliere
67098 Strasbourg
France

Juan A. Tovar
Department of Pediatric Surgery
Hospital Universitario "La Paz"
Paseo de la Castellana, 261
28046
Madrid
Spain

Jean Stephane Valla
Service de Chirurgie Pediatrique
Hopital Lenval
57 Avenue de la Californie
06200 Nice
France

Enrico Valletta
Pediatric Surgery
University of Verona
Verona
Italy

Yvan Vandenplas
AZ Kinderen-Vrije Universiteit Brussel
Laarbeeklaan 101
1090 Brussels
Belgium

David C. van der Zee
Wilhelmina Children's Hospital
University Medical Center Utrecht
Utrecht
The Netherlands

Biagio Zuccarello
Unit of Neonatal Surgery
Department of Medical and Surgical Pediatric Sciences
University of Messina
Messina
Italy

Part I
General

Chapter 1

Introduction

Guillaume A. Cargill

1

Gastroesophageal reflux (GER) is a frequent pathology in children, affecting as much as 30% of the pediatric population (very close to its incidence in adults). However, despite its frequency and, theoretically, its customary mildness, it has a complex pathology and is therefore not easily manageable. As a matter of fact, GER may give origin to disabling and even severe conditions: recurrent otitis – which may lead to decreased hearing ability and induced pulmonary pathology – which may result in severe disabling asthma and, as a consequence, respiratory failure, and specific pediatric diseases that may sometimes range from severe to extremely severe. Furthermore, this pathology may also lead to esophageal complications such as peptic esophagitis or even Barrett's esophagus – a potential cause of esophageal cancer. Lastly, we now know that reflux disease, independently of Barrett's esophagus, is a carcinogenic factor. Needless to say, such relevance requires accurate evaluation.

Its complexity may also derive from its multiple clinical presentations, which are in some cases obvious – as in the presence of postprandial regurgitations, although more often they are difficult to interpret – as in the case of painful colicky pain suggestive of esophagitis. The clinical manifestation may be more complex to interpret if the child seems to have no digestive symptoms at all. In addition, the clinical profile may become extremely complicated if upper respiratory or pulmonary symptoms prevail, or if more general symptoms, such as faintness, or allergic manifestations, such as rhinitis or asthma, are present. There are also more subtle forms, presenting as failure to thrive alone or associated with behavioral and/or feeding problems. In addition to these various clinical pictures, there are those described in patients with pathologies classically complicated by reflux disease: mentally and physically handicapped individuals, those affected by paraplegia, spastic conditions, where an insidious reflux is an important cofactor of morbidity.

The already long list of complications due to reflux disease continues to grow, since in addition to the classical ones described above we should add conjunctivitis, dental, lingual, gingival or vocal involvement, muscular conditions (torticollis) and probably some personality troubles. Moreover, we should keep in mind that stress can increase, or even give origin to reflux pathology. Lastly, some children aware of their condition may sometimes simulate aggravation of their symptoms in order to put pressure on their parents.

To further complicate things, the pathophysiology is also a bit different from the one in adults, at least in neonates, as a result of the shortness of the esophagus, and the nearly exclusive horizontal position and consumption of mainly liquid food at that age.

In addition to esophageal abnormalities such as transient lower esophageal sphincter relaxation (TLESR), poor sphincter tone, there may be problems in gastric emptying motility, esophageal motility, and upper esophageal sphincter motility. Nevertheless, we must also consider the possible association between food intolerance (intolerance to cow milk for instance) and weaning problems (perhaps introduced too early?) which may also modify gastric emptying. Along with these more or less detectable causes, the question of genetic transmission of the illness arises. The presence of reflux in first degree relatives of children (or adults) who are reflux carriers is indeed a common finding.

It is also complex for the diagnostic techniques required to assess its repercussions or explain its origin.

The radiological examination, which was for a long time the only (and imperfect) method of exploration, has given way to morphological and functional diagnostic techniques. Although the X-ray examination suffers from numerous limitations, it remains a useful tool. As a matter of fact, in some cases it remains useful, for instance, before deciding the appropriateness of surgery to search for an anatomical abnormality (malrotation, hiatal hernia, etc.). The imperfection of this method is partly linked to its achievement. There is nowadays no doubt that the distension of the gastric body favors the iterative relaxations of the lower sphincter, which can further aggravate the reflux. As a matter of fact, the radiological examination is performed during and after a barium swallow, which is, in any case, a meal. Moreover, the diagnostic methods for reflux disease are not physiological. In addition, it is not possible to establish whether the refluxes observed are physiological and thus due to TLESR, or pathological and thus due to an inefficient antireflux barrier. Against this background, it is not surprising that pH-metry developed. This test measures, through a probe, the concentration in H^+ ions in the esophagus. Initially it was employed over short periods, but it has become the gold standard in the diagnosis of reflux disease when it is performed in ambulatory conditions, thus evaluating the patient's reflux during normal living conditions over a 24-h period. There are nevertheless numerous points of debate. Firstly, there is controversy over which type of probe is more accurate, i.e., whether in antimony or glass. Secondly, there is a debate over the standards that vary according to the subject's age and which are not always properly applicable (e.g., neurologically impaired children).

As a matter of fact, when dealing with any type of reflux, it is advisable to define the problem as pathological as soon as it moves away from the standard or leads to pathological consequences. For example, I am reminded of the case of a child with unexplained faintness. The whole series of biological, cardiologic, and neurological explorations failed to explain the child's symptoms; the pH-metry was rigorously normal, although there was a distinct coincidence between faintness and reflux episodes. After three normal examinations which nevertheless consistently demonstrated the relationship between faintness and reflux symptoms, the child underwent surgery which put an end to the episodes of faintness.

In addition, there sometimes exists particular conditions. For example, we may see children with a clinically typical pathology with an esophagitis detected through endoscopy, an important reflux detected through radiological examination, but who show a normal pH-metry (because the reflux is not acid). The development of techniques such as impedancemetry, Bilitech, or examinations carried out over 2 or 3 days (cf. Bravo system in adults) will perhaps shed light on such false negative results. The endoscopy allows a simple and fast evaluation of the possible repercussions of reflux on the mucous membrane, to search for a cardiac gaping openness or a hiatus malposition, and to assess gastric integrity and pyloric permeability. Some indicators of severity may be severe malposition (hiatal hernia), intussusception of the stomach into the lower esophagus (it is often more visible with a simple sedation than with a neuroleptanalgesy), and Barrett's esophagus – where the presence of metaplasia or a dysplasia should be investigated by a whole series of biopsy samples according to a precise scheme of the taking site, which would be the first step of a long-term supervision.

The examination that still seems the most interesting to me to investigate a detected reflux is the manometry. At present, it is really the only available prospective examination to study this pathology. It enables the evalua-

tion of many parameters: the position of the lower sphincter, sphincter motility during and after swallowing, the action of the right pillar on the lower esophagus, the length of the sphincter, gastroesophageal gradient, beginning of esophageal motility [primary, linked to the deglutitions (wave amplitude, duration, speed of propagation, and morphotype), secondary or tertiary, spontaneous], upper sphincter tonus, amplitude of sphincter relaxation during swallowing, duration of the relaxation, appearance of pharyngeal contraction. This technique can be employed even in newborns if performed by a well-experienced team and with the proper equipment. The presence of severe malposition and/or hypotonicity may be indicators of significant reflux poorly amenable to medical treatment. However, while the techniques of endoscopy and pH-metry have gained ground, the manometric examination is still too much linked to the physician's experience. In a child with a clinically manifest reflux not amenable to treatment, it may seem more "profitable" to try to understand the reason of the resistance to treatment than to make a pH-metric examination that will simply confirm the reflux. The finding of a clinically severe reflux and a sphincter with a normal tone and motility in a child should suggest gastric emptying problems. Induced gastric distension could be at the origin of iterative, transitory, sphincteric relaxation (TLESR) even in a baby. Conversely, in a child affected by reflux treated with a combination of prokinetics and PPI (together with dietary and – possibly – postural treatment), with persisting reflux problems, the discovery of a sphincter with a low tonus (whether associated with malposition or not) will be at least an indication to increasing and continuing treatment, although we know that in the presence of collapsed tonus, withdrawing treatment will aggravate the problem. This is a case when the examination will help make the most suitable decision better than pH-metry or endoscopy. That decision will possibly be surgical, compatibly with the child's clinical condition. However, the value of the manometry goes much further since it is also a means to investigate possible motor troubles that represent a total or relative contraindication to surgery. It is able to detect abnormalities of the lower sphincter relaxation (achalasia), which can lead to severe swallowing problems. The condition of magaesophagus is a rare, but possible, event in children. As a matter of fact, the youngest case that has so far come to our attention was that of a 2-month-old infant. This may represent a diagnostic trap since lower sphincter abnormalities can translate into regurgitations that evoke "reflux." There are other pathologies which present contraindications to surgery: cartilaginous dysplasia of the lower esophagus, spastic motor troubles – indeed very rare in babies, hypoperistaltism in connection with a collagenosis (scleroderma) – a dysautonomia that can be combined with other motor impairments.

It is also complex as a result of its development. Indeed, the frequency of reflux is high in infancy, reaching about 30% – a rate close to that of adults in some studies (at the end of the 1970s, Sydney Cohen reported an incidence of 27% among the North American population). This observation raises a question that unfortunately still remains unanswered: is the presence of reflux in adults a consequence of a former reflux? If so, we must acknowledge that medical treatment and/or therapeutic abstention barely induce a transitory regression of the clinical outward signs, which reappear later in young adults after a decrease or a transitory period during adolescence. If not, does this suggest that as some abnormalities are corrected, others develop? Why? How?

Finally, this disease is complex also in terms of treatment, which may be only dietary, medical (prokinetic, PPI), or surgical, or a combination of these.

More suitable dietary habits consist of using meals with thicker consistency, and restricting the factors that favor reflux: parental addiction to smoking and unhealthy dietary habits (overfeeding, early weaning). We should adhere to the positional treatment. Thickeners may be either blended directly with milk or used as additives.

Prokinetic treatment is based on the use of xenobiotics that act on gastric motility, on the tonus of the lower sphincter of the esophagus, and on the contraction of the esophageal body – that is to say, on esophageal clearance. The five main products are:

1. Domperidone, which acts on gastric motility; the purely sphincteric and esophageal effect of gastric motility remains debated, but this treatment has the advantage of having few side effects.
2. Metoclopramide, which acts on motility by cholinergic, tryptaminergic, and dopaminergic mechanisms (5HT3 and 5HT4 receptors), quickens gastric emptying, improves the tonus of the lower sphincter and the motility of the esophageal body (these effects are also dose-dependent and basal-tonus-dependent); it is associated with neurological side effects.
3. Clebopride, which is not marketed in France, and has effects similar to those of metoclopramide.
4. Cisapride, which has been taken off the market in several countries for its possible association with arrhythmia; in France, it is still possible to prescribe it, even to children, under strict supervision that includes electrocardiogram and blood ionogram. This molecule is mainly active on 5HT4 receptors and, like the previous one, overcomes the clinical signs of reflux. It is as efficient as the previous one, and is dose-dependent and basal-tonus-dependent.
5. Cholinergic bethanechol is the last resort when other treatments fail. According to our experience, it seems able to correct a clear-cut hypotonicity of the lower sphincter. When prescribed for long periods it may induce lower sphincteral "maturation." For this reason, prokinetics is a logical medication for this pathology. Yet, they are often replaced by antisecretories, which mitigate or even eliminate the erosive action of gastric liquid. Nevertheless, although these treatments are useful in case of esophagitis, they do not correct the causes of reflux and do not treat non-acid regurgitations.

At last, other medical treatments, such as alginates, only have a slight effect on the reflux.

If medical treatment fails and the clinical condition is worrisome – for the presence of digestive, pulmonary, or ENT pathology – then surgery is an option. This last treatment option is still poorly accepted for its invasiveness, although the advent of coelioscopy has deeply modified the approach. Less invasiveness with identical efficacy, together with shorter hospitalization, are the current strong points of surgery. Of course, the indications for this type of treatment must be carefully evaluated to avoid failure or untoward effects. The operating technique requires the most accurate skill for permanent results. For these reasons specialized centers for this type of surgery are rather few. Nevertheless, when all the necessary conditions are met, the effects are outstanding, even on the child's psychological profile. Yet, it is important to bear in mind that the postoperative period can be marked by some difficulties, which may arise despite the surgeon's experience and the technique employed, but depend also on the careful evaluation of all indications and contraindications to the type of treatment.

On the basis of all the reasons briefly and simply described above, it seems of fundamental importance to consider the onset of such common pathology from every perspective. It should be reiterated that this condition is very often mild. It also seems useful to remember the different clinical presentations and types of investigation needed for its management as well as the medical and surgical treatment options available, which have really changed with the development of coeliosurgery. This is what the authors will do in the pages devoted to reflux disease and to its treatment. The authors will try to put the different elements of this clinical, pathophysiological, and therapeutic puzzle back in their true position.

■ **Acknowledgements.** With thanks to Marielle Audon and Jérôme J. Cargill.

Chapter 2

Anatomy of the Esophagogastric Junction

2

Giovanni Esposito · Giuseppe Amici

Contents

2.1
Introduction

The knowledge of the anatomy of the esophagogastric junction, of the contiguous structures (esophagus and stomach) and those that surround and sustain it (membranous and vascular formations, diaphragmatic pillars) is essential for understanding the physiopathology of gastroesophageal reflux disease (GERD) [5, 6].

It is therefore useful to review its morphologic characteristic, along with those of the esophagus and the stomach, not only because these organs are almost always involved to various extents in the esophagogastric junction's pathology responsible for GER, but also to understand the etiopathogenic mechanisms underlying the multifaceted symptomatology and the diverse clinical patterns of this disease, and to delineate the rudiments of the different approaches and techniques for their medical or surgical management.

2.2
The Esophagus

The esophagus (from Greek *oizo* and *phagein*) is a tubular channel basically of muscle tissue developed after the separation from the trachea, at about the third week of gestation, after the development of the cephalic primitive bowel [1, 7]. It is interposed between the pharynx, located above, and the stomach below, occupying since its origin the postero-inferior part of the neck, going down into the thorax to occupy the posterior mediastinum, finally passing through the diaphragm into the abdomen, where it ends into the stomach [2].

The opening through which the esophagus enters the stomach, called cardias, is located deep under the diaphragmatic cupola, 25 cm left of T11, although it may sometimes be at the level of T12, anteriorly to the aorta, which separates the cardias from the vertebral bodies [4].

The esophagus is ideally divided into four portions: the first, the cervical one, extends from the cricoid cartilage and the lower margin of the cricopharyngeus muscle to a horizontal plane going along the sternal fork; the second, or thoracic, portion goes from the former to the diaphragm; the third, the diaphragmatic portion, corresponding to the area across the diaphragm; the fourth, the abdominal one, is between the diaphragm and the stomach [3]. Its upper margin is at the level of the lower margin of the cricoid cartilage, corresponding backward to the lower margin of the VI cervical vertebra, whereas its lower margin corresponds to the left part of X-XI thoracic vertebra [1, 8].

The portion of its superior margin (the so-called mouth of the esophagus) changes with the position of the head, reaching the level of the V cervical vertebra when the neck is extended, and the VII cervical vertebra when it is bent [2, 4].

Its length varies with age, being about 8 cm in neonates, 13.5 cm in boys, to gradually reach, in adult age, 25 cm in length, with the cervical portion measuring 5 cm, the thoracic portion 16 cm, and the abdominal portion 4 cm [7].

During diagnostic procedures it is of utmost importance to know the distance from the upper incisor teeth to the cardias, which is of 40–42 cm in adults, 26–27 cm in a 10-year-old boy, 14–16 cm in neonates [6].

Also important is the distance between the upper incisor teeth and the lower esophageal sphincter (LES), which is for adults, boys, and neonates about 37–38 cm, 20 cm, and 12 cm, respectively [9].

Its course is not rectilinear but follows the curvature of the vertebral column, except in the abdominal portion, extending along an oblique direction from the front to the back. More exactly, on the frontal plane the course is sinuous, becoming oblique from left to right, from its origin to D4, then concave to the right from D4–D8 and back to the left at the level of the cardias and the vertebral column [4].

On the sagittal plane, the esophagus adheres to the vertebral column until D5, at which point it changes to a forward direction, with an anterior concavity curving at the level of its passage into the abdomen [3,10]. The caliber of the esophagus is also irregular: it has three strictures, the first one at the level of cricopharyngeal muscle and the cricoid cartilage (named cricopharyngeal narrowing or mouth of the esophagus); the second at the crossing point with the aortic arch and the left main bronchus (hence the name broncho-aortic narrowing); the third at the level of diaphragm (hiatal narrowing) [5].

Apart from these strictures, the diameter of the esophagus varies according to its tonus and measures approximately 2 cm.

Fixed above by the junction with the pharynx, down with its passage through the diaphragm, and continuing with the stomach, the esophagus has important attachments along its course.

The anterior part of the neck is adjacent to [3, 11]:

1. The posterior, membranous wall of the trachea from which it is separated by an areolar tissue and some muscular fibers.
2. The left lobe of the thyroid gland
3. The recurrent laryngeal nerves on the left, between the esophagus and the trachea, on the right along the lateral limit of the anterior wall of the esophagus

Posteriorly, the esophagus lies along the prevertebral muscles wrapped by the cervical deep fascia that separates it from vertebral bodies.

On each side of the esophagus we find the vascular-nervous branches and the sympathetic trunk, which passes along the esophagus posteriorly.

Lastly, at the roof of the neck on the left side of the esophagus we find the thoracic duct entering the left subclavian vein [8].

As to the thorax, in the posterior mediastinum the esophagus is adjacent posteriorly with the vertebral column from which it is separated by the aorta that descends inferiorly first on the left and then, at the VIII-IX vertebral body, behind the esophagus, forming the so-called aortic-esophageal crossing [5, 12]. Anteriorly, the esophagus is adjacent above to the trachea and inferiorly, below the carena, with the pericardial sac of Haller. On the upper left region, laterally, on each side of the esophagus there is the mediastinal pleura from which it is separated by the ascending portion of the left subclavian artery and in the lower left region by the azygos vein that crosses the esophagus laterally before flowing into the inferior vena cava [4]. The thoracic duct ascends first on the right and then on the left side of esophagus.

At the level of the abdomen, the esophagus is adjacent to the posterior margin of the liver, on which it leaves an impression, on the left to the stomach, and on the right to the caudate lobe of Spigelius; the posterior side is adjacent to the abdominal aorta and the diaphragmatic pillars that separate it from the vertebral column [2].

The anatomic structure of the esophagus consists of four layers: the mucosa – the innermost layer, the submucosa, the muscular layer, and the adventitia – the outermost layer [9]. In addition, the abdominal portion comprises also a serosa layer along most of its circumference. The mucosa, whose thickness is 300 μ, is lined by simple epithelium extending, on the bottom, to the cylindrical simple epithelium of the stomach along an irregularly indented line called the zigzag line [6, 10]. The mucosa is made of numerous little folds that form a sort of labyrinth of microgrooves filled with mucus to attenuate friction caused by chewed food.

In the submucosa there are numerous glands of various type: racemous and compound, located superiorly, simple or little stratified, located inferiorly, where they are named cardiac glands [11].

The muscular layer, which measures from 0.5 mm to 2 mm, according to age, is composed of striated fibers superiorly (1/4 of the length of the esophagus); in the intermediate zone by mixed, smooth, and striated fibers; in the lower half of the esophagus by smooth fibers. Concerning their disposition, it is plexiform on the superior esophagus while it is replaced, in the remaining esophagus, by a disposition in two layers: the outer longitudinal and the inner circular. The longitudinal musculature is not distributed uniformly over the esophagus, but forms on its each side two masses, while it is thinner over the anterior and posterior wall [1, 12].

As to the musculature of the esophagus, particular importance is played by two formations with sphincteric functions localized at the two extremities of the esophagus.

At level of cervical portion, the muscular striated fibers join to the cricopharyngeal muscle, part of the inferior constrictor of the pharynx, to form the upper esophageal sphincter. At the level of the inferior esophagus, a group of smooth muscular fibers, named claps, after embracing the cardias at the level of the little curvature of the stomach, joins anther groups of muscular fibers, named slings, (which derive from the posterior wall of the stomach, extend over the angle of His to end onto the anterior wall of the stomach), thus forming the inferior esophageal sphincter [7].

The adventitia, more than a true anatomic structure, is an extension of the connective tissue that surrounds the esophagus along its whole length. At last, concerning the serosa, which is present only on the abdominal portion of esophagus, it is formed by the peritoneum, which, after covering the anterior and the lateral walls of the esophagus, leaves its posterior wall uncovered to lie over on the vertebral bodies, thus forming a sort of mesoesophagus [4, 8].

Very important for the function of the esophagus is the innervation ensured by three types of innervations: parasympathetic, orthosympathetic, and intrinsic.

The parasympathetic innervation of the smooth musculature is ensured by fibers coming from the motor dorsal nucleus of the vagal nerve, localized in the bulb, and the striated musculature coming from the ambiguous nucleus [2].

The orthosympathetic innervation is ensured by preganglionic fibers coming from the intermediated lateral columns of the spinal cord across the communicating anterior branches that reach the sympathetic trunks, from which the postganglionic fibers to the esophagus derive [7].

The intrinsic innervation is ensured by two plexuses, one localized between the two muscle coats, named myenteric plexus of Auerbach, the other localized in the submucosa, named submucosal plexus of Meissner. Both contain parasympathetic and orthosympathetic motor fibers, and sensitive fibers [12].

Within the context of the myenteric plexus there are excitatory and inhibitory neurons: the former act to contract two muscle coats across muscarinic receptor (M2 and M3), while the latter operate on the circular musculature across the NO, a nonadrenergic, noncholinergic (nA nC) transmitter that inhibits the release of LES [5].

2.3
The Stomach

The stomach (from the Greek *stomakos*) is an enlarged and extensible bagpipe-shaped portion of the alimentary tube involved in the first stage of digestion; it is delimitated above by the cardiac opening, at the level of T10, at almost 2 cm left of the median line, and below by the pylorus, at the level of the superior margin of L1, at almost 2.5 cm right of the median line [2].

Morphologically, it is made of two walls, one anterior and another posterior; two curvatures (the little one on the right, the greater on the left); two incisures, the cardial, which extends from the junction of the abdominal esophagus with the greater curvature, and the angular one, at the level of the lesser curvature [7].

The stomach is formed by three portions: the *Fundus* extending from the cardial incisure at the bottom to the angular incisure; the *body*, between the fundus and a line extending from the angular incisure to the greater curvature; the antro-pyloric portion, that includes the

antral zone and the pyloric channel, extending from the body to the first duodenal segment [6].

The anatomy of the stomach comprises four layers, which are, from inside to outside, the *mucosa*, the *submucosa*, the *musculature* and the *serosa*.

The mucosa is covered by a single layer of columnar cells beginning at the cardias and continuing to the esophageal epithelium along an irregular line – the Z or Z–Z line; it is raised to form a plane of longitudinal folds that disappear when the stomach distends. These folds run parallel along the little curvature, and delimitate a gutter, called *gastric short way* or *Magenstrasse*, that connects the esophagus to the pylorus [4, 9].

In the mucosa there are three types of glands: the *cardiac glands*, around the cardiac orifice; the *fundic glands*, located in the fundus and the body of stomach; the *pyloric glands*, located at the pylorus [12].

The fundic glands, called also gastric glands, contain three types of cells, *mucoid, zymogenic*, and *parietal* cells; however, the argentaffin cells, normally present in the pyloric glands, may also be found [6].

The submucosa is formed by a loose connective tissue rich in elastic fibers. It is separated from the mucosa by the *muscolaris mucosae*, which contains the *plexus of Auerbach*.

The musculature of the stomach is formed only by smooth muscle fibers arranged into three layers: longitudinal-external, circular-median, and oblique-internal. The longitudinal layer, which is a continuation of the longitudinal musculature of the esophagus, is incomplete and arranged into two stripes: the first and stronger one follows the lesser curvature; the second extends along the greater curvature to reach the pylorus. In contrast, the circular musculature is a continuation of the esophagus; its fibers become very thick in the pylorus, where they form a muscular ring with a sphincteric function (the so-called pyloric sphincter). Lastly, the internal oblique musculature, which is more developed in the fundus, is formed by V-shaped loops [8].

The serosa is formed by the *peritoneum*, which covers the whole extension of the stomach except for the cardial region and the fundus, where the anterior and the posterior coat of the peritoneum join to form ligaments that connect the stomach to the contiguous organs.

From the anatomo-surgical point of view, the surgical treatment of GERD requires sound knowledge of the stomach, its contiguous organs, and peritoneal connections.

At the left hypochondrium, the anterior wall of the stomach is adjacent to the diaphragm, the left lobe of the liver and the spleen, while anteriorly to the peritoneum of the anterior abdominal wall, without interposition with the viscera.

Its posterior surface is in apposition to the lesser sac of the peritoneum (or omental bursa) and the viscera delimiting the postero-inferior wall of this cavity (pancreas, splenic vessels, left kidney, left suprarenal gland, diaphragm, transverse colon, and mesocolon); all this forms the so-called bed of the stomach.

Concerning the connections of the gastric curvature, the major convex one goes from the angle of His (formed by the left margin of the esophagus where it joins the stomach), to the pylorus. It is adjacent to the inferior surface of the liver and the formations contained in the duodenal ligament (hepatic artery, portal vein, and choledochus) [5, 8].

The lesser curvature, which is the concave, begins at the right margin of the esophagus, initially with a vertical course and then developing horizontally at the level on cardiac incisure. Its connections are with the aorta, the caudate lobe of Spigelius, the celiac artery, and the celiac plexus.

The peritoneal connections of the stomach consist of four ligaments named *epiploons*, which attach the circumference of the stomach to the contiguous viscera (Fig. 1):

1. The gastro-hepatic epiploon (the lesser omentum), extending from the lesser curvature to the lower surface of the liver, is divided into a larger and more proximal portion; the thinner one is called the *hepatogastric* ligament, whereas the thicker and more distal portion is called the *hepatoduodenal* ligament; the free margin of the hepatoduodenal ligament is the anterior margin of Winslow's foramen, through which it opens into the omental bursa [3].
2. The gastro-colic epiploon (the greater omentum) stems from the greater curvature of the stomach, goes down, as if suspended over the bowel, to the hypogastric region, where it is attached to anterior margin of transverse colon.
3. The gastro-splenic ligament extends from the fundus of the stomach to the hilum of the spleen.
4. The gastro-phrenic ligament extends from the fundus of the stomach to the inferior surface of the left hemidiaphragm and posterior parietal peritoneum.

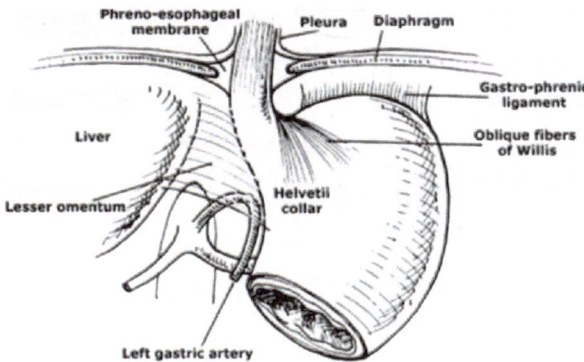

Fig. 1. The anatomic connections of the stomach (modified from Domini et al.)

When performing antireflux surgery, it is important to know the blood supply to the stomach, particularly the course of the short gastric arteries and veins; the former may vary in number from 2 to 8, and stem from the splenic artery or its branches to the superior portion of the greater curvature; the latter drain the blood from this region to the splenic vein. Also important is the knowledge of the innervation of the stomach, ensured by sympathetic and parasympathetic nerves containing afferent and efferent fibers and by intrinsic metasympathetic nerves [2, 10].

The orthosympathetic supply originates from the lateral cornual cells of the spinal cord located at the level of VI–X thoracic segment to enter the sympathetic trunks from which, through the splanchnic nerves, they reach the celiac plexus and its ganglions. From there, the formations reach the superior gastric plexus that passes through the left gastric artery, and the inferior gastric plexus that passes along the gastroepiploic artery [1].

The parasympathetic supply originates from the dorsal vagal nerves located at the floor of the IV ventricle and from two vagal nerves: the anterior one stemming from the left vagus, and the posterior one from the right vagus [3]. The anterior vagal trunk gives origin to Latarget's nerves, which reach the antral portion of the stomach. The metasympathetic or autochthonous innervation, is ensured by the myenteric plexus of Auerbach and the subcutaneous plexus of Meissner [7].

2.4
The Esophago-gastric Junction

As already mentioned, the knowledge of the esophago-gastric junction (EGJ), comprising the lower end of the esophagus and its junction to the stomach, is fundamental to understand the pathophysiology of GERD and thus enable its correction [4].

Normally located underneath the diaphragm, in relation with the dorsal vagus and the aorta posteriorly and the right pillar bilaterally, the EGJ may be situated in the thorax in the full posterior mediastinum – this is the case of congenital or acquired brachyesophagus.

The EGJ is an anatomo-functional system formed by the segment of the epicardial esophagus (the so-called epicardias), the functional esophagogastric vestibule – corresponding to the functional radiological dilatation of the esophagus below the cardiac narrowing of the esophagus and lastly by the cardia, which represents the lower orifice of the esophagus when it passes into the stomach [5].

The EGJ is anchored by various anatomic formations which, together with other functional elements, create an antireflux barrier that ensures its complete continence.

Before going on to describe these formations, it may be worthwhile to briefly overview the connections between the muscle coat of the esophagus and that of the stomach. The longitudinal muscle coat of the esophagus continues with the longitudinal outer muscle coat of the stomach, while the circular coat of the esophagus, appearing as a spiral at the level of cardia, is divided into two layers, one continuing with the circular intermediate coat of the stomach and the other with its oblique inner coat.

The oblique muscle fibers of the stomach cross the cardiac incisure and its circular musculature – which surrounds the stomach horizontally, making a muscle ring called the *collare* Helvetii, which is believed to have a sphincteric function [4, 11].

Also important to remember is that the inferior segment of the esophagus is characterized by a thickening of its entire musculature at the level of the esophagogastric vestibule, which extends for about 1–2 cm above the diaphragm to reach the cardia; this region is the inferior esophageal sphincter [1].

Another point to remember is how the mucosa passes from the esophagus to the stomach. The thin and pale mucosa of the esophagus becomes the deeper and redder gastric mucosa, characterized by an irregularly dentate transitional line, called line ZZ, or line Z. The transition from the squamous epithelium of the esophagus to the columnar epithelium of the stomach does not coincide with the anatomic level of the cardia, but is placed at a rather higher level, approximately between the cardia and the hiatus of the diaphragm [5].

Sometimes the columnar epithelium of the esophagus extends into the esophagus, even for a considerable length; this condition is known as Barrett's esophagus.

The last point to keep in mind regards the length of the abdominal esophagus, which is of about 2–3 cm in adults and almost 1–1.5 cm in children [9]. This portion is covered anteriorly and back by the peritoneum. Below the peritoneum, the esophagus moves freely due to lack of any cellular adipose tissue. This arrangement explains how the section of the peritoneal fold that covers the antero-superior part of the diaphragmatic pillars is useful to mobilize the esophagus downward.

The peritoneum that covers the esophagus is a continuation of the peritoneum that covers the anterior surface of the stomach; anteriorly and to the left it folds over the inferior surface of the diaphragm, while on the right toward the liver it folds to form the anterior leaf of the gastrohepatic ligament. The esophagus is thus covered by three peritoneal folds: the first extending from the left side of the esophagus to the diaphragm and at gastric fundus constitutes the superior portion of the gastro-phrenic ligament; the second and the third folds stem from the left side of the esophagus and consist of a superficial ligament and a deeper ligament [2, 11]. The superficial one – formed by two leaflets – extends from the esophagus to the liver and the diaphragm: it is merely the upper margin of the gastro-hepatic ligament. The

deep ligament, formed by only one leaflet, lines the right side of the esophagus in a forward to rear direction, and extends to line the aorta and the right diaphragmatic pillars – which is merely the deep leaf of the gastro-hepatic ligament.

The abdominal esophagus is adjacent anteriorly to the left vagal nerve and the posterior surface of the liver, posteriorly with the right vagal nerve, the diaphragmatic pillars, and the abdominal aorta, which separates it from the tenth vertebral bone; on the right with the caudate lobe of Spigelius and on the left with the fundus of stomach [4, 10].

We have already seen how the EGJ is kept in position by many anatomic structures that fix and anchor it to ensure perfect continence.

The factors of anchorage are intrinsic and extrinsic. The intrinsic ones consist of the so-called brace or Swiss tie and the angle of His and, probably, by Gubaroff's valve (Fig. 2). The extrinsic ones are the esophageal hiatus, the phreno-esophageal membrane of Laimer-Bertelli, the Juvara fibers, the Rouget fibers, and the Allison lace – also known as Allison's pliers or forceps (Fig. 3).

The factors of anchorage include the phreno-gastric ligament, the compact pars of the little epiploon and the so-called Moynihan anchor.

The physiological factors are the esophageal inferior sphincter and probably the valve of Gubaroff.

The most important factor of anchorage is certainly the esophageal hiatus (EH) by which the esophagus passes from the thorax into the abdomen [7]. The EH is a sort of very short and oblique S-shaped channel from forward to behind, from right to left, and from above to below, with a median antero-posterior length of 3–3.5 cm and a median transverse length of 1–2.1 cm [2, 8]. It is placed posteriorly to the caval hiatus, anteriorly to the aortic hiatus just a little on the left of the median line at the level of T10-T11. It is apparently delimited by two diaphragmatic main medial pillars.

Actually, the left pillar does not play any role in the constitution of the hiatus which, on the contrary, is formed only by a slightly larger right pillar. As matter of

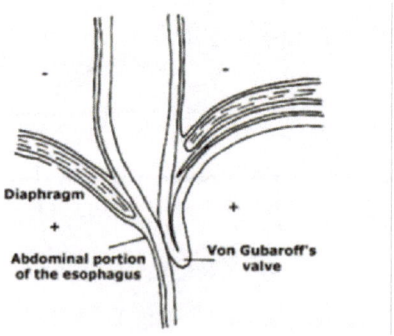

Fig. 2. The Gubaroff's valve it's an important factor for the continence of EGJ (modified from Domini et al.)

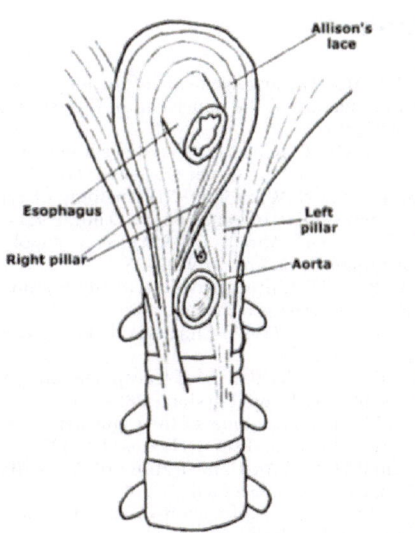

Fig. 3. The anatomic aspect of Allison's lace (modified from Domini et al. 1993)

fact, the right pillar encloses the esophagus by two bundles, the first passing on the right of the esophagus, whereas the second one, coming from behind, passes on the left of the esophagus. These two bundles are placed one above and across the another – as the blades of a scissor – and reach the tendinous center of the diaphragm [1, 11].

All the muscle fibers of the esophageal hiatus thus derive from the right pillar of the diaphragm: consequently, the passage of the esophagus occurs through the space within the right pillar, which thus plays an important role in the continence of the EGJ.

It is important to know that the fibers of the right pillar situated on the right of the esophagus are innervated by the right phrenic nerve, while those placed on the left side are innervated by the left phrenic nerve, as occurs for the left pillar [10].

It is also important to remember that, together with the esophagus, the hiatus is crossed by inferior esophageal vessels and vagal nerves.

An abnormal condition we may find is the so-called muscle of Low, constituted by a thin bundle of fibers that come from the left pillar, pass over the right pillar crossing its muscle fibers and become part of the tendinous center of the diaphragm at the level of the caval hiatus [3, 4].

Other abnormalities are the formation of a part of the left pillars from the fibers of the right pillar that delimit the hiatus on the left of the esophagus while, on in contrast, the fibers that delimit the hiatus on the right of esophagus derive from the left pillar.

Apart from the anatomic relevance of the hiatus, for the continence of EGJ, it is important also to remember that when the fibers of the hiatus contract, their action

on the GEJ is twofold because the compression of the esophageal walls is associated with an increase in the angle-shot of the esophagus [8].

The phreno-esophageal membrane of Laimer-Bertelli is another important anchoring factor for the esophagus; it is formed by folds that join laterally to form a sharp angle that wedges into the diaphragmatic ring with its medial basis (whereas the superior and inferior ones wedge into the supra and the infradiaphragmatic portions of the esophagus) (Fig. 4).

The zone delimitated on the two sides is the space in which the esophagus moves during breathing and swallowing.

The angle of His is an acute angle with the open side formed by the oblique entry of the esophagus into the stomach and mainly by the crossing between the left margin of the esophagus with the greater tuberosity of the stomach [5].

The brace or Swiss tie – also known as *collare Helvetii* – is constituted, as already mentioned, by a bundle of longitudinal muscle layers of the esophagus that bridge the anterior surface of the stomach to the posterior one and by another bundle of arciform fibers coming from the gastric musculature that cross the cardias incisure, known as the oblique fibers of Willis [8, 13].

The semilunar valve of Gubaroff is a sort of spur formed by the junction of the esophageal and the gastric mucosa, which corresponds externally to the angle of His. Many authors attribute to this area a valvular function, while others refuse such a role and consider it an incorrect appearance of the anatomic dissection, i.e., a false aspect.

The scythe of the coronary artery, corresponding to the initial portion of the coronaro-gastric artery called Moynihan's anchor, has an important role in the fixation of the cardias.

Lastly, the cellular-adipose tissue that extends for whole length (3–4 cm) and width of the posterior sur-

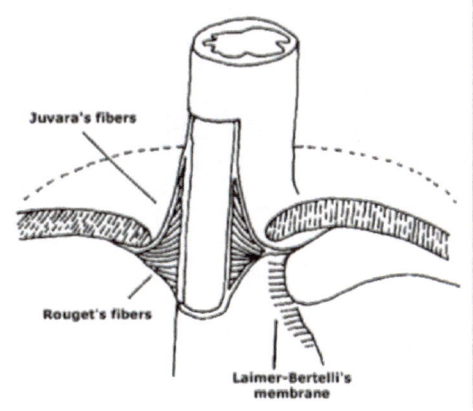

Fig. 4. The phreno-esophageal membrane of Laimer-Bertelli is an important anchoring factor for the esophagus (modified from Domini et al. 1993)

face of the esophagus is important for its fixation, considering that when dissected it produces the intrathoracic ascent of the esophagus [8, 10].

Although from the anatomical point of view the presence of a cardial sphincter is not demonstrated, there is a wealth of evidence suggesting the existence of a sphincteric mechanism at the level of the last 2–5 cm of the esophagus. When this sphincter does not carry out deglutition movements, it is in a state of tonic contraction, since the walls of the esophagus are tightly contracted. Within 1.5–2.5 s from the beginning of deglutition, this sphincter relaxes, while when the peristaltic wave reaches the inferior esophagus, the sphincter contracts to prevent the reflux of gastric contents; this does not occur when the intragastric pressure exceeds the resistance of the sphincteric contraction. All the functions of the esophageal sphincter presuppose the integrity of the vagal nerve and Auerbach's plexus.

References

1. Abel W (1913) The arrangements of the longitudinal and circular musculature of the upper end of the esophagus. J Anat Physiol 47:381
2. Allison PR (1951) Reflux esophagitis, sliding hernia and the anatomy of repair. Surg Gynec Obstet 92:419–431
3. Collis JL, Kelly N, Wiley T (1954) Anatomy of crura of diaphragm and surgery of hiatus hernia. Thorax 9:175–185
4. Collis JL, Satchell S, Abrams D (1954) Nerves supply to the crura of the diaphragm. Thorax 9:22–25
5. Domini R (1972) Chirurgia delle ernie diaframmatiche e del reflusso gastro-esofageo. Piccin, Padua
6. Domini R, Lima M (1993) Chirurgia delle malformazioni digestive. Piccin, Padua
7. Hwang K (1954) Mechanism of transportation of the content of the esophagus. J Appl Physiol 6:781–796
8. Jackson RG (1949) Anatomy of the vagus nerves in the region of lower esophagus and stomach. Anat Rec 103:1
9. Lendrum FC (1937) Anatomic features of the cardiac orifice of the stomach. Arch Intern Med 58:474
10. Netter FH (1983) Atlas of anatomy pathophysiology and clinics, vol 6, part II, Ciba-Geigy, Milan
11. Testut L (1943) Anatomia Umana. UTET, Turin
12. Testut L, Jacob O (1946) Trattato di Anatomia topografica. UTET, Turin
13. Willner V, Bandes F, Hollander F (1956) The normal anatomy and physiology of the esophagus. J Mt Sinai Hosp NY 23:3–13

Chapter 3

The Pathophysiology of Gastroesophageal Reflux

3

Peter J. Milla · Ciro Esposito

Contents

3.1
Introduction

Understanding the pathophysiology of gastroesophageal reflux (GER) is important in choosing the best diagnostic and therapeutic approach to adopt in children with GER [1, 9, 20]. GER is due to multiple factors which result in incompetence of the esophageal cardia, and allow reflux of gastric content into the esophagus. Competence of the esophageal cardia is due to both anatomical and physiological factors which form an antireflux barrier. GER is associated with the failure of these mechanisms against reflux [3, 6, 14, 15, 17, 19, 41, 44].

GER occurs to a very small extent in all people after eating, and to a greater extent in infants in the first year of life [48]. Under normal conditions food is swallowed and directed in an aboral direction by swallow-induced peristalsis down the esophagus. The lower esophageal sphincter (LES) is opened as the bolus of food passes the upper esophageal sphincter.

3.2
Mechanisms of Gastroesophageal Reflux

The competence of the cardia is due to the tone of the LES, the length of the abdominal esophagus, the diaphragmatic hiatus, the angle of His, the esophageal mucosa, the level of intra-abdominal pressure, and the ability of the stomach to empty [50, 51]. Reflux occurs when intragastric pressure exceeds the ability of the above factors to resist it and the gastric fluid then flows down a pressure gradient [14, 19, 23]. The nature of the refluxate may injure the esophageal mucosa due to acid and biliary secretions; defensive mechanisms include esophageal clearing, and salivary and mucous secretions of the esophageal mucosa.

3.2.1
Lower Esophageal Sphincter

The lower esophageal sphincter (LES) is not a true sphincter but a zone of high pressure, in adults 2–4 cm long (3.07±0.46 [mean±SD]), corresponding to a thickening of the circular esophageal muscle, and situated at the distal epicardial level of the diaphragm's esophageal hiatus [33, 38, 53]. In the superior part of the LES, pressure waves are positive in contrast to the inferior part, in which they may be negative. At birth, the LES is 0.5–1 cm long and grows gradually until at 3 months of age it is 2.5–3 cm. It is also important that the length of the abdominal part of the LES is at least 1 cm [8]. The upper limit of the LES coincides with the terminal segment of the phreno-esophageal ligament and it is, (like the inner sphincter of the anus) immature at birth, reaching a functional maturity after 7–8 weeks of life in normal newborns and after 10 weeks in premature infants [5]. GER is related to time and level of maturity, and this explains its frequency after feeding in the first weeks of life [35].

The LES has contractile activity and is able to respond to neuro-humoral stimuli. After a bolus of food is formed and swallowed, primary peristalsis is induced, which is characterized by an increase in intraluminal pressure. The peristaltic wave goes down the esophagus at a speed of approximately 3–5 cm/sec, resulting in progression of the swallowed food to the stomach. Relaxation of the LES occurs when the bolus passes the upper esophageal sphincter.

Under normal conditions, the pressure, or tone, of the LES ranges from 10 to 30 mmHg (13.2±4.7 mmHg [mean±SD]), increasing to 25–30 mmHg when intragastric pressure rises so that there is always a pressure gradient which prevents reflux, and then decreases down to gastric pressure level after deglutition, and at last returns to normal level after a peristaltic wave.

Thus, the function of the LES is coordinated with esophageal motor activity, opening a few seconds after the beginning of deglutition and closing after the swallowed food comes into the stomach.

Many chemical and humoral factors can influence the LES, increasing or decreasing its tone. LES tone is influenced by sympathetic and parasympathetic innervation. The first acts through alpha-adrenergic receptors which provoke a relaxation, while parasympathetic influences regulate basal LES tone and its increases related to intragastric pressure.

Those chemical agents which increase LES tone and can be used for pharmacological treatment of GER include cisapride, metoclopramide, domperidone, histamine, indomethacin, Ca-antagonists, nitrates, morphine and meperidine, antidopaminics, alpha-adrenergic substances, cholinergic substances, and prostaglandins E2 and A. Those which decrease tone include theophylline, dopamine, anticholinergics (atropine, etc.), benzodiazepines, vasopressin, alpha-adrenergic antagonists, beta-adrenergic agonists, and prostaglandins A2 and E2.

Hormonal factors which increase LES tone include secretin, glucagon, cholecystokinin, gastric inhibitory polypeptide, and progesterone. Also, some constitutional conditions like obesity may initiate reflux by causing increased intra-abdominal pressure.

Hormonal agents are also responsible for some interactions between stomach and LES. Gastrin secreted by gastric antrum causes an increase of LES pressure as demonstrated after administration of gastrin or pentagastrin, or production of gastrin following alkalinization of gastric contents, or the decrease of LES pressure after inhibition of gastrin production due to acidification of gastric content [31, 46].

In patients with GER, manometric studies have shown that the LES may behave abnormally in a number of different ways [13, 36, 43]. Currently, the following mechanisms are recognized:

1. A low basal pressure of the LES (under 6–8 mmHg) causes reflux. This condition is known as "hypotonic reflux."
2. An inadequate response of the LES, with low, late, or absent contraction, to an increase of intragastric and/or intra-abdominal pressure, especially when the increase is due to a physiological event such as sneeze, cough, physical effort, etc.
3. An increase of intragastric pressure, in patients with normal LES tone, due to delayed gastric emptying (pyloric stenosis, pyloric or antral membrane) or to an increase of intra-abdominal pressure caused by different effusions (ascites, hemoperitoneum, pneumoperitoneum).
4. Transient, inappropriate relaxation of the LES for 30 sec not preceded by normal peristaltic waves which come after deglutition. The characteristics of inappropriate relaxation are their independence from deglutition, and their longer length and faster opening of LES. Inappropriate relaxations are the commonest mechanism of GER in both children and adults.
5. A transient decrease of LES tone, in subjects with normal basal tone, due to motor incoordination caused by different types of esophageal anomalies (atresia, duplications, diverticula, etc.) [2, 10, 16, 37, 42, 51].

3.2.2
Intra-Abdominal Esophagus

The length of the intra-abdominal esophagus is another important factor of the antireflux barrier [8]. It is known that when the intra-abdominal esophagus is at least 1–2 cm in length it closes when intra-abdominal pressure increases.

A shortened length of this segment, as occurs in the case of hiatal hernia, may be responsible for the reflux shown by radiologic investigation of hiatus hernias.

The length of the intra-abdominal esophagus does not increase proportionally with LES growth; for this reason, at 2 months of life the length of the abdominal esophagus is longer than the total length of LES, thus exerting an antireflux action at this age. Fixing and anchorage of the gastroesophageal junction prevents reascending and helps to keep the length of the abdominal esophagus constant.

3.2.3
Esophageal Hiatus

The esophagus passes through the esophageal hiatus and goes from the thorax into the abdomen [40, 48]. This is one of the most important anatomical factors for the prevention of reflux and for anchorage of the gastroesophageal junction. Its right pillar and the corresponding area of the esophagus are surrounded by the esophageal membrane of Laimer-Bertelli, which marks the level of passage from thoracic into abdominal esophagus. The esophageal hiatus can be weakened and lose its ability to influence the competence of the cardia if the anatomy of the pillar, membrane, or length of the left gastric artery (anchor of Moynihan) is disturbed.

Muscle fibers of the diaphragm which surround the esophagus represent an important antireflux factor and are known as the crural diaphragm, crural sphincter, or outer esophageal sphincter [7]. This antireflux effect is due to the compression on the esophagus by the crural sphincter, which contracts during inspiration when the pressure gradient between abdomen and thorax increases, i.e., the intrathoracic pressure becomes negative. The way in which the crural diaphragm acts as an antireflux barrier is like that of a pinchcock and consists of increasing LES tone through the interaction between axial movement of the LES and crural diaphragmatic contraction [25, 32]. For these reasons, the anatomical or physiological incompetence of the crural sphincter may be responsible for reflux during LES relaxation.

3.2.4
Angle of His

The angle of His is another component of the antireflux barrier. It is an acute angle formed by the left margin of the esophagus and the fundus of the stomach [4]. It has an antireflux effect because the greater curvature of the stomach rises when intragastric pressure increases so that the angle of His decreases compressing the esophagus. On the contrary, if the angle of His becomes obtuse, as in some pathological conditions (organoaxial volvulus, hiatal hernia, esophageal atresia), the stomach changes into a funnel-shaped tube which diverts the gastric contents into the esophagus [28, 52].

3.2.5
Esophageal Mucosa

When the angle of His is normal, folds of the esophageal mucosa roll and become, at the level of the gastroesophageal junction, star- or rosette-shaped [44]. Hence, following increases of gastric pressure or decreases of esophageal thoracic pressure, these folds reduce the esophageal lumen and increase the antireflux function.

3.2.6
Abdominal Pressure

Abdominal pressure includes both abdominal and intragastric pressure. In order to retain competence of the LES, abdominal pressure must not exceed 6–8 - mmHg. Above these values the abdominal esophagus and the seal of the gastroesophageal junction are lost.

3.2.7
Gastric Emptying and Motor Activity of the Stomach

In patients with significant GER, delayed gastric emptying is very common. Gastric emptying occurs as a consequence of motor activity of the stomach and an understanding of this is required to appreciate its involvement in GER [18, 39, 45].

The stomach can be divided into two areas. The proximal half acts as a reservoir, exhibiting mainly tonic activity, which allows for large changes in intragastric volume. The distal region includes the lower half of the body, the antrum and the pylorus. Contraction here is phasic and organized to segment and break up food into small particles or to impart movement. In order to empty food from the stomach, gastric and duodenal contractions are coordinated, resulting in movement of lumenal contents in an aboral direction. When digestible food has been emptied from the stomach, the digestive phase ends and the fasting or interdigestive phase begins. Any remaining gastric contents are swept into the duodenum by bursts of forceful, rhythmic contractions, phase III of the fasting state, in both antrum and duodenum.

3.3
Proximal Stomach

3.3.1
Proximal Receptive Relaxation

Little contractile activity occurs in proximal regions of the stomach, where the predominant activity is receptive relaxation; on swallowing, the proximal muscle relaxes to accommodate the ingested food [34]. This mechanism is so efficient that the average full-term infant can accommodate 60–70 ml of feed with a rise in intragastric pressure of less than 5 mmHg. Receptive relaxation is mediated by a vagal reflex.

3.3.2
Tonic Contraction

Following ingestion of a meal, the proximal region of the stomach exhibits weak tonic contractions, which may play a role in passing intragastric contents to the antrum and pylorus.

3.4
Distal Stomach and Duodenum

3.4.1
Postprandial or Digestive Activity

The distal region of the stomach behaves quite differently from the proximal region, and together with the duodenum a separate pattern of activity occurs according to whether a meal has just been eaten or the individual is fasting. After a meal, rhythmic, phasic contractions which begin near the middle of the stomach are propagated toward the duodenum. The antral waves (about 3/min in humans) are constant in terms of frequency and propagation velocity and are determined by a pacemaker region on the greater curvature of the stomach. The timing and spread of the contractions are regulated by the slow wave activity of the smooth muscle cells and the pacemaking activity of interstitial cells of Cajal. Action potentials spread from the midstomach to the duodenum, but not to the fundal region of the stomach, ensuring that propagation of contractions with a maximum frequency and velocity of the action potentials occurs only in the aboral direction [12]. The occurrence, timing, amplitude, and spread of gastric contractions depend upon the integrity of the gastric muscle, its innervation, the activity of the interstitial cells of Cajal, and the endocrine balance.

These seemingly simple peristaltic contractions of the gastric body and antrum cause fairly complex movements of the intragastric contents, which result in mixing of the contents, mechanical breakdown of food particles, and gastric emptying. The antrum and pylorus are the sites of regulation for the emptying of solids. When a mixed meal is consumed, liquids empty more rapidly than solids, which are retained by antral contractile activity and passed through the pylorus only when they have been broken down into particles of approximately 1 mm.

When contraction begins, gastric contents are propelled toward the duodenum, but only a small amount enters the duodenum. As a consequence, pressure rises in the antrum and provides a continued driving force across the pylorus. As the pressure falls, retropulsion may occur, and the consequent mixing and shearing of flows that take place cause food particles to be broken down. Gastric emptying also occurs during the contractions, but the amount emptied depends upon the peristaltic contractions, tone of the proximal stomach, and contractile activity of the pylorus and duodenum. In the digestive phase, contraction of the pylorus and proximal duodenum is highly coordinated, up to 70% of antral contractions being linked to groups of 1–3 sequential duodenal contractions separated by periods of relative quiescence. This pattern of activity seems to be important for gastric emptying and is modulated not only be neural factors but also by nutrients via paracrine and endocrine polypeptide hormones. That both the nature of a meal and polypeptide hormones influence gastric emptying seems to be beyond doubt from a number of experimental studies in animals and the human infant. In the infant it is clear that increasing caloric density of feeds, with either carbohydrates in the form of glucose polymers vs. monosaccharides, or lipids in the form of long-chain triglycerides or medium-chain triglycerides, results in slower emptying.

3.4.2
Fasting or Interdigestive Activity

Toward the end of feeding activity, contractions become more forceful and propel any remaining undigested food into the duodenum, leaving the stomach empty. The pattern of activity then changes to that seen in the fasted state in both stomach and duodenum. In the interdigestive period the motor activity of several regions of the GI tract has a characteristic, specific, integrated cyclic pattern. This cyclic pattern of fasting activity was first shown in dogs by Szurszewski in 1969, and for the most part coordination of contractions between antrum and duodenum does not occur. The pattern is characterized by what he termed a migrating myoelectric complex (MMC).

It seems clear that where there is significant GER gastric emptying is delayed and a number of abnormalities of gastric motor activity occur, including loss of proximal compliance, incoordination of antroduodenal digestive activity, and loss of cyclical fasting activity [22, 24, 30]. However, whether the GER is part of a wider abnormality of foregut motor function as some have suggested or whether the GER occurs as a consequence of rises in pressure in the stomach which breach the antireflux barrier is at the present time not clear [51].

3.5
Gastric Content

The volume of gastric content plays an important role in gastroesophageal reflux, both quantitatively and qualitatively as discussed above. It is determined by a variety of factors, including the basal volume of gastric secretions, the volume and composition of food, the velocity of gastric emptying, and the amount of duodeno-gastric reflux. GER occurs more frequently after eating as feeds increase the volume of the stomach, which pushes it up against the diaphragm and thereby induces a reflex response resulting in relaxation of the LES [11].

Qualitatively, the composition of food varies and increased osmolarity and fat content all result in prolonged gastric emptying and increased GER [26].

3.6
Intra-Abdominal Pressure

Intra-abdominal pressure is one of the determinants of reflux. Increased pressure when the LES is open allows reflux to occur and results from cough, constipation, tumors, effusions, and extrinsic compression of abdominal wall. The reasons for the decrease in LES tone after increases of abdominal pressure are not entirely clear, but some studies have shown that compression of the abdominal wall leads to relaxation of the LES and diaphragm.

3.7
Gastric Compliance

Loss of compliance of the stomach, especially after feeds, results in increased intragastric pressure and shortening of the intra-abdominal esophagus.

3.8
Mucosal Damaging Factors

Hydrochloric acid and pepsin from the stomach and bile acids and pancreatic juices from the duodenum have all been invoked in the pathogenesis of esophagitis.

3.8.1
Gastric Secretion

Hydrochloric acid is the principal agent responsible for esophageal mucosal damage caused by reflux. The greatest damage is provoked by a high hydrogen ion concentration with pH ranging from 1 to 2, and results in necrosis of esophageal squamous epithelial cells and inflammation. This causes esophagitis. The esophagitis is influenced by the lumenal pH and the length of time that the mucosa is exposed to the acid.

The role of pepsin is not clear, but there is some evidence to suggest that it is also required.

3.8.2
Bile and Pancreatic Juices

Alkaline duodeno-gastric reflux, characterized by a pH>7, is another important factor, often underestimated, as demonstrated by Brigante [27, 29, 47]. This study of 56 patients showed that 48.21% had acid reflux, 19.64% alkaline, and 5.36% mixed reflux. Esophageal lesions were present in 100% of patients with mixed GER, in 36% with acid reflux, and 16% with alkaline reflux. Alkaline esophagitis is due to increased esophageal mucosal permeability to H^+ ions, to the detergent activities of bile acids, and the trypsin in pancreatic juices.

3.9
Mucosal Protective Factors

Factors which protect the esophageal mucosa include the clearing of refluxate by esophageal peristalsis, buffering of acid by swallowed alkaline saliva, and resistance factors of the esophageal mucosa such as mucous secretion [21].

3.9.1
Esophageal Clearance

Esophageal clearance is an important factor in decreasing the injurious effects of acidic gastric refluxate, and is dependant on effective secondary esophageal peristalsis.

Secondary peristalsis occurs in response to fluid refluxed into the esophagus from the stomach and is designed to clear the esophagus of the refluxed material. Clearance is favored by an upright position rather than a supine one. Where peristalsis is defective, clearance may be delayed and is an important factor in the development of esophagitis.

3.9.2
Mucosal Resistance

There are three levels of mucosal resistance [39].

The first level is pre-epithelial and is formed by a surfactant. The viscosity of the surfactant prevents pepsin from attacking epithelial cells and keeps the bicarbonate of the saliva in the lumen where it can neutralize lumenal acid.

The second level is epithelial and is formed by the cornified layer of the squamous epithelium lining the esophagus that prevents penetration of hydrogen ions into the epithelium.

The third level, postepithelial, is formed by factors that control cell trophism and blood circulation which result in oxygenation and neutralization of free radicals.

When these defense systems are inadequate, inflammation develops which may cause an ulcerative esophagitis and stricture formation; ultimately, the columnar metaplasia of Barrett's esophagus may appear. Conjugated bile acids cause damage at acid pH, while nonconjugated bile acids cause damage at alkaline pH.

3.9.3
Esophageal Peristalsis

The capacity of the esophagus to expel material coming from stomach is dependent on its peristaltic activity, which reduces the time that the mucosa is exposed to damaging substances. Mucosal damage is proportional to the time of exposure to such substances, especially at night when secretion of protective factors such as bicarbonate in saliva may be low.

References

1. Altorki NH, Skinner DB (1989) Pathophysiology of gastroesophageal reflux. Am J Med 86:685–689
2. Arnese V, Vantrappen G (2001) Disordini della motilità esofagea e patologie correlate. In: Gasbarini G, Greco AV (eds) Trattato di gastroenterologia. Min Med, Torino, pp 273–281
3. Ashcraft K (1993) Gastroesophageal reflux. In: Ashcroft K, Holder TM (eds) Pediatric surgery. Saunders, Philadelphia
4. Bardaji C, Boix-Ochoa J (1982) Contribution of the His angle to the esophageal antireflux mechanism. Pediatr Surg Int 1:172
5. Boix-Ochoa J, Canalis J (1976) Maturation of the lower esophageal sphincter. J Pediatr Surg 11:749–756
6. Boix-Ochoa J, Rowe M (1998) Gastroesophageal reflux. In: O'Neill A, Rowe MI, Grosfeld JL, Fonkalsurd EW, Coran AG (eds) Pediatric surgery. Mosby, St. Louis
7. Bombeck CT, Dillard DH, Nyhus LM (1966) Muscular anatomy of the gastroesophageal junction and role of phrenoesophageal competence. Ann Surg 164:643–654
8. Bonavina L (1986) Length of the distal esophageal sphincter an competency of the cardia. Am J Surg 15:25–34
9. Carcassonne M (1985) Surgery of gastroesophageal reflux. World J Surg 9:269–276
10. Cucchiara S (1980) Esophageal motor abnormalities in children with gastroesophageal abnormalities and peptic esophagitis. J Pediatric 198:20–27
11. Cucchiara S (1992) Reverse of gastric electrical dysrhythmias by cisapride in children. Dig Dis Sci 37:1136–1140
12. Cucchiara S (1993) Fasting and postprandial mechanism of gastroesophageal reflux in children with gastroesophageal reflux disease. Dig Dis Sci 38:86–92
13. Cucchiara S (1995) Real time ultrasound reveals gastric motors abnormalities in children investigated for dyspeptic symptoms. J Pediatr Gastroenterol Nutr 21:446–453
14. Cuomo R, Grasso R, Sarnelli P (2001) Role of diaphragmatic hernia and lower esophageal sphincter in gastroesophageal reflux disease: manometric and pH-metric study of small hiatal hernia. Dig Dis Sci 46:2687–2694
15. Dent J (1987) Recent views on the pathogenesis of gastroesophageal reflux disease. Baillieres Clin Gastroenterol 1:727–745
16. Dev NB, Boyle GT (1986) Phasic contraction of the diaphragm respiration impedes it role in the gastroesophageal antireflux barrier. Gastroenterology 96:120
17. Diener W, Patti MG, Malena D et al (2001) Esophageal dismotility and gastroesophageal reflux disease. J Gastrointest Surg 5:260–265
18. Di Gesu G (1993) La malattia da reflusso gastroesofageo. Med Prat II:62
19. Di Lorenzo C (1987) Gastric emptying with gastroesophageal reflux. Arch Dis Child 62:449–453
20. Fiorucci S, Morelli A (1998) La malattia da reflusso gastroesofageo: patogenesi. Ospedali Italiani Chirurgia 4:451
21. Gallone L, Pesi G (1976) Vedute attuali in fisiopatologia dello sfintere esofageo inferiore. Min Chir 31:408–414
22. Helm JF (1984) Effect of esophageal emptying and saliva on clearance of acid from the esophagus. N Eng J Med 310:284–288
23. Hillemeier AC (1981) Esophageal and gastric motor abnormalities in gastroesophageal reflux during infancy. Gastroenterology 84:741–746
24. Holloway RH (1985) Gastric distension: a mechanism for postprandial gastroesophageal reflux. Gastroenterology 89:779–784
25. Hyman SR (1999) Pediatric gastrointestinal motility disorders. New York Academy Professional Information Services, New York
26. Jackson C (1922) The diaphragmatic pinchcock in so-called "cardiospasm". Laryngoscope 32:139–142
27. Kahrilas PJ (1987) Effect of sleep, spontaneous reflux and a meal on upper esophageal sphincter presence in normal human volunteers. Gastroenterology 42:466–471
28. Kauer WK (1995) Does duodenal juice reflux into the esophagus of patients with complicated GERD? Evaluation of a fiberoptic sensor for bilirubin. Am J Surg 169:98–103
29. Lelli Chiesa PLP (1993) Ernia iatale e reflusso gastroesofageo. In: Domini R, Lima M (eds) Chirurgia delle malformazioni digestive: 1996. Piccin, Padova
30. Malthaner R (1991) Alkaline gastroesophageal reflux in infants and children. J Pediatr Surg 26:986–290
31. Milla PJ (1988) Disorders of gastrointestinal motility in children. John Wiley, New York
32. Mittal RK (1987) Do bile acid reflux into the esophagus? A study in normal subjects and patients with gastroesophageal disease. Gastroenterology 42:371–375
33. Mittal RK, Rochester DF, Mc Collum RW (1987) Effect of the diaphragmatic contraction on lower esophageal sphincter pressure in man. Gut 28:1564–1568
34. Moroz SP (1970) Lower esophageal sphincter function in children with and without gastroesophageal reflux. Gastroenterology 71:236–241
35. Muller-Lissner SA, Blum AL (1982) Fundic pressure rise lowers lower esophageal sphincter pressure in man. Hepatogastroenterology 29:151–152
36. Omari T, Barnett C, Shel A et al (1999) Mechanism of gastroesophageal reflux in premature infants with chronic lung disease. J Pediatr Surg 314:1795–1798
37. Orenstein SR (1992) Controversies in pediatric gastroesophageal reflux. J Pediatr Gastr Nutr 14:338–348
38. O'Sullivan C (1982) Interaction of lower esophageal sphincter pressure and length of sphincter in the abdomen as determinants of gastroesophageal competence. Am J Surg 143:40–47
39. Palterson GB, Bombeck CT, Nyhus LM (1980) The lower esophageal sphincter mechanism of open and closure. Surg 88:307–314
40. Pellicano R, Palmos F (2002) Malattia da reflusso gastroesofageo. Min Med, Torino
41. Perretin J, Moreaux J (1963) Chirurgie du diaphragme. Masson, Paris
42. Pauterson WG (2001) The normal antireflux mechanism. Chest Surg Clin N Am 11:473–483
43. Richter JE (2001) Esophageal motility diseases. Lancet 358:823–828
44. Romeo G, Zuccarello B, Proietto F (1982) Controllo manometrico dei risultati della chirurgia dell'esofago. Atti XVIII Congr Naz Chir Tor, vol I, pp 279–298
45. Rowe IM (1995) Essentials of pediatric surgery. Mosby, Philadelphia
46. Schwizer W, Hinder RA, Domesteer TR (1989) Does delayed gastric emptying contribute to gastroesophageal reflux disease? Am J Surg 157:74–81
47. Sturdevant RA (1974) Is gastrin the major regulator of lower esophageal sphincter pressure? Gastroenterology 67:551–553
48. Sutphen JL, Dillard VL (1989) Dietary caloric density and osmolarity influence gastroesophageal reflux in infants. Gastroenterology 97:601–604
49. Vanderplas Y, Loeb H (1991) Alkaline gastroesophageal reflux in infancy. J Pediatr Gastroenterol Nutr 12:448–452
50. Vantrappen G, (1960) The closing mechanism at the gastroesophageal junction. Am J Med 28:564–577
51. Vetterson GB, Bombeck CT, Nyhend M (1980) The lower esophageal sphincter mechanism of opening and closure. Surg 88:307–314
52. Werlin SL, DoddS WJ, Hogan WL et al (1980) Mechanism of gastroesophageal reflux in children. J Ped 97:244–249
53. Werlin SL (1981) Esophageal function in esophageal atresia. Dig Dis Sci 26:796–800
54. Zaninotto G (1998) The lower esophageal sphincter in health and disease. Am J Surg 155:104–111

Chapter 4

Clinical Aspects of Gastroesophageal Reflux in Infants and Children

4

Alessandro Settimi · Giuseppe Ascione · Ciro Esposito

Contents

4.1
Introduction

Presenting features of gastroesophageal reflux (GER) in infants and children are quite variable and follow patterns of gastrointestinal and extra-gastrointestinal manifestations that vary between individual patients and may change according to age [1]. Patients may be minimally symptomatic, or may exhibit severe esophagitis, bleeding, nutritional failure, or severe respiratory problems [2].

Any combination of the clinical consequences of GER may bring an infant or a child to the physician's attention.

The symptoms produced by GER in infancy and in childhood can best be divided into four groups: gastrointestinal, respiratory, systemic, and miscellaneous. Moreover, some children may have a particular clinical presentation.

As many as 65% of patients may present with multiple symptoms.

4.2
Gastrointestinal Features

Gastrointestinal clinical presentations vary with age: regurgitation or vomiting is the most common clinical findings in infants and small children, whereas in older children and adults GER presents more frequently with esophagitis and pain.

Painless regurgitation in otherwise healthy infants with normal growth and in the absence of pulmonary symptoms is the typical presentation of physiologic GER: approximately 60% of infants will become symptom-free by 18 months of age; for this reason, gastroesophageal reflux has been considered to be a self-limiting condition in infants and children [3].

In infants, pathogenic GER is clearly documented by frequent and severe vomiting, rumination, hematemesis, occult blood loss in stools, and rejection of food.

Digestive disorders may be differentiated from metabolic or neurological diseases, esophageal obstruction or achalasia, gastrointestinal obstruction (e.g., pyloric stenosis), urinary tract infection.

Emesis may be episodic or even projectile, but most episodes are effortless, usually temporally related to feeding, and often precipitated by physical or environmental stress such as viral infection, constipation, mother-infant conflicts, etc.

Generally, vomiting is of small entity, frequent, and may be considered as regurgitation. Occasionally, a pylorospasm may cause projectile vomiting, raising suspicion of pyloric stenosis, but the vomiting is usually less in volume and more frequent that in the latter condition. The repeated emesis may or may not be associated with growth impairment [4].

In children, vomiting is much less common, although symptoms of esophagitis prevail [5]. Pyrosis, epigastric, or thoracic pain, dysphagia and sensation of lump in the throat are clinical pictures of GER not much different from those affecting adults, and connote peptic esophagitis that may precede the development of a stricture. Inflammation of the esophageal mucosa causes a peristaltic dysfunction of the esophagus and a delayed acid clearance, as suggested by the high rate of GER in patients operated on for esophageal atresia [6].

Gastrointestinal features are summarized in Table 1.

Table 1. Gastrointestinal features

Painless regurgitation
Vomiting
Epigastric or thoracic pain
Pyrosis
Rumination
Rejection
Sensation of lump in the throat

4.3
Respiratory Features

Most infants and children with GER are referred for evaluation because of acute or chronic respiratory complications.

At present a causal relation between GER and respiratory disorders (Table 2) is not completely accepted, although the clinical experience reported by many authors seems to prove that treatment of GER can eliminate the respiratory symptoms in many patients.

Clinical experience strongly supports the theory that "GER can cause, contribute to, or be caused by all of the below-mentioned respiratory problems" [7]. At the present time there is no test capable of establishing the prognosis of a patient with GER associated with respiratory symptoms.

Recurrent aspiration [8] is a well-accepted mechanism for chronic pulmonary disease or recurrent pneumonia: pneumonias are frequent and involve different pulmonary lobes. Repeated episodes of acid aspiration may lead to chronic fibrotic pulmonary changes (pulmonary fibrosis) or to pulmonary abscesses and bronchiectasis. Aspiration leads to coughing, choking, dyspnea, and other respiratory complications, depending on the volume of refluxed fluid and the frequency of reflux episodes.

Central apnea [9], with or without bradycardia, is observed mainly in very young or premature infants and has been described as a symptom of occult GER. The presumed cause of apneic spells is a reflex laryngospasm following stimulation by aspirated reflux material of laryngeal and esophageal acid-sensitive receptors. Incomplete laryngospasm has been suggested to produce stridor.

The presence of apparent life-threatening respiratory events [10] (ALTE) in otherwise-healthy infants less than 6 months old has led to postulate GER as a cause for SIDS (sudden infant death syndrome), but the risks for sudden death from reflux should be limited to infants with a type I reflux pattern and a prolonged ZMD (mean duration of reflux during sleep).

Reactive airway disease, bronchospasm and asthma [11] may be exacerbated by GER: much of the evidence for these various manifestations as a result of GER is indirect, but it is unclear how many patients improve following medical or surgical treatment of reflux [14]. Respiratory features are summarized in Table 2.

4.4
Systemic Features

Insufficient weight gain or failure to thrive has been identified with GER/esophagitis. Reflux can be suspected after that other causes of growth retardation have been ruled out [11].

The first postulated mechanism for failure to thrive is a significant calorie deficit due to persistent vomiting, while the second is the child's refusal to eat as a consequence of the symptoms of esophagitis [12]. An alternative explanation for the failure to grow may be a protein-losing enteropathy secondary to the inflammatory changes in the esophagus. Such infants tend to be pale, thin, hypoactive, listless, and underweight: they are below the tenth percentile and usually improve promptly and dramatically by corrective surgery [13].

Constant irritability (infantile heartburn) or sleep disturbance are commonly related to esophagitis in infancy: these babies present as fussy, irritable, or "colicky." Crying is a very common complaint of parents.

Chronic anemia is a symptom less frequent due to esophageal bleeding with either hematemesis or occult blood loss in the stools. General features are summarized in Table 3.

Table 2. Respiratory symptoms

Wheezing
Chronic cough
Laryngospasm–stridor
Bronchospasm
Apnea
Asthma
Choking
Laryngitis
Bronchitis
Otitis media

Table 3. General features

Failure to thrive
Insufficient weight gain
Irritability
Sleep disturbance
Crying
Seizures
Hypotony

4.5
Miscellaneous

Various manifestations result related to GER, often without apparent explanation.

Reflux torticollis (Sandifer's syndrome) is a peculiar lateral tilting of the head, opisthotonic posturing, or head-cocking dramatically normalized by surgical elimination of reflux. In 1964, an association between hiatal hernia and contortions of the head and neck was first described [15].

A small number of patients have unusual neurological symptoms as seizures or hypotonia whose pathophysiology has not yet been elucidated satisfactorily.

Seizure activity may be secondary to hypoxia related to GER and, similarly, hypotonia could result from seizure activity. After successful treatment of GER, no further episodes of these entities persist.

4.6
Particular Clinical Presentations

Seventy to eighty percent of patients with severe neurological impairment have pathogenic GER with significant malnutrition and recurrent aspiration [16].

Predominance of supine position, uncoordinated swallowing mechanism, delayed gastric emptying, spasticity, seizures, aerophagia, chronic constipations, and scoliosis are conditions that may exacerbate the severity of signs and symptoms of GER. The need of feeding tube placement renders the neurologically impaired child more prone to GER and may also contribute to an increased recurrence of GER after fundoplication.

More than 30% (between 18% and 35%) of patients with esophageal atresia (EA) has symptoms of reflux [17]: recent pH-metry studies report significant GER in 59–82% of these children. Esophageal motility disturbances (uncoordinated peristalsis, absence of simultaneous contraction of low amplitude waves, incomplete relaxation of UES, decreased LES pressure) have been proposed to explain the significant occurrence of GER in EA and the higher recurrence rate of symptomatic reflux after fundoplication. GER in patients with EA may lead to anastomotic stricture.

References

1. Boyle J (1989) Gastroesophageal reflux in the pediatric patient. Gastroenterol Clin North Am 18:315–337
2. Fonkalsrud EW, Ament ME, Berquist W (1985) Surgical management of the gastroesophageal reflux syndrome in childhood. Surgery 97:42–48
3. Johnson DG, Jolley SG (1981) Gastroesophageal reflux in infants and children: recognition and treatment. Surg Clin North Am 61:1101–1115
4. Orenstein SR (1991) Gastroesophageal reflux. Curr Probl Pediatr 21:193–241
5. Hebra A, Hoffman MA (1993) Gastroesophageal reflux in children. Pediatr Clin North Am 40:1233–1251
6. Montgomery M, Frenckner B (1993) Esophageal atresia: mortality and complications related to gastroesophageal reflux. Eur J Pediatr Surg 3:335–338
7. Johnson DG (1985) Current thinking on the role of surgery in gastroesophageal reflux. Pediatr Clin North Am 32:1165–1179
8. Danus O, Larrain CC, Pope CE (1976) Esophageal reflux: an unrecognized cause of recurrent obstructive bronchitis in children. J Pediatr 89:220–224
9. Berger D, Bischof-Delaloye, Landry M, Roulet M, Micheli GL (1986) Bronchopulmonary aspiration syndrome and gastroesophageal reflux in infants and children. Pediatr Surg Int 1:168
10. Jolley SG, Halpern LM, Tunell WP, Johnson DG, Sterling CE (1991) The risk of sudden infant death from gastroesophageal reflux. J Pediatr Surg 26:691–696
11. Martin ME, Grunstein MN, Larsen G (1982) The relationship of gastroesophageal reflux to nocturnal wheezing in children with asthma. Ann Allergy 49:318–322
12. Descher WK, Benjamin SB (1989) Extraesophageal manifestations of gastroesophageal reflux disease. Am J Gastroenterol 84:1–5
13. Kibel MA (1979) Gastroesophageal reflux and failure to thrive in infancy. 76th Ross Conference of Pediatric Research, Columbus, pp 39–42
14. Sontag SG (2000) Gastroesophageal reflux disease and asthma. J Clin Gastroenterol 30:S9–30
15. Ramenofsky ML, Boyse M, Goldberg MJ (1978) Gastroesophageal reflux and torticollis. J Bone Joint Surg 60A:1140–1141
16. Flake AW, Shopene S, Ziegler MM (1991) Antireflux gastrointestinal surgery in the neurologically handicapped child. Pediatr Surg Int 6:92–94
17. Somppi E, Tammela O, Ruuska T, Rahnasto J, Laitinen J, Turjanmaa V, Jarnberg J (1998) Outcome of patients operated on for esophageal atresia: 30 years' experience. J Pediatr Surg 33:1341–1346

Chapter 5

The Gastroesophageal Reflux Secondary to Malformations

5

Mario Lima · Giovanni Ruggeri · Marcello Dòmini
Gabriella Pelusi

Contents

5.1
Introduction

The gastroesophageal reflux (GER) is a common problem in the neonatal period and in early infancy, when an effective maturation of the low esophageal sphincter (LES) [7] (with its definitive competence from the fifth to the seventh weeks of life) and an increasing length of the intra-abdominal esophagus, from 0.5–1 cm at birth to 2.5–3 cm at 3 months of age, have been demonstrated [8].

Therefore, vomiting and spitting up has to be considered physiologic to some degree in infants up to 6–8 weeks of life.

However, in healthy newborn and small infants, it could be difficult to determine whether GER should be considered normal or pathologic. Furthermore, GER can be consequent to disorders including anatomic defects, such as congenital diaphragmatic hernia (CDH), gastroschisis (G), omphalocele (O), esophageal atresia (EA), and tracheoesophageal fistula (TEF): the improvement in surgical techniques and peri-operative supports (both ventilatory and nutritional) decreased the mortality and morbidity and, at the same time, sparked new challenges for pediatric surgeons, who now face a set of unknown problems, such as late sequelae, considering the normal lifespan for most of the patients.

New "chronic" problems emerged while the most afflicted children survive: pulmonary and gastrointestinal ones are the most frequent among them.

The aim of this chapter is to summarize incidence, pathophysiology, clinical characteristics, and success of therapy in cases of GER associated with the mentioned congenital malformations.

5.2
GER in Children
with Congenital Abdominal Wall Defects

GER has been considered a common condition in children with a congenital abdominal wall defect. In both groups of patients with O and G, overall incidence of GER was found to be between 50% and 70%; that exceeds the data related to healthy children (estimated at 5–8%). Beaudoin measured an incidence of GER at 45.45% in O and 52.63% in G [4], whereas Koivusalo reported an incidence, in patients with congenital abdominal wall defect, that was normal (equal that of healthy children) in infancy, and higher in childhood [26].

Many studies have tried to determine the etiologic factors involved, the difference between patients with O and G, and the natural history of GER.

At the moment, the data suggest that there is no statistical correlation of GER with sex ratio, mean gestational age, and birth weight in patients with O and G.

Several factors are believed to be possible causes of GER:

1. Malposition of the stomach frequently associated with different degrees of nonrotation.

2. Increased intra-abdominal pressure after reduction of the intestinal viscera in an underdeveloped abdominal cavity [46]; the closure of the abdominal wall defect may be primary (with or without fascial repair) or staged (with the use of temporary prosthetic material); although this is the most important dilemma in the treatment of O and G, in all of the cases the decision whether to close or stage is based on hemodynamic and respiratory compromise (compression of the great vessels, reduction of venous return); Lacey et al. concluded that inferior vena cava pressures closely relate to intra-abdominal pressure and could be used as an index to primary repair and postoperative care [28] but some degree of abdominal hyperpressure (unable to cause hemodynamic changes) is almost always present.

3. Motility disturbance of the gastrointestinal tract [22] due to compression of the intestine at the neck of the abdominal defect [30] and intestinal changes caused by amniotic fluid exposure (ruptured O and G).

4. Neurological impairment (after prematurity or chromosome abnormality) [17] and associated anomalies (esophageal or duodenal atresia, congenital diaphragmatic hernia) are most frequent in O (an embryologically distinct defect from G; 35–80%) [19] and increase the risk of GER.

But none of these factors are sufficient to explain GER.

A study by Beaudoin et al. (1995) [4] and confirmed by Koivusalo and Rintala (1999) [26] found a higher risk of GER (in early infancy and later in childhood) in patients with large O, more than in those with small O or wide G. The authors analyzed 147 consecutive newborns with O and G to evaluate if GER was related to abdominal hyperpressure: in newborns with G, GER was found in 32/57 cases that had been primarily closed and in 8/19 that had been stage repaired (no statistical difference), whereas in newborns with O, GER was found in 18/45 versus 7/10; the conclusion was that the incidence of GER in G cases did not depend on initial closure, whereas in O cases it is related to staged repair. Those findings suggest that "abdominal hyperpressure alone does not induce GER" [4].

In conclusion, GER is a real complication in patients with abdominal wall defects, primarily involving O, in which morphogenetic and karyotypic anomalies could be parts of the multiple origins of the GER. It is important to note that, when present, the symptoms of GER are early and have a tendency to spontaneous improvement after infancy and a positive response to medical treatment [26].

Considering this data, as many authors suggest, since one baby out of two has GER, each case, including the asymptomatic patients, is to be assessed early with diagnostic workup, because early diagnosis of GER would allow avoidance of complications. As suggested by Fasching, the upper gastrointestinal series provides anatomical information (mucosal abnormalities, esophageal stenosis, hiatal hernia) and little functional information (esophageal dysmotility, gastric outlet obstruction); in combination with the provocation test it is diagnostic for detecting pathological GER. The 24-h pH-metry is considered the gold standard but, in such cases, GER may be missed by pH monitoring when the probe is placed too high, when food neutralizes the gastric content, or when there is insufficient contact with esophageal fluid for the impaction of the electrode tip (- with food or against the esophageal wall); the diagnosis also may be missed due to diminished activity of the patient during the period of the investigation [13].

In a study of asymptomatic patients, Fass and Sampliner demonstrated a frequent endoscopic and/or histologic evidence of GER disease in the presence of abnormal 24-h pH findings [15]. They suggested that this group of "silent refluxers" may present complications later in life such as strictures, Barrett's esophagus, and adenocarcinoma. Therefore, we suggest that all patients, including those who are asymptomatic, undergo the diagnostic work-up and the long-term followup.

The initial treatment should be medical and long-term followup should be arranged (with repeated studies). If symptoms persist (resistance to therapy) or there are morphological abnormalities (hiatal hernia) operative therapy (antireflux procedure) may be an option.

In cases of wide O, some authors suggest this procedure could be made at the time of primary closure of the defect.

There are no studies that evaluate the effectiveness of hemi- versus total fundoplication in GER associated with congenital abdominal wall defects. In our experience, we prefer the anterior hemifundoplication.

5.3
GER After Repair of CDH

At the same time, the survivors of congenital diaphragmatic hernia (CDH), especially those patients with large defects which require a prosthetic patch or are submitted to extracorporeal membrane oxygenation (ECMO), risked development of severe chronic lung abnormalities, recurrent herniation, and GER.

In comparison to the clinical challenges of compromised pulmonary status (pulmonary hypoplasia and persistent pulmonary hypertension), GER could be considered a minor problem; however, if only to prevent potential respiratory instability the possible occurrence of respiratory complications (due to GER) must be avoided.

The factors involved in development of GER are numerous: [24]

1. Lack of anatomic antireflux mechanisms (short abdominal portion of the esophagus, reduction of angle of His, malposition of the stomach) from incomplete maturation of gastroesophageal junction [52].
2. Changes in esophageal motility, resultant from compression of the esophagus by the herniated viscera in utero [57] and delayed gastric emptying.
3. Sliding of esophagus in thorax, in case of severe hypoplastic lung, deviation of the esophagus to the underexpanded lung and shortening of the abdominal esophagus or occurrence of hiatal hernia [40].
4. Thinning of the muscular component of left diaphragmatic crus: the repair of defect (especially in large defects) may require approximation under tension and lead to strain on the crus (predisposing to hiatal or peri-esophageal hernia) or direct suture of the patch to the esophageal wall (predisposing to manometric disturbances of the low esophageal sphincter) [24].
5. In the underdeveloped abdominal cavity, the reduction of hernial contents causes elevated intra-ab-

dominal pressures and high gradient with negative intrathoracic pressure, facilitating reflux of gastric material in thoracic esophagus [49].

6. Respiratory efforts during weaning from ventilation and regular tracheobronchial aspirations (siphon effect) [62]

The incidence of GER is about 60% [57, 63, 27]. Some authors reported an incidence of GER, during the first year of life, in patients with CDH, from 20% to 84% [37, 27, 49]. The incidence of GER in patients treated with ECMO is the same: from 39% to 81% [1, 6, 11, 29, 52, 61, 63].

Kieffer et al. have reviewed their 74 living patients (3): 46 had GER, 36 symptomatic and 10 asymptomatic (but with investigations-documented GER); comparing several parameters between the groups with and without GER, the author found that there was no significant correlation between GER and thoracic position of the left liver lobe, presence or absence of a hernia sac, size of the defect, gestational age, or birth weight, but there was significant correlation of GER with preoperative thoracic position of the stomach, prenatal diagnosis of CDH, duration of artificial ventilation and hospitalization (not for duration of total parenteral nutrition).

Fasching et al. have proved that the latter factors did not significantly influence the incidence of GER and, in particular, that the incidence of GER is equal between patients treated with or without ECMO [14], whereas NO inhalation is significantly higher in survivors without GER [23]. The authors hypothesize that reduced motility of hemidiaphragm (analyzed with M-mode sonography) relative to the contralateral side [14] may induce GER, but their data suggest "the patients with reduced motility of the diaphragm did not show any related clinical problems." [14]

In contrast, there is controversy about the correlation between GER and the use of diaphragmatic substitutes (Silastic, dura, muscle, fascia): the use of patches, in cases of large defects, allows avoidance of tension on crus and esophageal hiatus and reduces intra-abdominal pressures. This condition should ameliorate the prognosis of patients, but the percentage of GER did not appear to diminish [14].

The recurrence of the diaphragmatic hernia might increase the risk of GER: Fasching et al. reported the case of a patient with recurrent hernia that, at followup study, displayed severe GER [14].

In conclusion, at the moment, any parameter predictive of occurrence of GER (and it is probable that the etiology of GER can be found in CDH survivors) has multiple complex origins. It is generally clear that GER is not related to severity of defect, but to the repair techniques used.

In general, we should pay attention during the first operation to the anatomic reconstruction of antireflux mechanisms: the esophagus must be located with the wide intra-abdominal portion and fixed to prevent sliding into the thorax (which is very frequent in cases of severe hypoplasia of lung) [40]. In addition, an attempt must be made to create the angle of His (some authors propose a partial fundoplication) [52] and, in case of minimal left crus, to reconstruct a crus of 1–2 cm with diaphragmatic muscle or a portion of the right crus (shifting the location of the hiatus slightly to the right) [52]. In all cases, it is necessary to prevent tension in the closure of the defect.

The clinical signs indicative for GER are recurrent episodes of vomiting, regurgitation, bradycardia with oxygen desaturation and respiratory arrest, and bronchitis or pneumonia of the right lung. These symptoms also begin early after the enteral nutrition is administered. In the past, only symptomatic patients were screened for GER; more recently, most authors recommend investigating all patients to detect GER, because there are the "silent refluxers" [14]. The predictive value of symptoms in detecting esophagitis is relatively poor: in a followup study of adult patients operated on for CDH, Vanamo reported that only 54% of patients with typical symptoms of GER had endoscopic or histologic evidence of esophagitis (significantly higher than the estimated 2% prevalence of endoscopic esophagitis in the general adult population), and 27% of those with esophagitis were completely asymptomatic [60].

The diagnosis of GER is made by the classical investigations.

Management of GER, in general, follows normal guidelines which should include initial medical therapy (prokinetic and antiacid agents), antireflux posture, and diet. Many authors propose fundoplication if there is no response after 2–3 weeks of treatment [52]; others make the surgical procedure after a greater interval of time (from 1 to 36 months) [24]. There is a lack of data to determine whether there is an early indication for surgical antireflux operation and whether a single-step operation should be recommended (involving the hernia repair and antireflux). With regard to better techniques, it is widely accepted that Nissen fundoplication is recommended for good mobilization of lower esophagus (with careful attention to medial patch separation) and the reapproximation of the crura (which is the weakened anatomic region in these patients).

5.4
GER Occurring After Repair of Esophageal Atresia

GER is so common after surgical treatment of EA/TEF, that it is reasonable to consider it as a part of the disease. Extensive esophageal mobilization and anastomosis under tension are generally accepted as good explanations for gastroesophageal barrier insufficiency because partial denervation and traction on the cardia may weaken the lower esophageal sphincter. Acid reflux is also believed to increase the risk of esophageal anastomotic leak. Furthermore, persistent GER limits the ability to feed these patients orally, and often causes recurrent pulmonary aspiration.

The incidence of GER in these patients is an increasing problem: in a prospective evaluation of morbidity, Tibboel et al. found GER in 39% of children operated on between 1975 and 1984 and in 63% of those operated on between 1984 and 1985 [58]. Koch found the incidence of GER increased from 25% in 1958 to 75% in 1982 [25] and Okada found an overall incidence of 52%. This is probably related to an increased number of primary anastomosis to conserve the native esophagus. Persistent GER after esophageal anastomosis may bring gastric acid in contact with the esophageal suture line for prolonged periods, resulting in inflammation, edema, and eventual stricture.

Several reports suggest that abnormalities of vagal nerve innervation not related to surgical manipulation of the esophagus coexist with EA [12].

In addition to congenital abnormal esophageal clearance capacity, the anatomic and functional compromise secondary to operative repair must be considered.

First to be considered is the shortening of the intra-abdominal esophagus, due to extensive mobilization of the lower esophagus during intervention to perform anastomosis, either in case of EA with TEF or in case of long-gap isolated EA. Initially, the cases of isolated EA were treated with esophageal substitution with either gastric tube or colon; currently, many authors [32, 21, 45] confirm that delayed primary anastomosis (at 6–20 weeks of age) is feasible even in cases of isolated EA (such as EA Gross type III). This technique allows conservation of the patient's own esophagus and avoidance of cervical Barrett's esophagus [34] in gastric tube reconstruction and prolonged transit time in colon interposition [35]; the subjective long-term results are better in delayed primary anastomosis than in esophageal substitution. Despite these good results, there is a high incidence of stricture and GER. Lindahl and Rintala reviewed seven cases of isolated EA who underwent successful delayed anastomosis: at long-term followup, all patients underwent fundoplication because of symptomatic GER at a mean age of 6 months [36]. Montedonico and Diez-Pardo [38], "to test the hypothesis that one or more components of the gastroesophageal pressure barrier are weakened by esophageal anastomosis under tension," measured low esophageal sphincteric and crural sling pressure and the length of the intra-abdominal esophagus in 20 rats before and after resection of 15 mm of cervical esophagus and in eight rats of control group (before and after esophageal transection), to evaluate whether pure anastomotic tension accounts for

gastroesophageal barrier failure. The conclusion was that "anastomosis under tension decreases significantly the lower esophageal sphincteric tone and length of intra-abdominal esophagus but it does not change the crural sling pressure."

p1>The shortening of the esophagus is accompanied by a lack of permanently positive pressures on the intra-abdominal esophagus, lack of intermittent compression by diaphragmatic crural sling, and lack of anatomic peri-esophageal ligaments and angle of His.

Orringer et al. [43] observed that severe symptomatic GER developed in adult patients who underwent mobilization of more than 4 cm of the lower esophagus to perform anastomosis. It has furthermore been suggested that partial denervation of the esophagus during the dissection may disrupt esophageal peristaltic contractions and reduce esophageal clearance of acid reflux [48].

Secondarily, vagal iatrogenic injury may occur in case of extensive esophageal dissection.

Furthermore, the low esophageal sphincteric function must be considered: the evidence about it is conflicting. Shono [51] studied motility function of the esophagus before primary anastomosis and demonstrated upper pouch contractions and sphincteric relaxations in two babies (with incomplete relaxations after TEF-repair), whereas Romeo and Zuccarello showed lack of sphincteric relaxation [48]; the studies in the postoperative period revealed low pressures with normal relaxations [56], or normal [18] or increased pressures [31]. Therefore, although in patients with GER low pressure is a usual finding, in severe cases, reflux can occur when it is normal [59].

Ultimately, it must be considered the contractile activity of the esophagus (and stomach): the peri-anastomotic segment of esophageal body is aperistaltic, with low-amplitude and nonpropulsive contractions [59, 50]. Tovar et al. [59] reviewed 22 patients (adolescents and adults) previously operated on EA/TEF, submitting them to 24-h manometry and pH-metry: "the esophagus in patients with TEF has no peristaltic pump function (in presence or in absence of esophagitis), the propulsion of ingested material and clearance of refluxed fluid takes place mainly by gravity. In absence of conclusive sphincteric pressure data, the reflux probably is related to frequent extemporaneous nondeglutory relaxations. The finding of very long nocturnal episodes of GER sheds some light on the pathogenesis of long-term respiratory tract symptoms" [59].

Zuccarello et al. propose severe structural disorganization of the muscle layer and protein anomalies in an immunohistochemical study of atresic esophageal upper pouch [65]; Hokama found tracheobronchial remnants in unoperated cases [20]; Nakazato demonstrated the intramural ganglion cell and fiber paucity and absence of submucosal glands [41] not only in the esophagus but also extending to the stomach: this may be responsible for both esophageal dismotility and delayed gastric emptying.

Despite the data, the followup strategy is controversial: there are authors that perform screening investigations after EA/TEF repair in all of the cases (upper GI series, to investigate the anastomosis patency and gastroesophageal junction) [47], but there are also authors that submit their patients to radiologic postoperative evaluation based only on clinical request [2]. In our opinion, the early diagnosis of GER (even before the beginning of the symptoms) is important for the association and correlation between GER and esophageal perianastomotic stricture. The factors implicated in the pathogenesis of esophageal strictures include excessive tension anastomosis, ischemia at the ends of esophagus, anastomotic leak, and GER. In a review of Okada et al., it emerged that anastomotic strictures have a median incidence of 50% of the EA, of which about a half showed improvement within 6 months by dilatations, and 30% showed persistent stricture requiring repeated dilatations for 1–3 years [42]. A resistant stricture may be due to GER. The recognition of the GER role in the pathogenesis of strictures led to the realization that control of the GER is essential in the treatment of these strictures [39, 44]. Therefore, it is crucial to determine whether an esophageal stricture is associated with GER or not and, in that case, the patient should immediately start the treatment of GER, before the beginning of esophageal dilatation.

Bergmeijer and Tibboel [5] propose a postoperative treatment protocol with radiologic evaluation for GER at postoperative day 10, at 6 and 12 weeks, and at 6 and 12 months after atresia repair. If there is not GER, the followup includes X-ray only. If there is GER at postoperative day 10, the medical therapy must be initiated (prokinetic and/or antiacid agents), and successive investigations must include, besides X-ray, the 48-h pH monitoring (at 6 weeks) or the endoscopy (at 12 weeks). Until this point, the surgical therapy is indicated only in case of complications of GER (anastomotic stricture or pulmonary symptoms) or GER III/IV endoscopic grade (at 12 weeks). In absence of complications and also in cases of endoscopic reflux I/II grade, it is appropriate to continue the medical therapy for 6 months, at which point the authors repeat X-ray and pH-metry. The surgical therapy is indicated in case of persistent reflux.

This therapeutic strategy led to a substantial increase, year by year, in the number of antireflux procedures and to an important decrease in the number of stricture resection.

There are some reports that emphasize that "severity of GER, esophageal peristaltic abnormality, tracheal inflammation and impairment of pulmonary function seem to be alleviated with age" [55]. But, considering the congenital and acquired esophageal dismotility, the GER in EA/TEF must be suspected even in asymptomatic patients and there is no reasonable expectation of a benign natural course. Therefore, it must be treated early and an aggressive medical management can be the initial choice in cases of asymptomatic or mild GER; however, in symptomatic cases, it is suitable to propose a surgical treatment.

The need for fundoplication in patients who underwent prior EA/TEF repair have a reported incidence ranging from 6% to 64%: 6% [53], 26% [64], 27% [33], 45% [10], 64% [16].

The surgical treatment of GER after atresia repair remains a cumbersome issue. The Nissen has generally been considered the best choice and is the most widely applied operation in the past 20 years because it allows control of the low sphincteric relaxation and reconstruction of the gastroesophageal junction. However, the esophageal dismotility (with poor propulsive waves and aperistalsis in the peri-anastomotic segment), the inadequate clearance acid from the esophagus, the shortening of the esophagus, and the abnormally low esophageal sphincter pressures (all factors that predispose to GER) persist after the operation and lead to a higher failure rate. A circumferential wrap (that increases the low esophageal resistance) probably increases the risk of failure and prolonged dysphagia.

As reported by Lindahl [33], the results of Nissen fundoplication are good in the immediate postoperative period: all strictures responded to dilatations, no further recurrent pneumonias occur, vomiting ceased, eating problems decreased, distal esophagitis healed in each cases; but the long-term results show a high proportion of late failure. Recurrent respiratory symptoms are the main clinical manifestation of failed fundal wrap, whereas esophagitis (which was detected in all cases of failed fundoplication) manifests very few symptoms.

The recurrence rate of Nissen fundoplication varies from 15% to 38%: 15% [54], 25% [9], 33% [64], 38% [33]. Snyder [54] reports that breakdown of the wrap usually occurs 1 1/2 to 2 1/2 years after the surgical procedure, with wrap disruption (in half of patients) or slippage of an intact wrap. Therefore, the author suggested that partial wrap diminishes the problem of increased resistance associated with Nissen fundoplication, rendering the former (Thal or Toupet) theoretically more attractive. He analyzed the failure rate of Thal fundoplication performed for GER in EA/TEF population: he found a rate of 15% and, although it was higher than the non-EA/TEF patients, it was substantially better than data reported for Nissen fundoplication failure.

Lindahl et al. [33] reported that all surviving patients with failed fundoplication had gastric metaplasia (-Barrett's esophagus). For this reason, a long-term followup is essential.

It is important to note that the respiratory function may remain abnormal [3]. Sommpi found that the tracheal inflammation and the respiratory symptoms (especially cough during night) become "chronic" [55]: this is probably caused by tracheomalacia, vascular ring, and esophageal dysfunction related to aspiration.

References

1. Atkinson JB, Poon MW (1992) ECMO and the management of congenital diaphragmatic hernia with large diaphragmatic defects requiring a prosthetic patch. J Pediatr Surg 27:754–756
2. Bax NM, Zee DC (2003) Thoracoscopic repair of esophageal atresia with distal fistula. Surg Endosc 17:1065–1067
3. Beardsmore CS, MacFayden UM, Johnstone MS, et al (1994) Clinical findings and respiratory function in infants following repair of oesophageal atresia and tracheo-oesophageal fistula. Cur Resp J 7:1039–1047
4. Beaudoin S, Kieffer G, Sapin E, et al (1995) Gastroesophageal reflux in neonates with congenital abdominal wall defect. Eur J Pediatr Surg 5:323–326
5. Bergmeijer JHLJ, Tibboel D, Hazebroek FWJ (2000) Nissen fundoplication in the management of gastroesophageal reflux occurring after repair of esophageal atresia. J Pediatr Surg 35(4): 573–576
6. Bernbaum J, Schwartz IP, Gerdes M, et al (1995) Survivors of extracorporeal membrane oxygenation at 1 year of age: the relationship of primary diagnosis with health and neurodevelopmental sequelae. Pediatr 96:907–913
7. Boix-Ochoa J, Canals J. (1976) Maturation of the lower esophagus. J Pediatr Surg 11:749–756
8. Cohen S. (1978) Development characteristics of lower esophageal sphincteric function: a possible mechanism for infantile chalasia. Gastroenterology 67:252–258
9. Corbally MT, Muftah M, Guiney EJ (1992) Nissen fundoplication for gastroesophageal reflux in repaired tracheo-esophageal fistula. Eur J Pediatr Surg 2:332–335
10. Curci MR, Dibbins AW (1988) Problems associated with a Nissen fundoplication following tracheoesophageal fistula and esophageal atresia repair. Arch Surg 123:618–620
11. D'Agostino JA, Bernbaum JC, Gerdes M, et al (1995) Outcome for infants with congenital diaphragmatic hernia requiring extracorporeal membrane oxygenation: the first year. J Pediatr Surg 30:10–15
12. Davenport M, Mughal M, McCloy RF, Doig CM (1992) Hypogastrinemia and esophageal atresia. J Pediatr Surg 27: 568–571
13. Fasching G, Huber A, Uray E, et al (1996) Late followup in patients with gastroschisis. Pediatr Surg Int 11:103–106
14. Fasching G, Huber A, Uray E, et al (2000) Gastroesophageal reflux and diaphragmatic motility after repair of congenital diaphragmatic hernia. Eur J Pediatr Surg 10:360–364
15. Fass R, Sampliner RE (1994) Barrett's esophagus and other mucosal evidence of reflux in asymptomatic subjects with abnormal 24-hour esophageal pH monitoring. Dig Dis Sci 39: 423–425
16. Fonkalsrud EW (1979) Gastroesophageal fundoplication for reflux following repair of esophageal atresia. Experience with nine patients. Arch Surg 114:48–51
17. Fonkalsrud EW, Ament ME (1996) Gastroesophageal reflux in childhood. Curr Probl Surg 33:1–70
18. Gorostiaga L, Tovar JA, Arana J, et al (1991) La funciòn motora del esòfago operado de atresia. An Esp Pediatr 35:192–198
19. Haller JA Jr, Kehrer BH, Shaker IJ et al (1974) Studies of the pathophysiology of gastroschisis in fetal sheep. J Pediatr Surg 9:627–632
20. Hokama A, Myers NA, Kent M, et al (1986) Esophageal atresia with tracheo-esophageal fistula: a histopathological study. Pediatr Surg Int 1:117–121
21. Howard R, Myers NA (1965) Esophageal atresia: a technique for elongating the upper pouch. Surgery 58:725–727
22. Jolley SG, Tunell WP, Thomas S, et al (1985) The significance of gastric emptying in children with intestinal malformation. J Pediatr Surg 20:627–631
23. Kamiyama M, Kawahara H, Okuyama H, et al (2002) Gastroesophageal reflux after repair of congenital diaphragmatic hernia. J Pediatr Surg 37:1681–164
24. Kieffer J, Sapin E, Berg A, et al (1995) Gastroesophageal reflux after repair of congenital diaphragmatic hernia. J Pediatr Surg 30:1330–1333
25. Koch A, Rohr S, Plaschkes J, et al (1986) Incidence of gastroesphageal reflux following repair of esophageal atresia. Progr Pediatr Surg 19:103–113
26. Koivusalo A, Rintala R, Lindahl H (1999) Gastroesophageal reflux in children with a congenital abdominal wall defect. J Pediatr Surg 34(7):1227–1229
27. Koot VC, Bergmeijer JH, Bos AP, et al (1993) Incidence and management of gastroespphageal reflux after repair of congenital diaphragmatic hernia. J Pediatr Surg 28:48–52
28. Lacey SR, Bruce J, Brooks SP, et al (1987) The relative merits of various methods of indirect measurements of intra-abdominal pressure as a guide to closure of abdominal wall defects. J Pediatr Surg 22:1207–1211
29. Lally HP, Paranka MS, Roden J, et al (1992) Congenital diaphragmatic hernia stabilization and repair on ECMO. Ann Surg 216:569–573
30. Langer JC, Longaker MT, Crombleholme TM, et al (1989) Etiology of intestinal damage in gastroschisis, I: Effects of amniotic fluid exposure and bowel constriction in fetal lamb model. J Pediatr Surg 24:992–997
31. LeSouëf PN, Myers NA, Landau LI (1987) Etiologic factors in long-term respiratory function abnormalities following esophageal atresia repair. J Pediatr Surg 10:918–922
32. Lindahl H, Rintala R, Louhimo I (1987) Oesophageal anastomosis without bougienage in isolated atresia – Do the segments really grow with waiting. Z Kinderchir 42:221–223
33. Lindahl H, Rintala R, Louhimo I (1989) Failure of the Nissen fundoplication to control gastroesophageal reflux in esohageal atresia patients – Evaluation of lower esophageal sphincter function in infants and children following esophageal surgery. J Pediatr Surg 24:985–987
34. Lindahl H, Rintala R, Sariola H, et al (1990) Cervical Barrett's esophagus: a common complication of gastric tube reconstruction. J Pediatr Surg 25:446–448
35. Lindahl H, Rintala R, Sariola H, et al (1992) Long-term endoscopic and flow cytometric follow-up of colon interposistion. J Pediatr Surg 27:859–861
36. Lindahl H, Rintala R (1995) Long-term complications in cases of isolated esophageal atresia treated with esophageal anastomosis. J Pediatr Surg 30(8):1222–1223
37. Lund DP, Mitchell J, Kharasch V, et al (1994) Congenital diaphragmatic hernia: the hidden morbidity. J Pediatr Surg 29: 258–264
38. Montedonico S, Diez-Pardo JA, Possogel AK, et al (1999) Effects of esophageal shortening on the gastroesphageal barrier: an experimental study on the causes of reflux in esophageal atresia. J Pediatr Surg 34:300–303
39. Myers NA, Beasley SW, Auldist AW (1990) Secondary esophageal surgery following repair of esophageal atresia with distal tracheoesophageal fistula. J Pediatr Surg 25:773–777
40. Nagaya M, Akatsuka H, Kato J (1994) Gastroesophageal reflux occurring after repair of congenital diaphragmatic hernia. J Pediatr Surg 29:1447–1451
41. Nakazato Y, Landing BH, Wells TR (1986) Abnormal Auerbach plexus in the esophagus and stomach of patients with esophageal atresia and tracheo-esophageal fistula. J Pediatr Surg 11: 831–837
42. Okada A, Usui N, Inoue M, et al (1997) Esophageal atresia in Osaka: a review of 39 years' experience. J Pediatr Surg 32: 1570–1574
43. Orringer MB, Kirsh MM, Sloan H (1977) Long-term esophageal function following repair of esophageal atresia. Ann Surg 186:436–443

44. Pieretti R, Shandling B, Stephens CA (1974) Resistant esophageal stenosis associated with reflux after repair of esophageal atresia. A therapeutic approach. J Pediatr Surg 9:355–357

45. Puri P, Blake N, O'Donnell B, et al (1981) Delayed primary anastomosis following spontaneous growth of esophageal segments in esophageal atresia. J Pediatr Surg 16:180–183

46. Qi B, Diez-Pardo JA, Soto C, et al (1996) Transdiaphragmatic pressure gradients and lower esophageal sphincter after tight abdominal wall plication in the rat. J Pediatr Surg 31: 1666–1669

47. Rintala RJ, Schalamon J, Lindahl H, Saarikoski H (2003) Endoscopic follow-up in esophageal atresia – for how long is it necessary? J Pediatr Surg 38:702–704

48. Romeo G, Zuccarello B, Proietto F, et al (1987) Disorders of the esophageal motor activity in atresia of the esophagus. J Pediatr Surg 22:120–124

49. Schmittenbecher PP (1990). Die postoperative Kontrolle der Kardiafunktion in Neugeborener nach Oesophagus, Zwerchfell- und Bauchwandfehlbildungen. Z Kinderchir 45: 278–281

50. Schneeberger A, Scott R, Rubin, et al (1987) Esophageal function following Livaditis repair of long-gap esophageal atresia. J Pediatr Surg 22:779–783

51. Shono T, Suita S, Arima T, et al (1993) Motility function of the esophagus before primary anastomosis in esophageal atresia. J Pediatr Surg 28:673–676

52. Sigalet DL, Nguyen LT, Adolph V, et al (1994) Gastroesophageal reflux associated with large diaphragmatic hernias. J Pediatr Surg 29:1262–1265

53. Sillen U, Hagberg S, Rubenson A, et al (1988) Management of esophageal atresia: review of 16 years experience. J Pediatr Surg 23:805–809

54. Snyder CL, Ramachandran V, Kennedy AP, et al (1997) Efficacy of partial wrap fundoplication for gastroesophageal reflux after repair of esophageal atresia. J Pediatr Surg 32:1089–1092

55. Somppi E, Tammela O, Ruuska T, et al (1998) Outcome of patients operated on for esophageal atresia: 30 years' experience. J Pediatr Surg 33:1341–1346

56. Spitz L, Kiely E, Brereton RJ (1987) Esophageal atresia: five-year experience with 148 cases. J Pediatr Surg 22:103–108

57. Stolar CJ, Levy JP, Dillon PW, et al (1990) Anatomic and functional anomalies of the esophagus in infants surviving congenital diaphragmatic hernia. Am J Surg 159:204–207

58. Tibboel D, Pattenier JW, VanKrutgen RJ, et al (1988) Prospective evaluation of postoperative morbidity in patients with esophageal atresia. Pediatr Surg Int 4:252–255

59. Tovar JA, Diez-Pardo JA, Murcia J, et al (1995) Ambulatory 24-hour manometric and pHmetric evidence of permanent impairment of clearance capacity in patients with esophageal atresia. J Pediatr Surg 30(8):1224–1231

60. Vanamo K, Rintala RJ, Lindahl H, et al (1996) Long-term gastrointestinal morbidity in patients with congenital diaphragmatic defects. J Pediatr Surg 31:551–554

61. Van Meurs KP, Robbins ST, Reed VL, et al (1993) Congenital diaphragmatic hernia: long-term outcome in neonates treated with extracorporeal membrane oxygenation. J Pediatr Surg 122:893–899

62. Wang W, Tovar JA, Eisaguirre I et al (1993) Airway obstruction and gastroesophageal reflux: an experimental study on the pathogenesis of this association. J Pediatr Surg 28:995–998

63. West KW, Bengston K, Rescorla FJ, et al (1992) Delayed surgical repair and ECMO improves survival in congenital diaphragmatic hernia. Ann Surg 216:454–460

64. Wheatley MJ, Coran AG, Wesley JR (1993) Efficacy of the Nissen fundoplication in the management of gaastroesophageal reflux following esophageal atresia repair. J Pediatr Surg 28:53–55

65. Zuccarello B, Nicotina PA, Centorrino A, et al (1988) Immunohistochemical study on muscle actinin content of atresic esophageal upper pouch. It J Pediatr Surg Sci 2:75–78

Chapter 6

Conditions Mimicking Gastroesophageal Reflux

6

Mahmoud Sabri · Carlo Di Lorenzo

Contents

6.1
Introduction

Nissen fundoplication remains one of the three most common major surgical procedures performed in infants and children. However, despite its unquestioned value in preventing reflux and emesis, fundoplication is far from being an uncomplicated procedure. Dyspeptic symptoms such as fullness, early satiety, abdominal pain, or bloating may occur in up to 30% of patients who undergo surgery [4].

Failure of fundoplication to improve preoperative symptoms may be caused by an erroneous diagnosis of gastroesophageal reflux disease (GERD). Conditions mimicking GERD and associated with a high incidence of problems after surgery include dietary protein allergy, eosinophilic esophagitis, hypertrophic pyloric stenosis, rumination, and gastroparesis, entities which will be discussed in this chapter. Eliminating the ability to vomit in a child with any of these pathologies may lead to breakdown of fundoplication. Thorough preoperative evaluation aimed at recognizing the "wrong" patients for the procedure may give the child the best chance for an excellent prognosis.

6.2
Dietary Protein Allergy

Cow's milk allergy is an immunologically mediated adverse reaction to cow's milk proteins. Cow's milk is often the first major food protein ingested by formula-fed infants, which may lead to early sensitization. It may also occur in exclusively in breast-fed infants.

6.2.1
Epidemiology

In the developed world, cow's milk protein allergy has an incidence of approximately 2% in infants less than 2 years of age and is the most common food allergy in this age group [18, 46]. It is the most frequent parentally perceived adverse reaction to food with prevalence estimates based on parental perception between 12% and 15% in children under the age of 3 years. However, objective diagnostic testing has revealed that parents overestimate the role of milk as the cause of symptoms in their children. The actual reported prevalence is more likely to be 7.5% at 12 months of age and 5% at 24 - months of age [11].

6.2.2
Pathophysiology

Similar to other food allergies, cow's milk protein allergy may be divided into immunoglobulin (Ig) E-mediated and non-IgE-mediated food allergy, mainly type III (immune-complexes) and type IV (cell mediated) reactions [44]. In infants with cow's milk protein allergy, non-IgE- mediated mechanisms play an important pathophysiological role [43]. In addition, there is evidence that T-cell activation plays a role in cow's milk protein allergy in patients with atopic dermatitis [45], with increase in the T helper 2 (Th2) predominant cytokine profile, IL-4, IL-5, and IL-13. There are different proteins in cow's milk, the most important of which are α_{s1}-casein, one of the casein proteins, and β-lactoglobulin, one of the whey proteins, both responsible for the immunogenic-mediated reactions produced in patients with cow's milk protein allergy. Allergen-specific IgE and T-cells recognize peptides of varying sizes along the entire chain of α_{s1}-casein. T-cell recognition sites for β-lactoglobulin have been identified in children with cow's milk protein allergy [21].

There is increasing evidence that ingested cow's milk and other food antigens are secreted into human milk and can potentially sensitize the breast-fed infant [23]. IgA antibodies in human milk have a protective effect on the sensitization to food allergens as they may prevent antigen entry at the intestinal cell surface of infants. In a study of breast-fed infants, IgA concentrations in the colestrum and human milk were significantly lower in mothers whose infants developed milk protein allergy during the first 12 months of life, suggesting that IgA antibodies in human milk play a role in the sensitization to food allergens [22].

6.2.3
Presentation

Most infants with cow's milk protein allergy develop symptoms before 1 month of age, often within 1 week after the introduction of cow's milk-based formula. The majority of infants have two or more symptoms involving two or more organ systems. Cutaneous, gastrointestinal, respiratory, and even systemic reactions may occur in response to milk protein allergy [19].

Symptoms suggestive of cow's milk protein allergy may occur within a few minutes to 1 h after milk exposure or after 1 h and in some cases after several days. Anaphylaxis was reported in 9% of infants with cow's milk protein allergy. Cutaneous manifestations include atopic dermatitis, urticaria, angioedema, and contact rash. Gastrointestinal manifestations are in the form of local oral reactions, nausea, vomiting, colic, diarrhea, colitis, eosinophilic gastroenteritis, and protein-losing enteropathy. Respiratory reactions may occur in the form of asthma, laryngeal edema, or otitis media with effusion.

In young children, GERD and dietary protein allergy are difficult to differentiate on the basis of clinical presentation. Cow's milk protein allergy may cause delay in gastric emptying and has been associated with gastric dysrhythmias and may induce reflex vomiting or exacerbate symptoms of GERD [39]. The presence of other manifestations of cow's milk protein allergy, such as atopic dermatitis, eosinophilic esophagitis, enterocolitis, or constipation should alert the physician that the etiology of the infant symptoms is not simply GERD.

6.2.4
Diagnosis

The diagnosis of milk protein allergy relies upon a careful history, skin prick tests, in vitro measurement of food-specific IgE if applicable, an appropriate elimination diet, and blinded oral food challenges.

Skin prick tests are highly reproducible and are frequently used to screen patients with suspected IgE-mediated food allergies. The skin prick test may be considered an excellent means of excluding IgE-mediated food allergies, but is only suggestive of the presence of clinical food allergies. It is reliable for immediate food allergies, thus, it is more helpful to exclude immediate-type reactions caused by milk protein allergy. It is noteworthy that there are many false-positive skin prick tests with no clinical significance, so a positive skin test in isolation can not be considered a proof of clinically relevant hypersensitivity.

In vitro radioallergosorbent tests (RASTs) are also helpful in the evaluation of IgE-mediated food allergy. RAST negative results are very reliable in ruling out an IgE-mediated reaction to a particular food, but a positive result has low specificity. They are likely to be positive in syndromes that are acute in onset after ingestion of the causal protein and in patients with other manifestations of atopic disease.

A trial of elimination diet is a simple, practical, and definitive test to differentiate cow's milk protein allergy from GERD. A 1- or 2-week trial of a hypoallergenic formula is recommended by North American Society for Pediatric Gastroenterology and Nutrition guidelines for evaluation and treatment of GER in infants and children [40]. If symptoms resolve, an oral challenge testing with milk and other dairies may be considered. As tests for specific IgE antibodies are not relevant to milk protein allergy, oral challenges are often the only means of diagnosis. Oral challenge may cause severe allergic reactions; therefore, it should be performed under physician supervision and with the availability of emergency medications and equipment to treat allergic reactions.

A study by Iacono et al. found that 42% of patients with GER proven by intraesophageal pH monitoring study and endoscopic evidence of esophagitis had cow's milk protein allergy. During the 24-h esophageal pH monitoring study, the authors found that all the patients who had cow's milk protein allergy demonstrated a characteristic gradual decrease in esophageal pH between one meal and the next, the characteristic typical "phasic" pattern [20]. Another study failed to find any characteristic esophageal pH-metric pattern distinguishing patients with GER and cow's milk protein allergy from those patients with GER alone [32].

To differentiate GER from cow's milk protein allergy, a study was conducted on 25 infants with persistent vomiting, with the authors comparing a noninvasive test of small bowel permeability with more invasive tests involving endoscopy, mucosal biopsy, and esophageal pH monitoring. Each infant underwent a cellobiose/mannitol permeability study, upper endoscopy with small bowel biopsies and a 24-h pH study. Results of the permeability test were abnormal in only 6% of the patients with GER, but in 100% of those with GER and cow's milk protein allergy and in 100% of those with cow's milk protein allergy alone. This study suggested that such permeability test could avoid more invasive diagnostic tests in the evaluation of infants with persistent vomiting. However, adoption of this noninvasive test in clinical practice will not be established until further studies are conducted to prove its reproducibility [52].

6.2.5
Treatment

At present there is no effective therapy for IgE-mediated food allergy. The treatment of cow's milk protein allergy follows the general principles of allergen avoidance. Soy formula is often used as a cow's milk substitute. A significant proportion of infants with cow's milk protein allergy may also be sensitized to soy protein [61]. The introduction of highly allergenic food items (e.g., eggs, peanuts, and tree nuts) should be deferred in these patients until the second year of life. It has been estimated that approximately 10% of infants with cow's milk protein allergy are still intolerant to extensively hydrolyzed formulae [17]. In these infants, amino acid-based formula has proved effective and safe [49]. In breast-fed infants, maternal elimination of diet that contains milk, soy, and milk and soy products, is often effective. Dietary calcium supplementation to the mothers may be required. Approximately 85% of infants with milk protein allergy will develop tolerance to cow's milk protein by 3 years of age. Although allergen avoidance appears to hasten the subsequent development of antigen tolerance, it remains unclear to what extent dietary manipulations alter the course of food allergies.

6.3
Eosinophilic Esophagitis

Eosinophilic esophagitis (EE) is an increasingly recognized entity distinct from GERD. It is characterized by the presence in the esophagus of dense epithelial eosinophilic infiltrate with more than 15 eosinophils per high-power field.

6.3.1
Epidemiology

Eosinophilic esophagitis is a clinicopathologic disease entity that was initially described two decades ago [38]. This condition has now become frequent enough that new cases are not reported in the literature. It is diagnosed on a weekly basis in most major pediatric medical centers in the United States. There seem to be geographical differences in its incidence [12]. There is no sex or race predilection. A family history of allergic disorders such as bronchial asthma, hay fever, or eczema is not uncommon in patients with EE.

6.3.2
Pathophysiology

The pathophysiology of EE is not clearly understood. The observation that symptomatic and histologic response to restricted and elemental diets may occur in patients with EE has led to the speculation that food allergy may produce EE. Recent studies have shown that aeroallergens induce EE in animal models by cytokine-mediated mechanisms [33]. Eotaxin is an eosinophilic chemoattractant produced by epithelial cells at the site of inflammation. It has the propriety of controlling the recruitment of eosinophils to the tissue. Eotaxin generated at a site of allergic inflammation might contribute to eosinophil accumulation and activation [6]. Once activated, eosinophils release cytotoxic proteins in their granules, causing tissue damage.

6.3.3
Presentation

Symptoms of EE may overlap with symptoms of GER. Presentation is age-dependent and symptoms may vary in duration from a few days to years. Infants present with vomiting, irritability, failure to thrive, and even hematemesis. Older children and adolescents commonly present with dysphagia, food impactions, and strictures. Little is known about the natural history of this condition.

6.3.4
Diagnosis

The diagnosis of EE is based on the pathologic finding of more than 15 eosinophils/high power field (hpf) in the esophageal squamous epithelium, in contrast to 5 eosinophils/hpf or less found in esophagitis secondary to GERD [16, 36]. Other pathologic findings seen on histopathologic examination of the esophageal mucosa include the presence of eosinophil aggregation and degranulation, eosinophil abscess, and basal layer proliferation. Endoscopic findings are distinctive. The mucosa is extremely fragile, delicate, and inelastic, slightly contracted (corrugated rings) in a normal looking esophagus. Furrowing (Fig. 1) of the esophageal mucosa and microabscesses, which may be confused with yeast infection, are also peculiar findings typical of this condition [53] (Fig. 2).

Diagnostic work-up for EE include the search for food and environmental allergens by IgE-mediated RASTs or allergy skin testing, the recognition of drug reactions, and the exclusion of collagen vascular disease or autoimmune disorders.

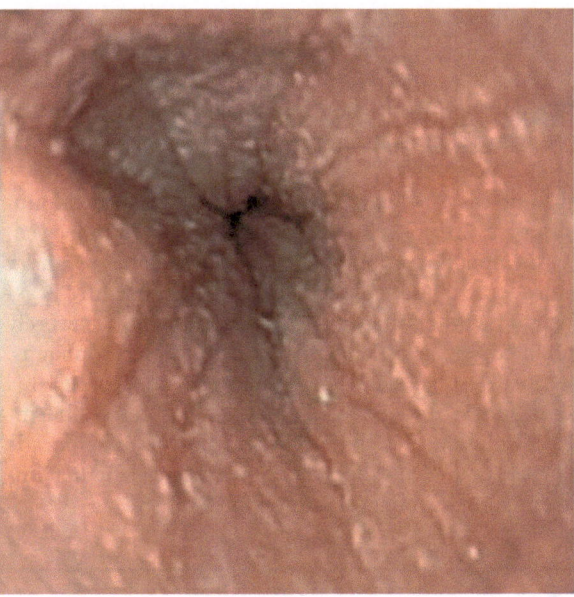

Fig. 2. Endoscopic photograph showing the presence in the distal esophagus of whitish lesions representing microabscesses, a finding typical of eosinophilic esophagitis

6.3.5
Treatment

Elimination of food proven to be antigenic by RASTs or skin prick tests is of great importance in the treatment of EE. Studies have shown that restriction of the common food antigens, milk, egg, peanuts, soy, wheat, tree nuts, and shellfish, along with introduction of elemental diet in children with EE for at least 6 weeks, will produce a remarkable clinical symptomatic response, even in the absence of positive allergy testing [51]. Food challenge may start when the patient is in a symptom-free state. This can be accomplished by the introduction of one type of food every 5–7 days with monitoring of symptoms in order to identify the offending foods.

Pharmacotherapy currently used for children with EE includes:

1. Systemic steroids:
   - Steroids cause symptomatic improvement within 1–2 weeks and histologic improvement in 4 weeks but are often associated with undesirable side effects.
2. Topical steroids:
   - This innovative usage of topical steroids was initially described 5 years ago [13]. The intake of the topical steroids (fluticasone propionate or beclomethasone) is done by swallowing, without inhaling. The inhaled steroids are associated with few side effects and should be used without a spacer. Anecdotally, a 6-week treatment period seems to be the optimal length of treatment.
3. Mast cell stabilizers:
   - They inhibit T-cell functions and the release of leukotrines and inflammatory cytokines. Their definite role in treatment of EE has not been established.
4. Anti-GERD therapy:
   - The use of H_2-blockers or proton pump inhibitors to treat GERD may give a synergistic effect along with the other therapy for EE.

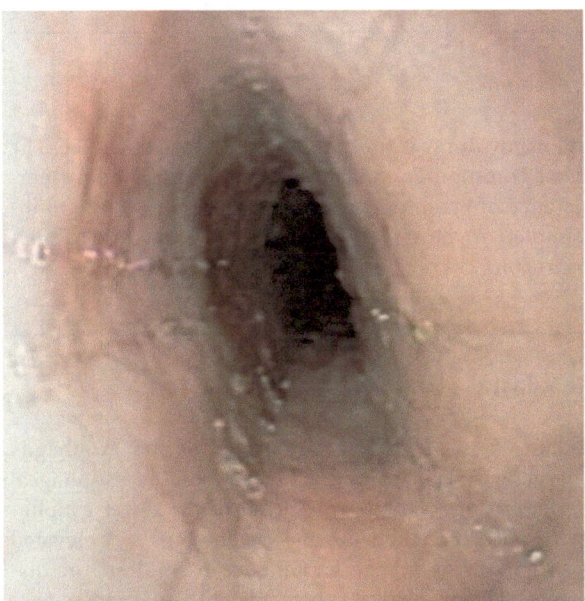

Fig. 1. Endoscopic photograph showing vertical lines in the distal esophagus (furrowing) suggestive of eosinophilic esophagitis

5. Leukotriene inhibitors:
   - The leukotriene inhibitor montelukast, mainly used for the treatment of bronchial asthma, has been proven in some reports to be useful in the treatment of eosinophilic gastroenteritis [34, 48].

In some cases when the swelling of the esophageal mucosa is severe, food impaction may ensue. In those cases, disimpaction and dilatation of the esophagus under endoscopic guidance is indicated. This procedure is associated with an increase risk of trauma to the severely inflamed, inelastic, and poorly distensible esophagus. Because dysphagia is such a prominent symptom of this condition, a fundoplication may be particularly harmful in individuals with EE. The addition of an antegrade block provided by the surgery may cause further impairment of esophageal emptying.

6.4
Hypertrophic Pyloric Stenosis

This is a condition that is characterized by thickening of the circular muscle at the pyloric sphincter resulting in gastric outlet obstruction.

6.4.1
Epidemiology

Hypertrophic pyloric stenosis (HPS) occurs predominantly in caucasians, with males being five times more affected than females. The incidence is reported to be 6–8 per 1,000 live births.

6.4.2
Pathophysiology

Hypertrophic pyloric stenosis is characterized by hypertrophy of the pyloric muscle, causing pyloric-channel narrowing and elongation. The etiology of HPS is not fully understood. There seem to be abnormalities in pyloric innervation, the intestinal pacemaker system, extracellular matrix proteins, smooth muscle cells, and growth factors. Recent studies have shown that marked alterations in cholinergic and adrenergic nerves occur in the hypertrophied pyloric muscle [26]. Other studies have demonstrated low levels of neuronal nitric oxide synthase mRNA in pyloric muscle in patients with HPS, with subsequent reduction of nitric oxide leading to excessive contraction of the hypertrophied circular muscle [27]. Abnormality or lack of the interstitial cells of Cajal has also been shown in patients with HPS [57].

6.4.3
Presentation

"Projectile" vomiting is very characteristic of the disease and may help in differentiating this entity from GERD, in which there is usually "effortless" regurgitation. Emesis usually begins in the second or third week of life. With successive episodes of vomiting, the infant becomes dehydrated and lethargic, with the development of hypochloremic metabolic alkalosis, a metabolic abnormality which would be unusual in babies with uncomplicated GERD. Infants with pyloric stenosis are typically hungry at the beginning of the feed then as the stomach fills they become irritable until vomiting occurs. Visible peristalsis can be noted in the upper abdomen [30]. An olive-like mass may be palpable in the upper abdomen. In patients with HPS, antireflux surgery may cause "closed-loop" obstruction with inability of the ingested food to be emptied either aborally or orally.

6.4.4
Diagnosis

Ultrasonography of the pylorus has become the diagnostic procedure of choice. Diagnostic criteria include muscle thickness of >4 mm and pyloric length of >16 mm. The specificity of this test is 100% and the sensitivity is 97%. Upper gastrointestinal series may show elongation of the pyloric canal, double tract of barium along the pyloric canal, and a prepyloric bulge into the distal antrum, giving a shouldering appearance.

6.4.5
Treatment

Pyloromyotomy is the surgical procedure of choice. The most common complications postoperatively are persistence of symptoms of pyloric obstruction due to incomplete myotomy and wound dehiscence due to malnutrition.

6.5
Achalasia

Achalasia is a functional disorder of the esophagus characterized by complete absence of the esophageal peristalsis, incomplete relaxation of the lower esophageal sphincter (LES) during swallowing, and elevated resting lower esophageal sphincter. In children, the disease usually presents at approximately 6–10 years of age.

6.5.1
Epidemiology

The incidence of achalasia is estimated to be 0.5/100,000 per year with a prevalence of 8/100,000 per year [31]. It is noteworthy that less than 5% of all symptomatic patients with achalasia are younger than 15 years of age [3].

6.5.2
Pathophysiology

Achalasia appears to be primarily due to impairment of LES relaxation. This impairment seems to be due to a decrease in the number and/or function of the inhibitory nerves supplying the LES. Histopathologic examination of the esophagus demonstrates a loss of inhibitory myenteric plexus ganglion cells. These impaired inhibitory nerves are probably nitric oxide- and/or vasoactive intestinal peptide-containing nerves [10, 1]. An inflammatory reaction may be the cause of the loss of nitrigenic inhibitory effect. The result of these pathophysiologic mechanisms is decrease in inhibitory innervation of the LES with preservation of excitatory cholinergic innervation leading to a predominance of the excitatory cholinergic tone. Esophageal aperistalsis in achalasia may be secondary to lack of inhibitory innervation throughout the esophageal body or be a sequela of long-term obstruction at the gastroesophageal junction.

6.5.3
Presentation

Less than 5.3% of children with achalasia present below 1 month of age, 15% between 1 month and 1 year, 22% between 1 and 5 years, and 57% present above 6 years of age [5]. The mean duration of symptoms is 23 months before diagnosis. Younger children have symptoms that simulate GERD, including refusal to eat, vomiting, and nocturnal regurgitation with vomiting being the most prominent symptom in 80% of the patients. The emesis is commonly manifested by food contents not mixed with gastric juice. In infants, the vomited milk is not curdled and is not being soured by acid. With frequent episodes of vomiting, failure to thrive ensues [42]. Respiratory symptoms include choking, recurrent pneumonia, and nocturnal cough. Older children and adolescents have symptoms of dysphagia and retrosternal chest pain. This dysphagia occurs initially with solids then worsens progressively with liquids. A typical complaint from adolescent patients is that the food is "stuck" in the chest and an effort is made to push the food down into the stomach by swallowing repeatedly. Triple A syndrome, a condition which includes also ala-

crimia and adrenocorticotrophic insensitivity, and the autosomal recessive syndrome of deafness, vitiligo, short stature, and muscle weakness have been associated with achalasia [35, 41].

6.5.4
Diagnosis

A plain chest radiography that shows the presence of an air fluid level in the widened mediastinum may suggest achalasia. Absence of air in the stomach may be suggestive of achalasia [5]. Barium swallow studies are considered essential for the diagnosis of achalasia. They typically demonstrate the presence of a dilated distal esophagus with typical "birds beak" appearance at the level at the gastroesophageal junction [28] (Fig. 3). Esophageal manometry is the preferred method of diagnosis in centers which have expertise in performing this test. Manometry provides information about the severity of achalasia as well as the response to treatment.

There are four manometric findings characterizing achalasia.
1. Lack of peristalsis in the esophageal body with low amplitude simultaneous pressure changes in the distal esophagus [8]. This is the hallmark of the disease and is the most constant finding. Occasionally, high amplitude, simultaneous contractions may be found in the initial stages of the disease, a condition named "vigorous achalasia."

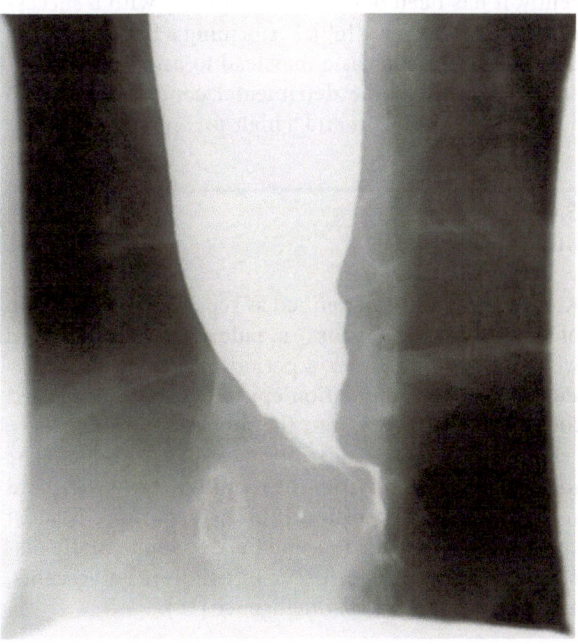

Fig. 3. Esophagogram showing the classic "bird-like beak" appearance in a child with achalasia

2. Incomplete LES relaxation is an important pathogenetic factor but not a constant finding in patients with achalasia [24, 58]. When it occurs, LES relaxation may decrease to less than 30% of the normal.
3. Increased LES basal pressure.
4. Intraesophageal pressure higher than intragastric pressure. Intraesophageal pressure was 6.1±0.7 mm Hg higher than the intragastric pressure in 90% of the patients with achalasia [56].

Endoscopy is usually used to diagnose conditions that may mimic achalasia and to insert a guide wire for positioning of a balloon for LES dilatation. The esophagus appears patulous and the LES does not open upon insufflation with air. The presence of esophagitis due to the stagnation of food material may occasionally make achalasia difficult to differentiate from GERD.

6.5.5
Treatment

The corner stone of treatment is to provide symptomatic relief of the mechanical obstruction at the LES. This can be accomplished with pharmacologic therapy, or with invasive procedures that include esophageal dilation, intrasphincteric injection of botulinum toxin, or surgical myotomy. Surgery usually provides better results and longer duration of remission. The choice for surgery versus pneumatic dilatation is based on the physician and patient preference. The modified Heller myotomy is the surgical procedure of choice [35]. Recently, it has been done laparascopically with a success rate of 90% at 5 years [60]. Performing a fundoplication in patient with achalasia may lead to catastrophic outcomes in view of the detrimental combination of an aperistaltic esophagus and a high-pressure LES.

6.6
Rumination

Rumination has been defined as repeated regurgitation of food, with weight loss or failure to gain expected weight, developing after a period of normal functioning. During the rumination episode, partially digested food is brought back into the mouth without nausea, retching, or associated gastrointestinal disorders. The food in then ejected from the mouth by rechewing and reswallowing or expulsion [2]. The syndrome is most commonly seen in infants and the developmentally disabled. However, it does occur in children, adolescents, and adults with normal intelligence [15].

6.6.1
Pathophysiology

The pathophysiology of rumination is not fully understood. It is believed to be due to coexistence of functional and psychiatric abnormalities [29]. Recently, it has been suggested that rumination syndrome is characterized by higher gastric sensitivity and decreased threshold for lower esophageal sphincter relaxation during gastric distension [54].

6.6.2
Diagnosis

Diagnosis is made mostly by observation, which may be difficult because rumination may cease as soon as the patient becomes aware of the observer. Characteristic features are the onset immediately after or even during feeding and the absence of esophagitis. Diagnosis can be based on the following Rome II ("symptoms-based") criteria which include:

For infants: At least 3 months of repetitive behavior, with contractions of the abdominal muscles, diaphragm, and tongue culminating into regurgitation of gastric contents into the mouth that are expectorated or rechewed and reswallowed in addition to three or more of the following:
1. Onset between 3–8 months
2. No response to management of GERD, anticholinergic drugs, formula changes, or gavage or gastrostomy feeding
3. Unaccompanied by signs of nausea or distress
4. No incidence during sleep or when the infant is interacting with individuals in the environment

For children and adolescents, the following are the proposed criteria for diagnosis [7]: at least 6 weeks of recurrent regurgitation of recently ingested food, in the preceding 12 months, which may not need to be consecutive, and:
1. Begins within 30 min of meal ingestion
2. Is associated with either reswallowing or expulsion of food
3. Stops within 90 min of onset or when regurgitant becomes acidic
4. Is not associated with mechanical obstruction
5. Does not respond to standard treatment for GER
6. Is not associated with nocturnal symptoms

Antroduodenal manometry shows a characteristic pattern with brief simultaneous pressure increases at all recording sites associated with the rumination episodes [25] (Fig. 4). Fasting manometry is characteristically normal.

Fig. 4.
Antroduodenal manometry showing brief, simultaneous increase in pressure at all recording sites ("r waves") marked by an asterisk, coinciding with rumination episodes

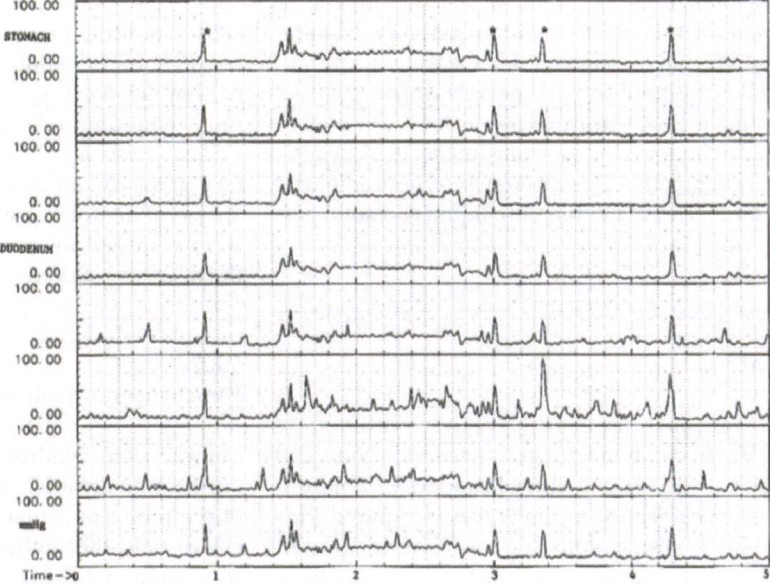

6.6.3
Treatment

Treatment is based on improving the bonding between the mother and the infant providing a nurturing environment to the infant. A multidisciplinary team approach is required for satisfactory recovery in adolescents. Parenteral nutrition or postpyloric tube feeding may be required. Nonadversive behavioral therapies, such as diaphragmatic breathing, have been effective in many adolescents. Because of the chronicity of the symptoms of regurgitation, some patients with rumination may mistakenly receive a fundoplication. After surgery, the stimulus to ruminate persists, and children develop recurrent episodes of retching, which may become quite fastidious.

6.7
Gastroparesis

Gastroparesis is a condition characterized by symptoms resulting from impaired emptying of intraluminal contents of the stomach into the duodenum in the absence of a mechanical obstruction. In older children, it may be found in association with other systemic diseases or after surgery. There are no data on the prevalence of gastroparesis in infants and children.

6.7.1
Pathophysiology

Any systemic disease or condition that leads to neuromuscular dysfunction of the gastrointestinal tract may lead to gastroparesis. The most common causes in infants and children include prematurity, viral infections, drugs such as opioids and anticholinergics, metabolic disturbances such as hypokalemia, acidosis, and hypothyroidism, eosinophilic gastroenteropathy, cerebral palsy, diabetes mellitus, vagotomy, pseudo-obstruction, and muscular dystrophy. Many patients have no apparent etiology and are diagnosed to have idiopathic gastroparesis. Postviral gastroparesis is a recently described entity in children, accounting for many forms of acquired gastroparesis. It follows a short viral illness, often rotavirus, and is associated with postprandial antral hypomotility [50].

6.7.2
Presentation

Nausea, vomiting, fullness, bloating, and early satiety are classically the predominant symptoms of gastroparesis. Some children with prolonged symptoms may have weight loss. The emesis characteristically occurs hours after eating, a differentiating feature from both GERD and rumination.

6.7.3
Diagnosis

Nuclear medicine scintiscan is the gold standard for the measurement of gastric emptying and can be used as a reliable screening test for abnormal gastric motility, although normal values for emptying of different meals at different ages are unknown. A normal gastric emptying of a solid meal by definition rules out gastroparesis.

Emptying of barium or liquid meals should not be relied upon for this diagnosis. In postviral gastroparesis, antroduodenal manometry demonstrates postprandial antral hypomotility with normal antral contractions during fasting. Ultrasonography has been used to evaluate gastric emptying in young infants [9]. The 13C-octanoic acid breath test is a newer, safe, nonradiologic test that has been used to measure liquid and solid gastric emptying [59].

6.7.4
Treatment

Postviral gastroparesis usually resolves within 6–24 months [50]. In children with prolonged symptoms and associated weight loss, nutritional support with nasoduodenal and nasojejunal feeding tubes is required. Various prokinetic medications such as cisapride, erythromycin, metoclopramide, and domperidone have been used to improve the gastric emptying. Erythromycin has proved to be the most effective gastrokinetic [55]. In patients with neurological impairment such as cerebral palsy, surgical pyloroplasty or pyloromyotomy remains a therapeutic option. Transpyloric feeding can be considered for a short period of time before pursuing surgery. Features differentiating common condition mimicking GERD are reported in Table 1.

6.8
Other Conditions

6.8.1
Intracranial Space-Occupying Lesions

Vomiting is a nonspecific symptom that may result from a disorder of any organ system, including the central nervous system. Elevated intracranial pressure commonly leads to vomiting. Tumors of the central nervous system are now thought to be the most common form of childhood malignancies [37]. Space-occupying lesions, particularly posterior fossa tumors, often have an insidious onset and a slow progression of symptoms. Similarly, hydrocephalus and subdural effusion may present with few manifestations other than vomiting. Space-oc-cupying lesions, especially brainstem gliomas, can also cause vomiting because of infiltration and damage to sensitive brain regions and are frequently unaccompanied by any focal signs [14]. Because vomiting is a common symptom, and since brain tumor or other structural lesions, such as Arnold Chiari malformation, need to be diagnosed and treated in a timely manner, appropriate use of neuroimaging, such as computed tomography (CT) scan and magnetic resonance imaging (MRI) of the head, in children with vomiting is mandated.

6.8.2
Munchausen's Syndrome by Proxy

Munchausen's syndrome by proxy (MSBP) or pediatric falsification disorder represents a persistent fabrication of symptoms or actual illness in young children by parents, usually the mother. The main benefit for the perpetrating parent lies in the leading role that he or she plays during repeated hospital admissions as the medical staff puzzles over the child's problem. The incidence of this syndrome is unknown because detection is inherently difficult. Vomiting may be the sole or part of the manifestations that gastroenterologists may observe when dealing with this syndrome. In specialist referral centers, gastroenterologists may be asked to evaluate young children who have recurrent vomiting, apnea, or a near-miss sudden infant death syndrome in which surgery for GERD is considered. Surgery in cases of MSBP is associated with frequent postoperative problems. The most important key for rapid diagnosis is heightened awareness. Assay for emetine in the body fluids is recommended if use of ipecac syrup is suspected. When the patient has serious, long-lasting, incomprehensible symptoms that do not respond to appropriate treatment and are at odds with the results of diagnostic testing, the clinician should always consider the possibility of MSBP [47].

6.9
Summary

Careful search for the etiology and pathophysiology of symptoms that mimic GERD may help to avoid unnec-

Table 1. Differentiating features of some clinical entities mimicking GER

	Vomiting	Esophagitis	Prokinetics	Antireflux surgery
GERD	Chronic, postprandial	Yes	Helpful	Helpful
Dietary protein allergy	Chronic, postprandial	At times	Not helpful	Not helpful
Eosinophilic esophagitis	Not common	Yes	Not helpful	Not helpful
Hypertrophic pyloric stenosis	Projectile	Yes	Not helpful	Not helpful
Rumination	During or minutes after meals	No	Not helpful	Not helpful
Gastroparesis	Hours after meals	No	Helpful	Not helpful

essary surgeries. Early detection of conditions that simulate GERD represents the best strategy to minimize complication from antireflux surgery.

References

1. Aggestrup S, Uddman R, Sundler F, Fahrenkrug J, Hakanson R, Sorensen HR, Hambraeus G (1983) Lack of vasoactive intestinal polypeptide nerves in esophageal achalasia. Gastroenterology 84:924–927

2. American Psychiatry Association (2000) Diagnostic and statistical manual of mental disorders, test revised. 4th edn. American Psychiatry Association, Washington DC, pp 105–106

3. Azizkhan RG, Tapper D, Eraklis A (1980) Achalasia in childhood: a 20-year experience. J Pediatr Surg 15:452–456

4. Baigrie RJ, Watson DI, Myers JC, Jamieson GG (1997) Outcome of laparoscopic Nissen fundoplication in patients with disordered preoperative peristalsis. Gut 40:381–385

5. Berquist WE, Byrne WJ, Ament ME, Fonkalsrud EW, Euler AR (1983) Achalasia: diagnosis, management, and clinical course in 16 children. Pediatrics 71:798–805

6. Bischoff SC (1996) Mucosal allergy: role of mast cells and eosinophil granulocytes in the gut. Baillieres Clin Gastroenterol 10:443–459

7. Chial HJ, Camilleri M, Williams DE, Litzinger K, Perrault J (2003) Rumination syndrome in children and adolescents: diagnosis, treatment, and prognosis. Pediatrics 111:158–162

8. Cohen S (1979) Motor disorders of the esophagus. N Engl J Med 301:184–192

9. Cucchiara S (1994) Ultrasound. In: Hyman PE, Di Lorenzo C (eds) Pediatric gastrointestinal motility disorders. Academy of Professional Information Services, New York, pp 313–318

10. De Giorgio R, Di Simone MP, Stanghellini V, Barbara G, Tonini M, Salvioli B, Mattioli S, Corinaldesi R (1999) Esophageal and gastric nitric oxide synthesizing innervation in primary achalasia. Am J Gastroenterol 94:2357–2362

11. Eggesbo M, Botten G, Halvorsen R, Magnus P (2001) The prevalence of CMA/CMPI in young children: the validity of parentally perceived reactions in a population-based study. Allergy 56:393–402

12. Elitsur Y (2002) Eosinophilic esophagitis – is it in the air? J Pediatr Gastroenterol Nutr 34:325–326

13. Faubion WA Jr, Perrault J, Burgart LJ, Zein NN, Clawson M, Freese DK (1998) Treatment of eosinophilic esophagitis with inhaled corticosteroids. J Pediatr Gastroenterol Nutr 27:90–3

14. Frank Y, Schwartz SB, Epstein NE, Beresford HR (1989) Chronic dysphagia, vomiting and gastroesophageal reflux as manifestations of a brain stem glioma: a case report. Pediatr Neurosci 15:265–268

15. Fredericks DW, Carr JE, Williams WL (1998) Overview of the treatment of rumination disorder for adults in a residential setting. J Behav Ther Exp Psychiatry 29:31–40

16. Furuta GT (2002) Eosinophilic esophagitis: an emerging clinicopathologic entity. Curr Allergy Asthma Rep 2:67–72

17. Hill DJ, Heine RG, Cameron DJ, Francis DE, Bines JE (2001) Cow's milk protein allergy and possible means for its prevention. Nutrition 17:642–651

18. Hill DJ, Hosking CS (1996) Cow milk allergy in infancy and early childhood. Clin Exp Allergy 26:243–246

19. Host A (1994) Cow's milk protein allergy and intolerance in infancy. Some clinical, epidemiological and immunological aspects. Pediatr Allergy Immunol 5:1–36

20. Iacono G, Carroccio A, Cavataio F, Montalto G, Kazmierska I, Lorello D, Soresi M, Notarbartolo A (1996) Gastroesophageal reflux and cow's milk allergy in infants: a prospective study. J Allergy Clin Immunol 97:822–827

21. Inoue R, Matsushita S, Kaneko H, Shinoda S, Sakaguchi H, Nishimura Y, Kondo N (2001) Identification of beta-lactoglobulin-derived peptides and class II HLA molecules recognized by T cells from patients with milk allergy. Clin Exp Allergy 31:1126–1134

22. Jarvinen KM, Laine ST, Jarvenpaa AL, Suomalainen HK (2000) Does low IgA in human milk predispose the infant to development of cow's milk allergy? Pediatr Res 48:457–462

23. Jarvinen KM, Suomalainen H (2001) Development of cow's milk allergy in breast-fed infants. Clin Exp Allergy 31:978–987

24. Katz PO, Richter JE, Cowan R, Castell DO (1986) Apparent complete lower esophageal sphincter relaxation in achalasia. Gastroenterology 90:978–983

25. Khan S, Hyman PE, Cocjin J, Di Lorenzo C (2000) Rumination syndrome in adolescents. J Pediatr 136:528–531

26. Kobayashi H, Puri P (1994) Abnormal adrenergic innervation in infantile pyloric stenosis. The VII International Symposium Pediatric Surgical Research, Heidelberg, Germany

27. Kusafuka T, Puri P (1997) Altered messenger RNA expression of the neuronal nitric oxide synthase gene in infantile hypertrophic pyloric stenosis. Pediatr Surg Int 12:576–579

28. Lemmer JH, Coran AG, Wesley JR, Polley TZ Jr, Byrne WJ (1985) Achalasia in children: treatment by anterior esophageal myotomy (modified Heller operation). J Pediatr Surg 20:333–338

29. Levine DF, Wingate DL, Pfeffer JM, Butcher P (1983) Habitual rumination: a benign disorder. Br Med J (Clin Res Ed) 287:255–256

30. Mackay AJ, Mackellar A (1986) Infantile hypertrophic pyloric stenosis: a review of 222 cases. Aust N Z J Surg 56:131–133

31. Mayberry JF (2001) Epidemiology and demographics of achalasia. Gastrointest Endosc Clin N Am 11:235–248

32. Milocco C, Torre G, Ventura A (1997) Gastroesophageal reflux and cow's milk protein allergy. Arch Dis Child 77:183–184

33. Mishra A, Hogan SP, Brandt EB, Rothenberg ME (2001) An etiological role for aeroallergens and eosinophils in experimental esophagitis. J Clin Invest 107:83–90

34. Neustrom MR, Friesen C (1999) Treatment of eosinophilic gastroenteritis with montelukast. J Allergy Clin Immunol 104:506

35. Nihoul-Fekete C, Bawab F, Lortat-Jacob S, Arhan P, Pellerin D (1989) Achalasia of the esophagus in childhood: surgical treatment in 35 cases with special reference to familial cases and glucocorticoid deficiency association. J Pediatr Surg 24:1060–1063

36. Orenstein SR, Shalaby TM, Di Lorenzo C, Putnam PE, Sigurdsson L, Mousa H, Kocoshis SA (2000) The spectrum of pediatric eosinophilic esophagitis beyond infancy: a clinical series of 30 children. Am J Gastroenterol 95:1422–1430

37. Packer RJ (1999) Brain tumors in children. Arch Neurol 56:421–425

38. Picus D, Frank PH (1981) Eosinophilic esophagitis. Am J Roentgenol 136:1001–1003

39. Ravelli AM, Tobanelli P, Volpi S, Ugazio AG (2001) Vomiting and gastric motility in infants with cow's milk allergy. J Pediatr Gastroenterol Nutr 32:59–64

40. Rudolph CD, Mazur LJ, Liptak GS, Baker RD, Boyle JT, Colletti RB, Gerson WT, Werlin SL (2001) Guidelines for evaluation and treatment of gastroesophageal reflux in infants and children: recommendations of the North American Society for Pediatric Gastroenterology and Nutrition. J Pediatr Gastroenterol Nutr 32:S1–31

41. Rozycki DL, Ruben RJ, Rapin I, Spiro AJ (1971) Autosomal recessive deafness associated with short stature, vitiligo, muscle wasting, and achalasia. Arch Otolaryngol 93:194–197

42. Samarasinghe DA, Nicholson GI, Hamilton I (1991) Dilation of achalasia in the young: a useful alternative. Gastrointest Endosc 37:568–569

43. Sampson HA (1999) Food allergy. Part 1: immunopathogenesis and clinical disorders. J Allergy Clin Immunol 103:717–728

44. Sampson HA, Anderson JA (2000) Summary and recommendations: classification of gastrointestinal manifestations due to immunologic reactions to foods in infants and young children. J Pediatr Gastroenterol Nutr 30:S87–S94

45. Schade RP, Van Ieperen-Van Dijk AG, Van Reijsen FC, Versluis C, Kimpen JL, Knol EF, Bruijnzeel-Koomen CA, Van Hoffen E (2000) Differences in antigen-specific T-cell responses between infants with atopic dermatitis with and without cow's milk allergy: relevance of TH2 cytokines. J Allergy Clin Immunol 106:1155–1162

46. Schrander JJ, van den Bogart JP, Forget PP, Schrander-Stumpel CT, Kuijten RH, Kester AD (1993) Cow's milk protein intolerance in infants under 1 year of age: a prospective epidemiological study. Eur J Pediatr 152:640–644

47. Schreier HA, Libow JA (1994) Munchausen by proxy syndrome: a modern pediatric challenge. J Pediatr 125:S110–S115

48. Schwartz DA, Pardi DS, Murray JA (2001) Use of montelukast as steroid-sparing agent for recurrent eosinophilic gastroenteritis. Dig Dis Sci 46:1787–1790

49. Sicherer SH, Noone SA, Koerner CB, Christie L, Burks AW, Sampson HA (1999) Hypoallergenicity and efficacy of an amino acid-based formula in children with cow's milk and multiple food hypersensitivities. J Pediatr 135:118–121

50. Sigurdsson L, Flores A, Putnam PE, Hyman PE, Di Lorenzo C (1997) Postviral gastroparesis: presentation, treatment, and outcome. J Pediatr 131:751–754

51. Spergel JM, Pawlowski NA (2002) Food allergy. Mechanisms, diagnosis, and management in children. Pediatr Clin North Am 49:73–96

52. Staiano A, Troncone R, Simeone D, Mayer M, Finelli E, Cella A, Auricchio S (1995) Differentiation of cows' milk intolerance and gastroesophageal reflux. Arch Dis Child 73:439–442

53. Straumann A, Rossi L, Simon HU, Heer P, Spichtin HP, Beglinger C (2003) Fragility of the esophageal mucosa: a pathognomonic endoscopic sign of primary eosinophilic esophagitis? Gastrointest Endosc 57:407–412.

54. Thumshirn M, Camilleri M, Hanson RB, Williams DE, Schei AJ, Kammer PP (1998) Gastric mechanosensory and lower esophageal sphincter function in rumination syndrome. Am J Physiol 275:G314–321.

55. Tomomasa T, Miyazaki M, Koizumi T, Kuroume T (1993) Erythromycin increases gastric antral motility in human premature infants. Biol Neonate 63:349–352.

56. Uribe P Jr, Csendes A, Larrain A, Ayala M (1974) Motility studies in fifty patients with achalasia of the esophagus. Am J Gastroenterol 62:333–336

57. Vanderwinden JM, Liu H, De Laet MH, Vanderhaeghen JJ (1996) Study of the interstitial cells of Cajal in infantile hypertrophic pyloric stenosis. Gastroenterology 111:279–288

58. Vantrappen G, Janssens J, Hellemans J, Coremans G (1979) Achalasia, diffuse esophageal spasm, and related motility disorders. Gastroenterology 76:450–457

59. Veereman-Wauters G, Ghoos Y, van der Schoor S, Maes B, Hebbalkar N, Devlieger H, Eggermont E (1996) The 13C-octanoic acid breath test: a noninvasive technique to assess gastric emptying in preterm infants. J Pediatr Gastroenterol Nutr 23: 111–117

60. Zaninotto G, Costantini M, Molena D, Portale G, Costantino M, Nicoletti L, Ancona E (2001) Minimally invasive surgery for esophageal achalasia. J Laparoendosc Adv Surg Tech A 11: 351–359

61. Zeiger RS, Sampson HA, Bock SA, Burks AW Jr, Harden K, Noone S, Martin D, Leung S, Wilson G (1999) Soy allergy in infants and children with IgE-associated cow's milk allergy. J Pediatr 134:614–622

Infant Regurgitation

Paul Hyman

7

Contents

In healthy infants, regurgitation is a symptom commensurate with the expected range of behavior for the stage of development. The upper gastrointestinal tract is free of disease, despite discomfort in the infant or caretakers. The most important message in this chapter is that uncomplicated regurgitation in an otherwise healthy infant should be treated as a developmental issue rather than a disease.

The pediatric Rome 2 working team defined infant regurgitation as one of thirteen pediatric functional gastrointestinal disorders. Functional disorders include "a variable combination of chronic or recurrent symptoms not explained by structural or biochemical abnormalities [1]." Functional symptoms are those that occur in the absence of anatomic abnormality, inflammation, or tissue damage, and within the expected range of behaviors for the body. Like a runner's cramp in the back of the leg, or shivering on a cold day, the symptoms of functional gastrointestinal disorders are real, but there is no easily distinguished disease. Functional gastrointestinal disorders are diagnosed by symptoms; for most of them, no medical testing is necessary or desirable.

7.1
Definitions

Regurgitation is the involuntary return of previously swallowed food or secretions into or out of the mouth or nose. Regurgitation is distinguished from *vomiting*, which is defined by a central nervous system reflex involving both gastrointestinal smooth and skeletal muscles. In vomiting, gastric contents are forcefully expelled through the oro-and naso-pharynx because of coordinated movements of the small bowel, stomach, esophagus, and diaphragm. Regurgitation is also different from *rumination*, the voluntary return of small volumes of gastric contents into the pharynx and mouth, with subsequent reswallowing or expectoration. Regurgitation, vomiting, and rumination are all examples of *gastroesophageal reflux* (GER), defined as the retrograde movement of gastric contents back into the esophagus. *Gastroesophageal reflux disease* (GERD) refers to symptoms or tissue damage caused by GER. GERD is covered in other chapters in this volume.

7.2
Epidemiology

In the United States, approximately half of all mothers with healthy infants 2–10 months of age reported that their infants regurgitated two or more times daily [2]. The numbers of affected infants peaked at about 4 - months of age. Most had improved by 7 months of age, and symptoms resolved by 1 year in almost all. Occasional regurgitation may persist until the third year in a few healthy children.

Although regurgitation is common in healthy infants, parents frequently perceive it as a problem, particularly if the infant is irritable and fussy around mealtimes, or if regurgitation is large in volume or frequent. If half of all healthy infants meet symptom-based criteria for infant regurgitation, and half of their caretakers believe that regurgitation is a medical problem, then 25% of all infants may be evaluated for infant regurgitation during the first year of life. Infant regurgitation may be considered the most common of the pediatric functional gastrointestinal disorders, and its evaluation and treatment has enormous impact on economic and health care utilization issues.

7.3
Diagnostic Criteria

Infant Regurgitation was defined as [3]:
1. There is a history of regurgitation 2 or more times per day for 3 or more weeks.
2. There is no retching, hematemesis, aspiration, apnea, failure-to-thrive, or abnormal posturing.
3. The infant must be 1–12 months of age and otherwise healthy.
4. There is no evidence of metabolic, gastrointestinal, or central nervous system disease to explain the symptom.

Neither the forcefulness of the regurgitation nor its outflow through the mouth or nose carries diagnostic relevance.

7.4
Evaluation

The diagnosis of infant regurgitation is based on history. A thorough physical examination including assessments of growth and development aids the clinician in confirming health, and reassures parents that the clinician has taken the presenting complaint seriously. Diagnostic testing is unlikely to change the management or prognosis.

Risk factors for GERD include premature birth, developmental delay, and congenital abnormalities of the oropharynx, chest, lungs, central nervous system, and gastrointestinal tract. Physical signs that may indicate a systemic disorder include eczema for protein allergy, and an abnormal neurological examination. Failure-to-thrive, occult blood in the stool, or food refusal should prompt an evaluation for GERD.

7.5
Anatomic Features

Infant regurgitation is most often a transient problem, in part due to growth and maturation of anatomy and physiology, respectively. The infant's esophageal volume is 1/20th of the adult volume, or about 2 ml. With episodes of reflux in infants, volumes greater than 1 or 2 ml spill into the pharynx. As the infant grows, the esophagus becomes a reservoir for refluxed material. In adults, GER is rarely associated with regurgitation, because the esophageal volume holds the full volume of refluxed material.

The intra-abdominal esophagus is an important barrier to GER. With increases in intra-abdominal pressure, for example from coughs, sneezes, or straining to defecate, the lumen of the intra-abdominal esophagus collapses, preventing GER. In infants, the intra-abdominal esophagus may be too short to provide an effective barrier to GER caused by increased intra-abdominal pressure.

In preterm infants, large volumes and high osmolarity meals delay gastric emptying by inducing postprandial duodenal hypomotility [4–6]. Delayed gastric emptying, in turn, may increase postprandial GER. A full gastric fundus increases the number of transient lower esophageal relaxations, the most common motor event associated with GER. Postprandial duodenal motility changes over the first weeks and months of life to a mature pattern in which meal volume does not affect the rate of gastric emptying. With maturity, duodenal motility increases with larger, more complex meals, and the rate of gastric emptying remains constant for each formula.

7.6
Psychological Features

It may be difficult to discern at the first meeting whether a parent is anxious because a regurgitating infant is fussy and difficult to feed, or if the anxious parent is the source of the infant's distress, and regurgitation and food refusal are symptoms of the infant's emotional distress. There is little evidence that GER causes irritability in infants. (For a review, see [7]) Variations in the parent's perception of excessive crying often complicate the clinician's assessment. Infant temperament and environmental stressors may interact and alter the parent-child interaction.

Communications between the clinician and the parents are critical to maintaining the health of the child. Well-meaning clinicians may unintentionally create a parent's perception of the vulnerable child by using words that medicalize the problem, rather than keeping to a developmental or functional explanation for the symptom. Simply using the term "gastroesophageal reflux" instead of "infant regurgitation" medicalizes the symptom for the parents.

7.7
Treatment: The First Visit

The natural history of infant regurgitation is one of spontaneous improvement in a large majority of infants [7]. Therefore, treatment goals are to provide effective reassurance and symptom relief while avoiding complications. Effective reassurance includes (a) an empathetic, satisfactory response to the stated and unstated fears of the parents: What is wrong with the baby? Is it dangerous? Will it go away? What can we do about it? and (b) a promise of continuing clinician availability [8].

Primary care clinicians educate and reassure for the first complaint of daily regurgitation. They counsel parents that there may be an immaturity responsible for regurgitation in healthy infants, because the symptoms disappear after a few months. If there are warning signs or symptoms of disease such as failure-to-thrive, hematemesis, or nonatopic reactive airway disease, then evaluation and referral to a pediatric gastroenterologist may be appropriate. In the absence of alarming symptoms, the clinician may choose a diagnostic and therapeutic trial of time.

The clinician explains that because there is an expectation for spontaneous resolution of infant regurgitation, there is a choice to avoid medical interventions. Effective reassurance is based on the clinician's prior discovery of the experiences, fears, and other emotional factors driving parents to seek medical care for their infant. The clinician offers continuity and accessibility so that in the unlikely event that the symptoms worsen, there can be a prompt reassessment from the clinician who knows the baby and family, and who is always ready to reconsider the diagnosis if symptoms change. This management style almost always relieves parents' worries, and establishes an alliance between parent and clinician. Parents who may have started the interview with a demand for "something to be done" may leave the office grateful that their child did not experience and will not require additional stress or discomfort. These communications may take more than the conventional 20–40 min, but this style eliminates a costly, premature medical work-up. The choice to use time as a diagnostic and therapeutic test ("Let's wait and see...") requires acceptance by the clinician and parents. The clinician must feel safe about the working diagnosis of infant regurgitation, and the parents must be relieved of the worry that a serious problem exists. The clinician has an opportunity to help the parents to a sense of well being by addressing the symptom in a serious and compassionate way. When a parent's chief complaint to the pediatric gastroenterologist is "my baby has reflux" the referring clinician has inadvertently communicated a bias toward viewing regurgitation as pathological. The tendency to think of the symptom as abnormal may mislead the parent to seek premature and unnecessary procedures and interventions. Moreover, the adverse long-term consequences of calling regurgitation a disease include creating the parent perception of a vulnerable child, and the potential for family stress and guilt. The clinician reinforces the message at the end of the visit. "Remember: It's infant regurgitation, a functional symptom that is within the expected range of behaviors for a healthy infant. It is not dangerous. It will go away.

There are things we can do to reduce the symptoms if we choose to do so. I am available to you by phone or, better yet, by email if the symptoms change or you have new questions."

7.8
Followup Evaluation and Treatment

When infant regurgitation persists, the clinician senses a growing concern in the parents. Often clinicians will change the infant's formula, assuming that the switch will serve as a therapeutic trial for formula protein sensitivity. Switching formulas may have a placebo effect. It may satisfy the parent's need to do something and the clinician's desire to please the parent, and allow a period of time to elapse before there are more phone calls or visits. The week or two of continued observation following a formula change may provide sufficient time for a spontaneous improvement or resolution of infant regurgitation. However, it is unlikely that a formula switch treats protein sensitivity for a majority of regurgitating infants. Up to 40% of infants with sensitivity to one formula protein will have sensitivity to others [9], so that if a clinician truly suspects a protein sensitivity it is prudent to prescribe a hydrolyzed protein formula. True formula protein allergy affects only 1–2% of infants [10], but regurgitation affects a majority of otherwise healthy infants. Formula protein allergy most often causes more than one symptom or sign – failure-to-thrive, diarrhea, colicky pains, anemia, and hematochezia – and is often associated with reactive airway disease and eczema. In contrast to uncomplicated infant regurgitation, formula protein allergy is a disease: symptoms arise from the inflammatory response. Changing formulas may send a message to the parents that something is wrong with their baby, and may heighten rather than relieve anxiety. Parents who change formulas in infancy may believe erroneously that their child has a milk allergy for years after.

A working group sponsored by the European Society for Pediatric Gastroenterology and Nutrition recommended that the initial treatment for infants with regurgitation and no alarming signs or symptoms should be "lifestyle" behavior changes, including prone positioning, formula thickened with cereal, and small, frequent feedings [11].

Positioning infants face down reduces the time that the esophageal contents are acidic [12, 13]. Prone positioning makes sense when one considers the anatomy of the stomach and lower esophageal sphincter. The sphincter enters the gastric cardia on its dorsal aspect. When the infant is in an infant seat, the effect of gravity is to shift the gastric contents so that they cover the lower esophageal sphincter. Relaxations of the sphincter not accompanied by a peristaltic esophageal wave might be expected to cause an episode of GER. Indeed, transient lower esophageal sphincter relaxations are the most important cause of GER episodes in adults and children [14]. In contrast to supine positioning, when the infant is prone, the gastric contents shift ventrally, away from the lower esophageal sphincter. The American Academy of Pediatrics has excluded infants with recurrent regurgitation from their recommendations for supine positioning [15].

Thickened feedings decrease emesis, crying, and improve caloric intake in infants with GER [16]. Feedings are usually thickened by adding 1 tablespoon of rice cereal to each ounce of formula. This step increases the caloric density of standard formulas from 0.67 to 1.0 Kcal/mL. Small, frequent feedings are a traditional recommendation. There is indirect evidence supporting a role for small, frequent feedings in some infants with GER. In preterm infants, duodenal motility is decreased and gastric emptying slowed by increasing the feeding volume above a critical threshold, which varies from infant to infant [17, 18]. This effect may represent a duodenal "brake" mechanism that may serve a protective function for the immature intestine, by preventing nutrients from entering the bowel at a dangerously fast rate. Perhaps this transient postprandial duodenal hypomotility may respond to small, frequent feedings. Conversely, overfeeding might cause an increase in the frequency and volume of emesis, as the duodenal brake takes effect. As infants mature, the duodenal brake disappears, and so does vomiting.

Above all, healthy infants eat for pleasure. If their feedings are interrupted, they get fussy and irritable. Moreover, preventing infants from feeding to satiety may result in an iatrogenic lag in weight gain, which in turn might be misinterpreted as being caused by GER. In healthy infants with recurrent regurgitation, it is most important to focus on maintaining mother-infant comfort, and not on limiting the volume of feedings. Thus, frequent feedings may prevent overfeeding after a prolonged fast, but feedings should not be interrupted before the infant reaches satiety.

Although the European Working Group suggested antacids for infant reflux as an early intervention, there seems to be no rationale for their use in the absence of esophagitis. Formula feedings buffer gastric acid for an hour or two, and it would seem more desirable to neutralize gastric acid with a nutrient rather than a medication. A gastric pH greater than 4 is maintained for an hour or two after a formula feeding.

If there is no response to lifestyle changes after 1 or 2 weeks, but no acceleration in the disease trajectory, then the European Working Group suggested a trial of the prokinetic drug cisapride. Cisapride binds to serotonin receptors within the myenteric plexus to facilitate the release of acetylcholine and so increase the number and strength of contractions throughout the gastrointestinal tract. The dose range for oral cisapride suspension is 0.2–0.3 mg/kg/dose three or four times a day. Transient diarrhea is common, but resolves spontaneously within several days. Other side effects are unusual. In trials with pediatric patients, cisapride improved esophageal peristalsis, increased basal lower esophageal sphincter pressure, and decreased acid reflux time [19].

In many babies with chronic emesis, persistent postprandial duodenal hypomotility may be the cause. As noted previously, Berseth and colleagues described a decrease in the duodenal motility index of healthy preterm neonates as feedings increased [17, 18]. In fact, six toddlers presenting with a life-long history of vomiting necessitating special means of nutritional support had persistent postprandial duodenal hypomotility [20]. All six of these toddlers had excellent responses to cisapride, advancing from parenteral or tube feedings to oral feedings. These toddlers suffered from postprandial gastroparesis and vomiting, much as preterm infants do.

It is possible that in infants with uncomplicated GER and a normal temperament and maternal-child interaction, there is a persistent duodenal brake that is activated by large or complex feedings. Since cisapride increases duodenal motility in children [21], it should work for regurgitating infants with a persistent duodenal brake. Over-feeding tends to exacerbate the symptoms, because it activates the brake. Smaller, frequent feedings work better. The natural history of the hypothetical duodenal brake reflex is that in the vast majority of infants, it spontaneously disappears over the first weeks and months of life, corresponding to the disappearance of emesis. Cisapride, which increases the number and strength of duodenal contraction, is the correct drug for this physiology, and improves the symptom in these infants.

Excessive serum concentrations of cisapride prolong the cardiac QT interval and predispose to the drug-induced ventricular tachycardia torsade de pointes. The clinician prescribing cisapride educates parents to avoid coadministration of drugs that interfere with cisapride metabolism. The most likely setting is the need for erythromycin or clarithromycin for infection in an infant treated with cisapride for regurgitation. Clinicians should not prescribe cisapride concurrently with other drugs known to prolong the QT interval.

In countries where cisapride is no longer available, the dopamine receptor antagonists metoclopramide or domperidone may be prescribed instead of cisapride. Both improve esophageal peristalsis and speed liquid gastric emptying, as well as having antiemetic effects in the chemoreceptor trigger zone. Metoclopramide is effective when dosed at 0.2–0.3 mg/kg per dose TID or QID. About 30% of patients using a therapeutic dose will develop central nervous system side effects that limit metoclopramide's use. Moreover, drug tolerance develops after 4–6 weeks of metoclopramide. However, in many patients with infant regurgitation, treatment is needed for just a short time, until the upper gastrointestinal tract matures. Like cisapride, tegaserod is active at serotonin receptors that increase acetylcholine release and reduce afferent pain signals. There is no data yet on tegaserod for infant regurgitation.

Because infant regurgitation is a symptom related to impaired motility, it is logical to treat with a motility drug. However, a weak argument might be made that gastric acid antisecretory drugs may be indicated to prevent complications of acid reflux. H2-histamine receptor antagonists have an unsurpassed safety profile. Proton pump inhibitors have the advantage of once-daily dosing. The effectiveness of antisecretory drugs in reducing infant regurgitation is unknown.

In contrast to the calm parents, anxious parents convey their ambivalent, uncomfortable feelings to their vomiting infants, who may not have postprandial hypomotility. These infants may have pylorospasm and delayed gastric emptying as one of many potential physiologic responses to their emotional arousal. Pylorospasm often is observed radiographically and manometrically in such infants [22]. Emesis as a consequence of pylorospasm does not respond to cisapride, which increases the number and strength of contractions. The overaroused infant responds to comfort.

It is incumbent upon the clinician to recognize the behavioral reverberations of recurrent regurgitation in infants, because appropriate early intervention may prevent disease acceleration, especially in families with aberrant caretaker-child interactions. A therapeutic trial of comfort may seem incomprehensible because this is an area in which we receive no formal training. Even so, early and appropriate interventions by the primary care clinician are more likely to achieve success than later tries by the specialist, following months of apparent illness. For improving a troubled caretaker-child interaction, the clinician prescribes comfort for the caretaker and child. The steps to provide therapeutic comfort include (a) relieving the parents' fears about the condition of the infant; (b) aiding the parents in identifying sources of physical and emotional distress: make a plan to reduce or eliminate them. Ask for a description of the scene as the infant is fed. Is there turmoil and interruption? The clinician writes a prescription to the family: "Every feeding to include 30 minutes for the caretaker and infant alone in a dimly lit room, with a comfortable chair, and some peaceful music;" and (c) assurance that the clinician will be available for regularly scheduled followup. In selected cases in infants older than 6 months, when both parents and infant are fussy, colicky, and sleep disordered but with no signs or symptoms other than frequent regurgitation, low doses of the tricyclic antidepressant imipramine may reduce visceral pain, arousal, and irritability and regulate the infant's sleep cycle. Imipramine may improve appetite, and reduce regurgitation episodes by reducing

Table 1. Checklist for the regurgitating infant

1. Assess historical risk factors for gastroesophageal reflux disease: prematurity, delayed development, and congenital disorders of the oropharynx, chest, lungs, central nervous system, or gastrointestinal tract.

2. Assess physical signs that may indicate a systemic condition associated with chronic regurgitation: for example, eczema (milk allergy) or abnormal neurologic exam (cerebral palsy).

3. Assess the effect of the symptom on the emotional state of the caretaker and the family.

4. Assess for the presence or absence of alarm symptoms: failure-to-thrive, hematemesis or occult blood in the stool, and pulmonary disease.

5. Provide comfort through the formation of a therapeutic alliance. Hear both the spoken and unspoken distress in the caretaker, then educate, reassure, and ensure continuity of care.

6. At a second visit, add lifestyle changes to effective reassurance: prone position, thickened feedings, and frequent feedings without overfeeding.

7. At a third visit, consider adding a drug in addition to effective reassurance and lifestyle changes: cisapride, metoclopramide, domperidone, tegaserod, H2-histamine receptor antagonist, proton pump inhibitor, imipramine, gabapentin.

8. Re-evaluate symptoms and their impact on the family at each visit. The presence of alarm symptoms triggers evaluation for gastroesophageal reflux disease.

arousal or visceral pain. Dosing begins at 0.2 mg/kg hs, and increases by 0.2 mg/kg each week until the infant sleeps comfortably through the night, or the dose reaches 1.0 mg/kg hs, whichever comes first. One in 10 infants will become dysphoric when treated with imipramine. In these infants, gabapentin 50 mg BID may be a safe and effective alternative for treating arousal and chronic visceral pain.

If we assume that regurgitation in an otherwise healthy infant is a functional disorder, commensurate with the normal age-related experience, then are we doing a disservice by empirically treating the condition with lifestyle changes, prokinetic or antisecretory drugs? Will those instructions confer a subliminal message that the infant is ill? Perhaps it would be useful to think of these instructions much as we think of car seats or immunizations–as part of routine pediatric care designed to avoid injury or disease. Table 1 summarizes the steps in the approach to treating infant regurgitation.

7.9
Re-Evaluation

On the first visit that includes a complaint of regurgitation, the clinician asks about associated symptoms that might suggest a disease–fevers, diarrhea, urinary frequency, abnormal breathing patterns, weight loss, peculiar movements, etc. The physical examination provides important information to complement the history. If there is no evidence of disease (i.e., regurgitation is the only complaint in a child with a normal examination), then the clinician provides effective reassurance, including education, comfort, and a promise of availability.

During each visit, the clinician asks about the emotional impact of the infant's regurgitation on the mother and family. A chronically regurgitating infant may make the primary caretaker feel guilty and depressed, anxious, or angry. Family members may view the caretaker as less than competent. If the house smells from baby vomit, relatives and friends may choose not to visit. In such cases, these psychosocial aspects of infant regurgitation are the most relevant and require the most guidance.

If there is no change in 1–3 weeks, the clinician may re-evaluate. In the absence of new symptoms or signs, the clinician should repeat the messages of effective reassurance, and may suggest thickened feedings, prone positioning, frequent feedings (but no overfeeding), and a calm mealtime and postprandial environment for parent and infant. If these behavioral changes work, they may be continued for several months. If the parent phones to report no change after 1–3 weeks of behavior changes, the clinician may re-evaluate. In the absence of new symptoms or signs, clinician should repeat the messages of effective reassurance and may add a drug, in a therapeutic trial. Parents are informed that drugs do not cure regurgitation, but may improve the symptoms even as the infant's digestive system is maturing. Drugs that improve esophageal and gastric motility reduce GER parameters [23]. Although prescribing drugs for a functional disorder might increase the parents' perception of their child's vulnerability, this effect may be outweighed by symptom resolution. Parents are reminded that, analogous to acetaminophen for fever, the medicine treats a symptom, not disease.

7.10
When to Refer to the Specialist

The pediatric gastroenterologist has the tools and the interest for evaluating GER. Enthusiasm for referring regurgitating infants must be tempered with the knowledge that the majority, especially those with no pre-existing medical conditions, do not develop disease. Subjecting otherwise healthy regurgitating infants to unnecessary evaluations results in expense, worry, and occasional iatrogenic illness. Effective reassurance should be part of the repertoire of the primary care provider.

Indications for a consultation with your pediatric gastroenterologist are listed in Table 2.

■ **Acknowledgements.** The author thanks David R. Fleisher, MD for sharing ideas.

References

1. Drossman D (ed) (2000) The functional gastrointestinal disorders. Degnon Associates, McLean, VA
2. Nelson SP, Chen EH, Syniar GM, Kaufer Christophel K (1997) Prevalence of symptoms of gastroesophageal reflux during infancy: a pediatric practice-based survey. Arch Pediatr Adolesc Med 151:569–571
3. Rasquin-Weber A, Hyman PE, Cucchiara S, Fleisher DR, Hyams JS, Milla PJ, Staiano A (1999) Childhood functional gastrointestinal disorders. Gut 45(Suppl II): II60–II68
4. Tawil YA, Berseth CL (1996) Gestational and postnatal maturation of duodenal motor responses to intragastric feeding. J Pediatr 129:374–381
5. Knapp E, Berseth CL (1996) Immature duodenal motor responses to bolus feedings are associated with delayed gastric emptying in preterm infants. Pediatr Res 39:313A
6. Baker JH, Berseth CL (1997) Duodenal motor responses in preterm infants fed formula with varying concentrations and rates of infusion. Pediatr Res 42:618–622
7. Rudolph C, Mazur LJ, Liptak GS, Baker R, Boyle JT, Colletti RB, Gerson W, Werlin S (2001) Evaluation and treatment of gastroesophageal reflux in infants and children. J Pediatr Gastroenterol Nutr 32:S1–31
8. Fleisher DR (1994) Integration of biomedical and psychosocial management. In Hyman PE, Di Lorenzo C, (eds) Pediatric gastrointestinal motility disorders. Academy Professional Information Services, New York, pp 13–31
9. Gryboski J and Walker WA (1983) Gastrointestinal problems in the infant. WB Saunders, Philadelphia, pp 593–596
10. Halpern SR, Sellars WA, Johnson RB et al. (1973) Development of childhood allergy in infants fed breast, soy, or cow milk. J Allergy Clin Immunol 51:139–151
11. Vandenplas Y, Ashkenazi A, Belli D et al. (1993) A proposition for the diagnosis and treatment of gastroesophageal reflux disease in children: a report from a working group on gastroesophageal reflux disease. Eur J Pediatri 152:704–711
12. Orenstein SR, Whittington PF, Orenstein DM (1983) The infant seat as treatment for gastroesophageal reflux. N Engl J Med 309:709–710
13. Orenstein SR, Whittington PF (1982) Positioning for preventing infant gastroesophageal reflux. Pediatrics 69:768–772
14. Mittal RK, Holloway RH, Penagini R, Blackshaw LA, Dent J (1995) Transient lower esophageal sphincter relaxation. Gastroenterology 109:601–610
15. AAP Task Force on Infant Sleeping Position and SIDS (1994) Commentary. Pediatrics 93:820
16. Orenstein SR, Magill HL, Brooks P (1987) Thickening of infant feedings for therapy of gastroesophageal reflux. J Pediatr 110:181–186
17. Koenig WJ, Amarnath RP, Hench V, Berseth CL (1995) Manometrics for preterm and term infants: a new tool for old questions. Pediatrics 95:203–206
18. Jadcherla SR, Berseth CL (1995) Acute and chronic intestinal motor activity responses to two infant formulas. Pediatrics 96:331–335

Table 2. Warning signs: indications for specialist consultation

Red flags	Pink flags
Gastrointestinal bleeding	Failed empiric therapy
Dysphagia	Daily regurgitation past the first year
Aspiration pneumonia	
Failure to thrive	

19. Cucchiara S, Stainano A, Boccieri A, et al. (1990) Effects of cis-apride on parameters of esophageal motility and on the prolonged intraesophageal pH test in infants with gastroesophageal reflux disease. Gut 31:21–25

20. Hyman PE, DiLorenzo C, McAdams L, Flores AF, Tomomasa T, Garvey TQ (1993) Predicting the clinical response to cisapride in children with chronic intestinal pseudo-obstruction. Am J Gastroenterol 88:832–836

21. DiLorenzo C, Reddy SN, Villanueva-Meyer J, Mena I, Martin S, Hyman PE (1991) Cisapride in children with chronic intestinal pseudo-obstruction: an acute, double- blind crossover placebo-controlled trial. Gastroenterology 101:1564–1570

22. Fleisher DR (1994) Functional vomiting disorders of infancy: innocent vomiting, nervous vomiting, and infant rumination syndrome. J Pediatr 125:584–594

23. Scott RB, Ferreira C, Smith L, et al. (1997) Cisapride in pediatric gastroesophageal reflux. J Pediatr Gastroenterol Nutr 25(5):499–506

Chapter 8

The Gastroesophageal Reflux in Patients with Respiratory Symptoms

8

Alberto Ottolenghi · Francesco S. Camoglio
Enrico Valletta · Anna Pasquini · Luca Giacomello

Contents

Gastroesophageal reflux (GER), i.e., the backward flow of gastric content into the esophagus, may be regarded, within limits, as a physiologically normal event, especially in the first few months of life and after feeding.

North American epidemiological studies have shown how regurgitation and gastroesophageal reflux are conditions that tend to resolve themselves without treatment in 80% of cases during the first 18 months of the infant's life. 15% of cases resolve themselves by the age of 2 years and only 5% of patients present symptoms that require specific treatment [1].

It is well known that the signs and symptoms for which GER is considered responsible do not affect only the upper digestive tract (with inflammation of the mucosa that can lead to actual erosion of the esophagus, which may cause anemia, hematemesis, and possible esophageal stenosis), but also the respiratory apparatus. Respiratory tract symptoms in children with GER may include asthma attacks or respiratory symptoms other than those of asthma. In the youngest children, stridor, choking fits, and apnea predominate, while among children of 1 year, chronic coughs, wheezing, chronic bronchitis, relapsing pneumonia, hoarseness, recurrent earache, and chronic sinusitis are more commonly encountered [2, 3].

Despite the work of many researchers, the mechanisms that lead to and cause pulmonary disease in patients affected by GER remain unknown. It is not easy to define GER precisely as a pathological event nor to satisfactorily explain its relationship to any lung condition; 24-h esophageal pH-monitoring has shown that, though common in infants and children, GER is not always ac-companied by respiratory symptoms or lesions to the esophagus [4–6]. It would be useful if there were highly sensitive and specific tests available that could detect disorders of the two systems involved (gastroenteric and respiratory), particularly if these were of real predictive value. That is, it would be useful if they could clearly distinguish respiratory problems definitely correlated to GER (i.e., responsive to medical or surgical antireflux treatment) from those where the two pathologies coexist but have causes that are independent of each other. There is at the present time no test capable of establishing the prognosis of a patient with GER associated with respiratory symptoms. Neither medical treatments for reflux in the form of antacids or prokinetic drugs, nor the surgical treatments of the condition are able to eliminate the respiratory symptoms of all the affected patients [7].

Assessment of a child with GER and respiratory symptoms starts by careful study of the patient's medical history, with due attention paid to all symptoms presented by the patient, including those not apparently reflux-related.

One important factor to consider when analyzing symptoms is the moment in which such symptoms first manifested. It has been observed that when a respiratory condition (e.g., asthma) precedes the gastrointestinal symptoms of GER, it is probable that the two conditions do not have a common pathogenesis. If, on the other hand, the gastrointestinal symptoms associated with GER preceded the respiratory ones by some years, there is a greater likelihood that the two conditions are closely related.

The diagnostic tests available for gastroesophageal reflux today are many, but they are quite diverse as regards sensitivity and specificity, leaving a wide area for the doctor's own interpretation of the results [8].

Among the diagnostic tools used for children with GER, *echography* of the distal tract of the esophagus and the gastroesophageal junction is a noninvasive method that makes accurate reflux assessment possible, since such examinations can be extended up to a period of about 15 min. The method is used today both for screening and followup in patients with respiratory symptoms with a likely GER correlation. It does, however, have a number of limitations, such as being unusable, for example, with obese patients. Echography enables viewing of the reflux and examination of the anatomy of the gastroesophageal junction (including measurement of the intra-abdominal tract of the esophagus and the acuteness of the His angle). The only drawback of this method of investigation is the not insignificant number of resulting false positives, especially in the youngest of patients. Crying and abdominal contraction may lead to a greater number of refluxes than is really the case. A scoring system has thus been worked out based on the number of refluxes occurring during the 15-min period in which the esophageal echography probe is in position (Table 1). It can be seen that the degree to which GER is considered a true disease condition depends not only to the number of episodes but also on the patient's age.

Radiographic examination of the upper primary digestive paths is not an ideal method for examining for GER, but it does nevertheless provide useful information on the presence or nonpresence of any esophageal lesions (certainly more clearly identified by endoscopy) and especially for highlighting any lack of deglutition motor coordination. Contrastography is also very useful in identifying any mechanical or functional obstacles to food transit in the proximal tract of the digestive apparatus (Ladd's bands in patients with intestinal malrotation; annular pancreas; Roviralta syndrome, etc.) that may be the cause of GER, but is quite unable to show any correlation between GER and the possible aspiration of material of gastric origin into the bronchial tree. Long term *pH-monitoring in the esophagus* is a highly sensitive technique that permits, among other things, correlation between gastroesophageal reflux episodes with physiological (alimentation) or pathological (cough, apnea, stridor, or asthma attacks) situations.

The very slim and well-tolerated probes now available are able to detect (as regards extent and number) only those refluxes capable of effecting changes in esophageal pH levels. Minor refluxes that are still capable of reaching the bronchial tree and causing respiratory symptoms could, however, elude this examination [9, 10, 11].

Table 1. GER esophageal echography severity

Severe	5 or more GER up to the age of 6 months
	4 GER between 7 months and 2 years
	2 GER after 2 years
Medium severity	4–5 GER up to the age of 6 months
	3–4 GER between 7 months and 2 years
	1–2 GER after 2 years
Light	2–3 GER up to 6 months of age
	1–2 GER between 7 months and 2 years
	1 GER after 2 years

As well as identifying gastroesophageal reflux, pH monitoring also reveals the following:

1. The so-called reflux index, or the total esophageal mucosa exposure time to gastric acidity (pathological levels being where 5% is exceeded in the 24-h period)
2. The "symptom index" (relationship between symptoms referable to GER and reflux itself)
3. The "sensitivity index" (relationship between the number of refluxes associated with GER symptoms and the total number of GER over the 24-h interval)

Currently, an instrument with acidity-detecting electrodes is used in the proximal esophagus to seek any correlation between the gastroesophageal reflux and any concomitant respiratory condition. Patients with GER and respiratory symptoms with positive test results should certainly be considered as having respiratory disease that is secondary to GER.

Where there is alkaline GER (bile acids, trypsin), respiratory symptoms may be no less significant than those found with acid reflux. In this case, pH monitoring provides no diagnostic assistance.

Esophageal scintigraphy with technetium^{99m} colloid-sulfide is indicated where hypo-acid refluxes are suspected, were often postprandial and not revealed by pH monitoring. Such a test may in fact show radioactive traces in the bronchial tree. Unfortunately, a negative test does not exclude all cases either of bronchial reflux or bronchial aspiration.

Endoscopic examination and *esophageal manometry*, though so important in determining the degree of damage suffered by esophageal mucosa from the reflux, as well as lower esophageal sphincter (LES) pressor parameters at the preoperative stage, do not permit the identification of any correlation between GER and respiratory disease [12, 13].

It is often said how difficult it is to demonstrate, in infants and young children, the aspiration of material of gastric origin into the respiratory system, just as it is difficult to attribute the presence of any respiratory signs and symptoms there may be to such aspiration. It was demonstrated some time ago that patients who have aspirated gastric material (with aspiration pneumonia) into the bronchial tree, have *lipid Laden macrophages* in the alveoli that can be seen in the broncho-alveolar lavage fluid. In the past this was attributed to the aspiration of milk, which has a high concentration of lipids, but it is now seen that the alveolar macrophages have lipid inclusion even in patients where there is no documented evidence of any reflux (healthy controls). It has been observed that alveolar macrophages not only have exogenous (aspirated material) but also endogenous lipid inclusions (derived from the metabolism of membrane phospholipids or the destruction of tissue elements such as surfactant). There is no way of distinguishing between the two lipid types and so such a test obviously can have no diagnostic significance [14].

The only relevant factor here is that children with GER and associated lung disease have a higher concentration of lipids in their alveolar macrophages than that found in healthy controls or in patients with chronic or recurrent respiratory disease without GER [15].

The *Bernstein test,* which assesses patient pain on infusion of acid (HCl 0.1 N) into the distal esophagus compared with that caused by normal saline, is of little use in the case of infants and young children due to low (or zero) patient cooperation. The test has been changed to meet the needs of pediatric patients whereby the infusion of diluted HCl into the esophagus, and the saline control, must induce coughing, stridor, or wheezing for there to be concrete reasons for supposing the GER and respiratory symptoms to be correlated. Also, in the case of this test, a negative result cannot necessarily completely exclude that there is a correlation between the two conditions [16].

8.1
Gastroesophageal Reflux and Asthma

The association between GER and asthma in children is one of the most hotly debated issues in pediatrics and also among specialists in adult pneumology and gastroenterology. This is due to the great difficulty in proving a correlation between the two diseases. For such a correlation to be considered established, the following must be demonstrated:

1. That the patients affected by asthma exhibit a greater prevalence of GER as compared with nonasthmatic individuals
2. That there is a scientifically valid explanation of the cause of both diseases and the mechanism by which the two conditions interact
3. That when asthma patients suffering from GER are treated medically or surgically, their respiratory symptoms, such as asthma, also disappear

The correlation between asthma and gastroesophageal reflux cannot easily be proven. The incidence of asthma in European infants and children stands at 10% of the population. In the same population, esophageal pH monitoring gives positive results in 10% of breast-feeding infants. The incidence of the two diseases in association is therefore about 1% in an unselected population. If the rates of GER in a pediatric population affected by asthma is considered (i.e., a selected population), it is found that 57% of asthmatic patients are subject to gastroesophageal reflux when pH-monitored. This incidence is similar to that found among adults [17–20].

Several diagnostic tests have been carried out with the aim of correlating GER and asthma among pediatric patients, but none with a specificity level. *Reflux scintigraphy with technetium[99]* does not always settle the question, as false negatives are possible due to fact that a very slight reflux may be sufficient to induce bronchial spasm and may be rapidly removed by muco-ciliary clearance. Furthermore, aspiration of refluxed gastric material may be sporadic, in which case the scintigraphy should, if negative, be repeated on successive days, something which is clearly unacceptable.

In conclusion, all investigative methods aimed at showing the presence and severity of GER in patients with asthma or similar symptoms may provide indicative results that are not, however, able to correlate the two diseases with any degree of certainty. Asthma and GER are two frequently occurring conditions, especially among infants and young children, that may coexist in the same patient without one necessarily being caused by the other [21–23].

It has been suggested that some asthma patients may suffer from GER as a result of the effects of certain medicines used to treat their respiratory condition. Bronchodilators, in particular, could negatively affect SLE tone and thus favor gastric reflux into the esophagus, however, this view is not supported by evidence that GER in asthmatic patients treated with bronchodilators is similar in extent to that of patients with the same respiratory symptoms who have not undergone specific therapies for their condition [22, 24].

It is therefore reasonable to state that the association between GER and asthma constitutes a self-sustaining condition and one in which the gastroesophageal reflux, usually the first to present itself clinically, could be a cause of the appearance of the patient's asthma. The asthma, in its turn, due to the frequent respiratory attacks involving forced inspiration and especially expiration, could aggravate the GER. Over time this could lead to the establishment of hyperactivity of the bronchial tree and a tendency for the asthma condition to become chronic.

Finally, the variable clinical attention afforded to the patient with asthma and GER must also be taken into account, in the sense that the doctor may decide to specifically treat the more dominant disease while paying little attention to possible diverse causes.

To conclude, the role of GER therapy in demonstrating the dependence of asthma on the reflux continues to be controversial, bearing in mind that: (a) the two conditions can certainly be correlated where the respiratory symptoms are resolved with medical or surgical treatment for reflux, and (b) some patients treated for GER show no significant improvements in their respiratory condition.

8.2
Gastroesophageal Reflux and Nonasthmatic Respiratory Disease

Supra-esophageal symptoms, mostly referable to respiratory disease of the upper and lower airways, usually require diagnostic investigation for the presence of any GER.

The clinical picture may concern the area of otolaryngology or pneumology, and may involve varying degrees of complexity (see obstructive apnea or *sudden infant death syndrome*) [25, 26].

There remain many areas of controversy surrounding the association of GER with these respiratory diseases.

The first of these regard the mechanism by which GER could involve the respiratory system even in the absence of clinical signs of reflux (silent reflux). Two events have been put forward as explanations:

1. Direct contact between gastric content and the respiratory mucosa
2. Provocation of a vagal nerve reaction caused by the presence of acid in the esophagus

There are few certainties about the respective role of either proposed mechanism. The direct action of gastric acid or acidity in the proximal esophagus are not thought to be essential for the occurrence of respiratory symptoms, while nervous stimulation of the distal esophagus or the activation of chemical mediators could have a prime role in the development of the respiratory condition.

It is important to emphasize that there are no satisfactory explanations for individual sensitivity to GER in terms of respiratory symptoms. It has been suggested that different types of reflux could stimulate, with different degrees of effectiveness, the respiratory tract's protection systems. It is also possible that esophageal clearance mechanisms and airways' protection systems play an important role in determining the extent to which the reflux may cause disease [27, 28].

The question of cause and effect is another, and crucial, aspect which modern diagnostic methods fail to clarify.

The medical literature is full of reports indicating the relevance of GER to numerous diseases of the upper airways.

The relationship between GER and *disease of the larynx* is extensively covered in the literature, particularly with regard to the adult population. Patients with chronic disease and laryngoscope results ranging from light erythema to ulceration of the mucosa or even stenosis [29].

Laryngeal symptoms in children, especially when recurrent, lead to the suspicion of GER, a suspicion supported by the pH monitoring results, which show high reflux indices in as many as 50–60% of cases.

The authors would nevertheless cast doubt on the importance of this connection where no causal relationship is given.

The association between GER and *recurrent otitis media* would seem to be less frequent, as is that between GER and *chronic sinusitis*. In this case, the population affected is a selected group of children with chronic symptoms that fail to respond to conventional treatment and that are sufficiently severe for a surgical approach to be seriously considered.

According to the literature, after asthma, *recurrent pneumonia* represents the pulmonary disease that is most often attributed to GER. The mechanism in this case involves the aspiration of gastric content with resulting bronchial obstruction, atelectasis, and chemical pneumonia. Repeated inhalation even of small quantities of gastric juices may lead to bronchitis and recurrent bronchopneumonia, bronchiectasia, and pulmonary fibrosis [30, 31].

There would, however, seem to be only a modest causal connection (on the order of about 5%) and mostly found in neurology patients.

Chronic coughing secondary to GER may be a result of repeated micro-aspiration into the bronchopulmonary system, laryngeal exposure to acid, or the stimulation of the distal esophago-bronchial reflex. The cough may sometimes be accompanied by infection of the lower airways or by signs of inflammation of the larynx, or it may simply appear as an isolated symptom [32].

A good deal of literature, not surprisingly, considers the possibility of a relationship between GER and *apnea, "apparent life threatening events" and "sudden infant death syndrome."*

Initial observations seemed to confirm the pathogenic role of reflux, but these were followed by studies showing that it was not possible to establish a time connection between the two events, this despite the existence of experimental evidence that, in the newborn child, fluids instilled in the pharynx or the presence of acids in the esophagus can cause apnea and brachycardia [33].

Vinocur et al. [34] pointed out that eight of 40 newly diagnosed infants with *cystic fibrosis* had significant GER, characterized by vomiting (7 infants), recurrent pneumonia (7 infants), and failure to thrive (4 infants). Three infants had rapid and permanent alleviation of symptoms after standard medical therapy; in five infants, therapy failed and they required a Nissen fundoplication. All children had complete relief of their preoperative symptoms. The group that required surgery presented earlier (mean 7 weeks of age) to the cystic fibrosis center than either the medically treated group (mean 5 months of age) or the group free of gastroesophageal reflux symptoms (5 1/2 months of age). The pulmonary manifestations of cystic fibrosis are extremely variable, and evaluation of the effect that any intervention has on the natural history of the disease is difficult. Gastroesophageal reflux should be managed as aggressively as it is in any child with reflux, and a successful and safe reduction of symptoms can be expected with intensive management.

8.3
Medical Therapy

Gastroesophageal reflux is an important (causative) factor in chronic recurrent respiratory disease. This entity is often resistant to "classical" respiratory treatment, but can often be treated with an antireflux therapy [35]. Malfroot et al. [36] thought GER was probably the cause of the respiratory disease in 63% of patients, since treatment of GER was followed by disappearance of the respiratory complaints in most of them.

Early diagnosis and antireflux therapy in cases with GER-related respiratory complaints can result in significant improvement in symptoms. Antireflux therapy (cisapride 0.2 mg/Kg q.i.d.) resulted in an improvement of the symptoms in 84.6% of the patients [35]. A prokinetic drug (cisapride) significantly decreased the percentage of time during which the pH was 4 or less (versus placebo; total period, –60%; sleep, –80%) and reduced the number of reflux spells of at least 5 min (–64%; –92%). No adverse effects of cisapride were observed [37].

A significant ($p<0.01$) decrease was noticed in the number of further episodes in children with GER-related recurrent bronchopneumonia and reactive airway disease after starting antireflux therapy [38].

Five hundred patients [39], who presented with respiratory symptoms including apnea, cyanosis, or "near miss" sudden infant death syndrome (36%), poorly controlled asthma (28%), recurrent bronchopneumonia (13%), bronchiolitis (9%), and miscellaneous symptoms such as intermittent dyspnea, chronic cough, and stridor (12%) underwent 20-h pH monitoring to assess GER: severe reflux was present in 156 patients (31%) and moderate reflux in 159 patients (31%). All patients were treated for a minimum of 8 weeks. The majority of patients (81%) had resolution of their symptoms with change in position, thickened feedings, and, when indicated, additional therapy with metoclopramide, cisapride, or domperidone. Most of these patients were found to have a specific position, usually prone, which decreased reflux.

Treatment of reflux with recommended doses of H_2 blockers and prokinetic agents has a high failure rate in asthmatic patients [40].

Three of six trials of proton pump inhibitors documented improvement in asthma symptoms with treatment; benefit was seen in 25% of patients. Half of the studies reported improvement in pulmonary function, but the effect occurred in fewer than 15% of patients [41].

Other studies showed no objective improvement by spirometry of asthmatics treated for gastroesophageal reflux, but recognized improvement in asthma symptoms and decreased use of asthma medication.

8.4
Surgical Approach

Twenty-one of 23 patients with repeated bronchopulmonary infections showed abnormal GER with 24-h pH monitoring[42]. Twenty children received medical therapy. Three out six patients who failed to show improvement with medical therapy received fundoplication and had marked improvement of reflux and symptoms postoperatively.

Of 36 patients with recurrent pneumonias (and/or clinical asthma) and GER followed for response to therapy [43], 32 patients attempted medical therapy and four had fundoplications. Ten of 32 (31%) patients on medical therapy had improvement in symptoms but none became asymptomatic. Twenty patients who failed a trial of medical therapy also had fundoplications for a total of 24 patients surgically treated. Of these, 22 (92%) had improvement or became asymptomatic.

Fundoplication has been consistently shown to ameliorate reflux-induced asthma; results are superior to the published results of antisecretory therapy [41].

Andze et al. detected that 18% of patients with respiratory symptoms treated initially by medical therapy had documentation of persistent reflux by pH monitoring and underwent an antireflux procedure [39].

Infants and children with severe symptoms and poor response to medical treatment may benefit from operation. Children who do not respond to 6 weeks with aggressive medical treatment should be referred to surgery [44].

Nissen fundoplication is the most commonly used procedure. Alternatively, partial fundoplication according to Toupet or Boix-Ochoa was usefully performed. In some patients, gastroesophageal scintiscan showed slow gastric emptying and it was necessary to add a pyloroplasty to the fundoplication.

Our thirty-year behavior towards GER with or without respiratory symptoms, in infants and children, was the following:

1. Toupet or Dor partial fundoplication was performed in primary GER with adequate LES pressure
2. Nissen partial fundoplication was chosen when lower esophageal sphincter is incompetent (LES pressure lower than 10 mm Hg)
3. Nissen total fundoplication (with or without pyloroplasty) was made in gastroesophageal reflux associated (or secondary) to esophageal atresia, congeni-

tal diaphragmatic hernia, intestinal malrotation, Roviralta syndrome or other neurological impairment

Eighteen per cent of patients who had undergone Nissen fundoplication for GER with respiratory tract disease were symptomatic in spite of the control of GER [45]. Ninety-two per cent of children had at least partial relief of respiratory symptoms postoperatively.

However, Rothenberg et al. [46] reported that 85.7% of patients who had undergone laparoscopic Nissen fundoplication noted significant improvement in their respiratory symptoms in the first week.

Of 43 children, 91% with preoperative recurrent aspiration pneumonia had no additional episodes after Nissen procedure [47].

The complete relief of these symptoms was more likely in patients without major associated disorders (97% versus 59% $p=0.0009$). It appears that a significant number of affected infants and children may have respiratory difficulties unrelated to the presence of GER [48].

8.5
Conclusions

1. Respiratory disease associated with GER can be divided into that involving or not involving asthma. In the latter group of patients, the clinical picture may be otolaryngological (laryngitis, otitis media, or sinusitis) of pneumological (chronic coughing, chronic bronchitis, bronchopneumonia, or sudden infant death syndrome).

2. The association between GER and respiratory disease in children is the subject of much debate given the extreme difficulty in proving a correlation between the two. Generally speaking, it is held that the two conditions can be correlated when: (a) the gastrointestinal symptoms precede the respiratory symptoms by a number of years; (b) the respiratory symptoms are resolved by medical or surgical treatment for reflux.

3. Surgical correction of GER consists of a traditional partial or total fundoplication, if necessary associated with pyloroplasty (in patients with difficulties in gastric emptying). Surgical intervention required in about 25% of patients who undergo protracted medical treatment, results in remission of symptoms in 85–92% of cases.

References

1. Castro M, Lucidi V (1998) Reflusso gastro-esofageo e altre malattie dell'esofago. In: Castro M (ed) Gastroenterologia pediatrica. McGraw-Hill, Milano
2. Kern W Descher, Bensamin SB (1989) Extraesophageal manifestations of gastroesophageal reflux disease. Am J Gastroenterol 84:1–5
3. Vijayaratnam V, Simpson LC, Tolia PV (2000) Lack of significant proximal esophageal acid reflux in infants presenting with respiratory symptoms. Pediatr Pulmonol 27:231–235
4. Simpson H, Hampton F (1991) Gastroesophageal reflux and the lung. Arch Dis Child 66:277–283
5. Hillemeier AC (1996) Gastroesophageal reflux. Diagnostic and therapeutic approaches. Pediatr Clin North Am 43(1):197–212
6. Sondheimer JM, Hoddes E (1992) Gastroesophageal reflux with drifting onset in infants: a phenomenon unique to sleep. J Pediatr Gastroenterol Nutr 15:418–425
7. Shi G, Kahrilas PJ (1999) Asthma: reflux-induced or reflux-associated?. Ital J Gastroenterol Hepatol 31:376–377
8. Herbst JJ (1999) Gastroesophageal reflux and respiratory disorders. Pediatr Pulmonol 27:229–230
9. Colletti RB, Ghristie DL, Orenstein SR (1995) Indications for pediatric esophageal pH monitoring. J Pediatr Gastroenterol Nutr 21:253–262
10. Barabino A, Costantini M, Ciccone MO, Pesce F, Parodi B, Gatti R (1995) Reliability of short-term esophageal pH monitoring versus 24-h study. J Pediatr Gastroenterol Nutr 21:87–90
11. Vendenplas Y, Goyvaerts H, Helven R, Sacre L (1991) Gastroesophageal reflux, as measured by 24-h pH monitoring, in 509 healthy infants screened for risk of sudden infant death-syndrome. Pediatr 88(4):834–840
12. Vandenplas Y, Derde MP, Piepsz A (1992) Evaluation of reflux episodes during simultaneous esophageal pH monitoring and gastroesophageal reflux scintigraphy in children. J Pediatr Gastroenterol Nutr 14:256–260
13. Vandenplas Y, Ashkenazi A, Belli D, Boige N, Bouquet J, Cadranel S et al. (1993) A proposition for the diagnosis and treatment of gastroesophageal reflux disease in children: a report from a working group on gastroesophageal reflux disease. Eur J Pediatr 152:704–711
14. Colombo JL, Hellberg TK (1999) Pulmonary aspiration and lipid-Laden macrophages: in search of gold (standards). Pediatr Pulmonol 28:79–82
15. Bauer ML, Lyrene RK (1999) Chronic aspiration in children. Evaluation of the lipid Laden macrophages index. Pediatr Pulmonol 28:94–100
16. Orstein SR (1993) Gastroesophageal reflux. In Wylie R, Hyams JS, (eds) Pediatric gastrointestinal disease: pathophysiology, diagnosis and management. WB Saunders, Philadelphia, pp 337–369
17. Putnam PE, Ricker DH, Orenstin SR (1999) Gastroesophageal reflux. In: Beckerman R, Brouilette R, Hunt C (eds) Respiratory control disorders in infants and children. Williams et Wilkins, Baltimore, p 322
18. Ninan TK, Russel G (1992) Respiratory symptoms and atopy in Aberdeen school children: evidence from two surveys 25 years apart. BMJ 304:873–875
19. Vendenplas Y, Goyvaerts H, Helven R, Sacre L (1991) Gastroesophageal reflux, as assessed by 24-h pH monitoring, in 509 healthy infants screened for SIDS risk. Pediatrics 88:834–840
20. Tucci F, Resti M, Fontana R, Novembre E, Adami Lami C, Vierucci A (1993) Gastroesophageal reflux and bronchial asthma: prevalence and effect of cisapride therapy. J Pediatr Gastroenterol Nutr 17:265–270
21. Balson M, Kravitz EKS, McGleady SJ (1998) Diagnosis and treatment of gastroesophageal reflux in children and adolescents with severe asthma. Ann Allergy Asthma Immunol 81:159–164
22. Sontag SJ (2000) Gastroesophageal reflux disease and asthma. J Clin Gastroenterol 30(suppl):S9–30
23. Willing J, Furukawa Y, Davidson GP, Dent J (1994) Strain induced augmentation of upper esophageal sphincter pressure in children. Gut 35:159–164
24. Sontag SJ, O'Connell S, Khandelwal S, Miller T, Nemchausky B, Schnell TG et al. (1990) Most asthmatics have gastroesophageal reflux with or without bronchodilator therapy. Gastroenterology 99:613–620

25. Booth IW (1992) Silent gastroesophagal reflux: How much do we miss? J Br Pediatr Assoc 67:1325–1327
26. Irwin RS, French CI, Curlej FJ, Zawacki JK, Bennett FM (1993) Chronic cough due to gastroesophageal reflux. Chest 104: 1511–1517
27. Shaker R, Dodds WJ, Ren J, Hogan WJ, Arndorfer RC (1992) Esophago-glottal closure reflex: a mechanism of airway protection. Gastroenterology 102:857–861
28. Helm JF, Dodds WJ, Pele LR et al. (1984) Effect of esophageal emptying and saliva on clearance of acid from the esophagus. N Engl J Med 310:284–288
29. Cherry J, Margulies SI (1968) Contact ulcer of larynx. Laryngoscope 73:1937–1940
30. Malfroot A, Vandenplas Y, Verlinden M et al. (1987) Gastroesophageal reflux and unexplained chronic respiratory disease in infants and children. Pediatr Pulmonol 3:208–213
31. Owayed AF, Campbell DM, Wang EE (2000) Underlying causes of recurrent pneumonia in children. Arch Pediatr Adolesc Med 154:190–194
32. Irwin RS, Boulet LP, Cloutier MM et al. (1998) Managing cough as a defense mechanism and as a symptom: a consensus panel report of the American College of Chest Physicians. Chest 114(suppl):133s–181s
33. Davies AM, Koenig JS, Thach BT (1989) Characteristics of upper airway chemoreflex prolonged apnea in human infants. Am Rev Dis 139:668–673
34. Vinocur CD, Marmon L, Schidlow DV, Weintraub WH (1985) Gastroesophageal reflux in the infant with cystic fibrosis, Am J Surg 149(1):182–186
35. Blecker U, De Pont SM, Hauser B, Chouraqui JP, Gottrand F, Vandenplas Y (1995) The role of "occult" gastroesophageal reflux in chronic pulmonary disease in children. Acta Gastroenterol Belg 58(5–6):348–352
36. Malfroot A, Vandenplas Y, Verlinden M, Piepsz A, Dab I (1987) Gastroesophageal reflux and unexplained chronic respiratory disease in infants and children. Pediatr Pulmonol 3(4):208–213
37. Saye ZN, Forget PP, Geubelle F (1987) Effect of cisapride on gastroesophageal reflux in children with chronic bronchopulmonary disease: a double-blind cross-over pH-monitoring study. Pediatr Pulmonol 3(1):8–12
38. Jain A, Patwari AK, Bajaj P, Kashyap R, Anand VK (2002) Association of gastroesophageal reflux disease in young children with persistent respiratory symptoms. J Trop Pediatr 48(1):39–42
39. Andze GO, Brandt ML, St Vil D, Bensoussan AL, Blanchard H (1991) Diagnosis and treatment of gastroesophageal reflux in 500 children with respiratory symptoms: the value of pH monitoring. J Pediatr Surg 26(3):295–299
40. Balson BM, Kravitz EK, McGeady SJ (1998) Diagnosis and treatment of gastroesophageal reflux in children and adolescents with severe asthma. Ann Allergy Asthma Immunol 81(2):159–164
41. Bowrey DJ, Peters JH, DeMeester TR (2001) Gastroesophageal reflux disease in asthma: effects of medical and surgical antireflux therapy on asthma control. Ann Surg 234(1):130–131
42. Chen PH, Chang MH, Hsu SC (1991) Gastroesophageal reflux in children with chronic recurrent bronchopulmonary infection J Pediatr Gastroenterol Nutr 13(1):16–22
43. Berquist WE, Rachelefsky GS, Kadden M, Siegel SC, Katz RM, Fonkalsrud EW et al. (1981) Gastroesophageal reflux-associated recurrent pneumonia and chronic asthma in children. Pediatrics 68(1):29–35
44. Berstad T (1995) Gastro-esophageal reflux and chronic respiratory disease in infants and children: surgical treatment. Scand J Gastroenterol Suppl 211:26–28
45. Eizaguirre I, Tovar JA (1992) Predicting preoperatively the outcome of respiratory symptoms of gastroesophageal reflux. J Pediatr Surg 27(7):848–851
46. Rothenberg SS, Bratton D, Larsen G, Deterding R, Milgrom H, Brugman S, Boguniewicz M, Copenhaver S, White C, Wagener J, Fan L, Chang J, Stathos T (1997) Laparoscopic fundoplication to enhance pulmonary function children with severe reactive airway disease and gastroesophageal reflux disease. Surg Endosc 11(11):1088–1090
47. St Cyr JA, Ferrara TB, Thompson T, Johnson D, Foker JE (1989) Treatment of pulmonary manifestations of gastroesophageal reflux in children two years of age or less. Am J Surg 157(4):400–403
48. Jolley SG, Herbst JJ, Johnson DG, Matlak ME, Book LS (1980) Surgery in children with gastroesophageal reflux and respiratory symptoms, J Pediatr 96(2):194–198

Chapter 9

Gastroesophageal Reflux and Barrett's Esophagus

9

Moti M. Chowdhury · Nigel Hall · Agostino Pierro

Contents

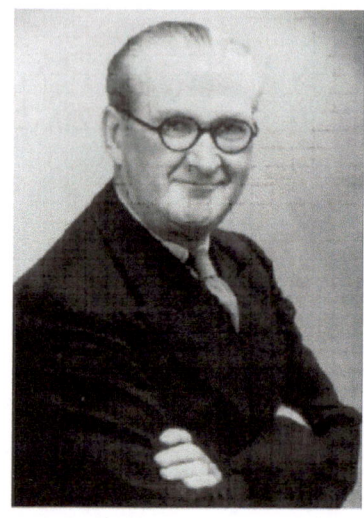

Fig. 1. Norman R. Barrett (1958)

In 1950, Norman Rupert Barrett, an Australian-born thoracic surgeon (Fig. 1; 1903–1979), described ulcers in the lower esophagus, previously attributed to gastroesophageal reflux (GER) by Allison [3], as in fact "chronic peptic ulcers" within an intrathoracic stomach assuming a tubular form secondary to a "short esophagus" [10]. Three years later it was Allison [4] that corrected Barrett's misinterpretation and described the condition as we now understand it, namely columnar metaplasia replacing the normally squamous epithelium of the esophagus, and termed this "Barrett's Esophagus." Over the last 50 years this definition of Barrett's esophagus (BE) has continued to evolve, and in spite of his original erroneous description, to this day the condition remains eponymous to Norman Barrett. We describe the advances that have been made over these 50 years that have contributed to our understanding of the pathophysiology and management of this very difficult condition in adults and then focus on aspects of the disease specific to the pediatric population.

9.1
Epidemiology

The subclinical nature of most patients with BE means that its true incidence among the general population is difficult to quantify. Figures reported between 2.5–44% are likely to be overestimated, reflecting the selective populations in whom endoscopic assessment is performed [14, 27, 50, 52, 60, 89, 109, 180, 207, 217, 232, 238, 240, 250, 268]. The highest prevalence of 44% was observed in patients with chronic GER complicated by peptic strictures of the esophagus [239, 250]. The true population prevalence is likely to be closer to 0.02–3.9%, when examining all individuals undergoing endoscopy for any etiology [19, 27, 34, 36, 50, 109, 168, 180, 207, 232, 269]. The largest such review by Wong [269] of 16,606 patients found an incidence of BE in 0.06%. The incidence of BE has been reported to be increasing over the past 30 years [191]. However, Conio et al. attributed this apparent epidemiological rise predominantly to increased diagnosis [47]: whist the incidence of BE increased 28-fold from 0.37/100,000 person years during 1965–69 to 10.5/100,000 person years during 1995–1997, endoscopic examinations also increased 22-fold in the same period. The incidence of BE increases with age, with a bimodal age distribution [22, 26, 29, 106, 109, 167, 232]. Most adults are affected during the late peak of 50–80 years, but this is preceded by an earlier peak affecting children between 0–15 years. BE is predominantly a condition affecting Caucasian males, with the ratio of male to female being up to 4:1 [20, 34, 35, 47, 102, 147, 207, 230, 232, 240, 266] and the ratio of white to black patients estimated to be up to 20:1 [199].

9.2
Pathophysiology

9.2.1
Definition of BE

A consistent diagnosis of BE has proved difficult owing to the controversy surrounding its pathophysiology and definition, which has evolved over time from Allison's early description. In 1976, Paull [185] demonstrated that the columnar metaplasia of the lower esophagus consisted of a mixture of gastric and intestinal lining (goblet) cells, leading some to believe there exists two types of BE, one replaced with gastric-type cells only, and the second by intestinal cells. Later, the definition in adults evolved further, requiring the metaplasia to extend 3 cm or more beyond the gastroesophageal junction [233]). Currently, BE is recognized in the presence of intestinal metaplasia of the lower esophagus, without specification of the length. Instead, some authors have attempted to subclassify this current definition into "short segment" (<3 cm) or "long segment" BE (>3 cm) according to the length of the intestinal metaplasia [122, 164, 264]. The prevalence of "short segment" BE (2–12%) is thought to be much higher than that of "long-segment" BE (0.3%) [35, 237]. The term "micro-Barrett's" or "ultra-short" segment BE has also been used to describe intestinal-type goblet cells localized to the Z-line of the gastroesophageal junction or gastric cardia, referred to as "cardiac intestinal metaplasia." There is some disagreement as to whether this is appropriate as up to 30% of biopsies taken from this junction in GER patients with no macroscopic evidence of BE will demonstrate intestinal type goblet cells. Secondly, cardiac intestinal metaplasia in GER seems to occur with similar frequency in women and Africans as in white males, yet their risk of overt BE is much lower than that of white males. Thirdly, the term *Barrett's* implies an increased risk of cancer, and there is currently no evidence to suggest that cardiac intestinal metaplasia is associated with an increased cancer risk.

9.2.2
Etiology

The presence of BE has been recognized for over half a century, yet our understanding of its pathogenesis remains limited to the following:

9.2.2.1
Lifestyle Factors

In adults, a positive association between BE and smoking and alcohol have been found by some [48, 50, 157, 180, 237, 266] but not all [45, 99, 102, 141, 203, 205] groups. However, indirect evidence from the known link between Barrett's adenocarcinoma and smoking and alcohol [26, 45, 61, 98, 99, 123, 156, 191, 259, 274] as well as obesity [138] supports the association between these lifestyle factors and BE, a known premalignant condition.

9.2.2.2
Drug-Induced BE

The development of BE following chemotherapy has been described in adults and children [59, 218]. It is thought that chemotoxicity may induce erosive ulceration of the lower esophageal epithelium, leading to columnar metaplasia [59, 218].

9.2.2.3
Helicobacter Pylori Infection

The role of Helicobacter Pylori in the development of BE remains unclear. Although the organism has been found in the mucosa of patients with BE [20, 80, 114, 124, 146, 186, 248, 260], no significant differences in its prevalence were found when compared to control populations [80, 172, 186]. Furthermore, given the known link between GER and BE, it is possible that the Helicobacter Pylori may have originated from an associated gastritis in these patients [20, 146].

9.2.2.4
GER and Esophagitis

BE is found in 3–12% of patients undergoing endoscopy for symptoms of GER [35, 93, 143, 268], the single most important factor attributed to the pathogenesis of BE. Repeated injury from gastric acid induces columnar metaplasia of the esophagus. This is thought to be an adaptive response as the columnar epithelium is more resistant to acid injury than normal esophageal squamous epithelium. However, the constituents of the refluxate differ significantly in patients with BE compared to those with GER without BE. Direct measurement of bile and pancreatic enzymes have shown that duodeno-esophageal reflux is significantly more frequent in those with BE than in those with GER without BE [8, 33, 40, 79, 90, 117, 128, 129, 145, 171, 175, 241]. As we will discuss later, this may have an important bearing on the success of medical and surgical antireflux treatments for BE compared to those with GER without BE. The risk of BE from reflux is also dependent on the duration of insult. Lieberman found that patients with chronic GER symptoms for 5 or more years had a 10% chance of finding BE on endoscopy while those with symptoms for 10 or more years had a 20% chance of finding BE [143]. Furthermore, Lagergran et al. found that patients with longstanding GER had a 43-fold higher risk of esophageal adenocarcinoma [137] compared to the general population, giving more weight to this association between BE and GER. The link between GER and BE and concerns raised from the increasing incidence of Barrett's adenocarcinoma have driven the need for surveillance of patients with longstanding GER for BE.

9.2.2.5
Family History

According to Giuli, 1% of patients with BE have a positive family history [229]. The first report of a family with BE was described by Lehman [140]: a father and his five children all had BE and the mother who had a hiatal hernia, a predisposing factor. Similar findings by others of families with BE [39, 54, 73, 76, 77, 87, 88, 121, 193], equivalent to 28% risk of family members being affected [206], have suggested a genetic predisposition. While a specific gene has not been linked to the development of BE, Hu [115] found a locus on chromosome 13 (13q14 position) linked with a phenotype they identified as "severe pediatric GER," the major risk factor for BE development. Using linkage analysis, they found a 21-cM region of chromosome 13 to be strongly linked to their reflux phenotype. In addition, a number of genetic links between BE and Barrett's adenocarcinoma have been reported, which are discussed in Sect. 9.2.3.

9.2.3
Barrett's Esophagus and Malignant Disease

BE did not gain popular attention until the mid-1970s when a number of case-reports [13, 67, 154] and two case-series [100, 168] reported a strong association between adenocarcinoma of the esophagus and BE. In a series of 140 patients with BE, Naef reported a 10% incidence of esophageal adenocarcinoma [168], while a review by Haggitt of 14 patients with esophageal adenocarcinoma found that 12 (86%) arose in a Barrett's epithelium [100]. This period also saw a sharp increase in the incidence of esophageal adenocarcinoma relative to other malignancies [17, 32, 65, 187]. The reported prevalence of adenocarcinoma in BE since then has been

widely variable (0–64%) [1, 21, 25, 34, 35, 50, 102, 107, 157, 159, 160, 167, 195, 197, 202, 207, 217, 219, 230, 237, 240, 266, 268], and is equivalent to 30–125 times increased risk in patients with BE relative to the general population [35, 101, 132, 156]. Malignant transformation, however, is primarily associated with the intestinal type of BE [185, 251]. Barrett's adenocarcinoma develops from dysplasia of the metaplastic esophagus. The grading of dysplasia in BE (Table 1) is based on the system developed for ulcerative colitis [201] that makes use of standardized terminology.

A number of chromosomal aberrations potentially contributing to the pathogenesis of esophageal carcinomas have been identified. Cytogenetic analysis by Rodriguez et al. of nine patients with adenocarcinoma of the esophagus and gastroesophageal junction demonstrated a rearrangement of a specific region of chromosome 11 in 8 of these patients, including all three with Barrett's adenocarcinoma [204]. The absence of such a rearrangement involving chromosome 11 in nonneoplastic Barrett's mucosa [86] suggests that such a rearrangement is a late event in the biology of Barrett's adenocarcinoma development. Meanwhile, Blount, et al. [18] found allelic deletions of chromosome 17p in 92% of patients with Barrett's adenocarcinoma, but this time the deletions were observed in early and advanced lesions, suggesting a possible role for such deletions in the progression from metaplasia to carcinoma. Chromosome 17p is the site of the tumor suppressor gene p53, which encodes a 293-amino-acid phosphoprotein that is involved in cell cycle regulation [66], DNA repair [136] and apoptosis [272]. Loss of p53 gene expression, either by mutation and/or deletion, facilitates genomic instability and malignant transformation [5, 125]. Indeed, p53 heterozygosity is the most dominant genetic link identified for Barrett's adenocarcinoma, found in 40–60% of cases [38, 196]. Interestingly, some groups

Table 1. Grading dysplasia for Barrett's Esophagus

Grade of Dysplasia	Histological features
Negative	Inflammatory and regenerative lesions without any dysplasia (i.e., neoplastic epithelial changes)
Indefinite	Epithelial changes that appear to exceed the limits of ordinary regeneration but are insufficient for an unequivocal diagnosis of dysplasia or are associated with other features that prevent such unequivocal diagnosis
Positive – low grade	Low-grade neoplastic epithelial changes
Positive – high grade	High-grade neoplastic epithelial changes (i.e., marked architectural and nuclear abnormalities, e.g., mitosis, hyperchromatism)

have reported overexpression of p53 being associated with increased risk of malignancy [190, 196, 263, 273].

Other genetic markers for Barrett's dysplasia and adenocarcinoma reported include "Ki-67" and "Proliferative Cell Nuclear Antigen," both markers of proliferation, which are observed in dysplastic tissue epithelium. Polkowski et al. demonstrated that an increased Ki-67 labeling index correlated with increased p53 expression and increasing grades of dysplasia [190]. These findings were not reproduced by Iftikhar, et al. [118]. Immunohistochemical studies demonstrate Proliferative Cell nuclear Antigen Index to be highest in adenocarcinoma and high grade dysplasia (25%), followed by intestinal-type mucosa (20%) and gastric type metaplasia (12%) [120].

The role of the cyclo-oxygenase (COX)-2 gene, which has the capacity to exactitude replication, has also been realized. In 1998, Wilson et al. demonstrated that COX-2 RNA was expressed in squamous and adenocarcinoma of the esophagus but not in normal gastric epithelium [267]. Furthermore, Shirvani, et al. [228] subsequently demonstrated that COX-2 was increasingly expressed as one progressed farther along the carcinogenic pathway (squamous epithelium – intestinal metaplasia – dysplasia – carcinoma). The ability to modulate COX-2 expression has therefore attracted interested in COX-2 inhibitors that may alter the transformation of metaplastic epithelium to cancerous epithelium, which are discussed in Sect. 9.5.5.5.

9.3
Clinical Features

Barrett's esophagus has no pathognomonic symptoms. At least 30% of patients with BE and Barrett's adenocarcinoma have GER symptoms [119], i.e., heartburn, nausea and vomiting, water brash. Chronic reflux, particularly in children, may result in new onset asthma, bronchitis, or if complicated by aspiration, pneumonia and apnoeic episodes may ensue. Reflux with esophagitis may cause chronic bleeding detected incidentally with anemia, or less commonly acute GI hemorrhage (hematemesis or malena). In many adult cases, however, the condition remains subclinical until it becomes complicated by stricture, resulting in dysphagia. This stricture may be benign from esophagitis with fibrosis or from malignant transformation of the Barrett's mucosa. The lack of reliable symptamotology indicative of BE before the development of complications has necessitated the need for regular surveillance with endoscopy and biopsy.

9.4
Diagnosis and Screening

9.4.1
Diagnosis

BE is a histological diagnosis made almost exclusively on endoscopic assessment and biopsy, and requires the demonstration of intestinal metaplasia. However, as mentioned earlier, intestinal metaplasia of esophageal origin (BE) may histologically resemble cardiac intestinal metaplasia. Given the difficulty of determining the precise site of a biopsy taken at the site of the gastroesophageal junction, and the higher risk of dysplasia and carcinoma with intestinal metaplasia of BE compared to cardiac intestinal metaplasia [92, 163, 226], there is a need to distinguish these two forms of intestinal metaplasia by means other than simple histology. A number of endosopic staining techniques have been used to enhance the recognition of BE, including Lugol's iodine [270], Toluidine blue [44], Indigo Carmine [245], and Methylene Blue [37, 134]. These findings have so far demonstrated only limited reproducibility in the recognition of BE. Meanwhile, Ormsby, et al. [177] used immunohistochemical stains for the cytokeratin (CK) subsets CK7 and CK20, and demonstrated that Barrett's intestinalized mucosa was characterized by superficial and deep CK7 immunoreactivity but only superficial staining for CK20. In contrast, cardiac intestinal metaplasia was characterized by superficial and deep CK20 staining and patchy or absent staining for CK7. These findings have been supported by others [227, 261], including Glickman [91], who found this "Barrett's CK7/20 pattern" to be similar for both short and long segment BE.

The use of fluorescence techniques as a tool to aid endoscopic diagnosis has also been described [158, 244]. The technique, which allows targeted areas to be marked for subsequent biopsy or removal, is particularly useful for early carcinomas and severe dysplasia that cannot be recognized macroscopically on endoscopy alone. The technique involves exogenous administration of a photosensitizing agent (e.g., sodium porfimer) which is taken up selectively by dysplastic cells. Approximately 48 h later a Xenon gas lamp is used to illuminate bright red areas of porphyrin fluorescent cells in areas of dysplasia and carcinoma.

In patients with dysplasia, imaging techniques such as computed tomography and endoscopic ultrasound may allow assessment of the extent of submucosal dysplasia or carcinoma. Endosonography is superior to computed tomography for local tumor assessment as it identifies individual wall layers and can therefore precisely delineate the extent of the tumor spread into the surrounding area. Indeed, Scotiniotis, et al. [221] reported that endoscopic ultrasound had a sensitivity and specificity of 100% and 94%, respectively, for detecting submucosal involvement of Barrett's dysplasia and adenocarcinoma.

9.4.2
Screening and Surveillance

The primary objective of screening patients with BE is to detect the development of dysplasia or malignancy. However, whether routine surveillance is effective, and if so who should be screened and at what frequency are questions that remain unresolved. The argument for surveillance is that if a patient with high-grade dysplasia or cancer is identified early before the development of symptoms of dysphagia, the chance of cure of esophageal adenocarcinoma may be as high as 90%. In contrast, without endoscopic screening these patients may not be diagnosed until they develop dysphagia, when the cure rate is as low as 10%. This is supported by a number of authors [188, 246, 258], who demonstrated that patients treated for Barrett's adenocarcinoma detected by surveillance had significantly better outcomes than those that presented incidentally, with patients detected by surveillance also significantly more likely to have earlier stage disease. Conversely, the low incidence of adenocarcinoma in BE of less than 1% annual risk [19, 68, 71, 101, 116, 148, 159, 174, 222, 254] is used by some authors to counter the necessity for surveillance [169, 234, 256]. Indeed, esophageal cancer is an uncommon cause of death (2.5% of deaths) even among patients with BE not undergoing surveillance [256]. The problem is, however, that less than 5% of all patients with esophageal adenocarcinomas have had an endoscopy to demonstrate that they had BE before their can-

cer was found [53]. Thus, the challenge is to identify those GER patients who have Barrett's by screening patients with chronic GER [62, 133, 199, 235, 236]. Previous recommendations of annual endoscopies have been seen as uneconomical and unjustified given the increasing data showing an annual risk of malignant transformation from BE at less than 1% [19, 68, 71, 101, 116, 148, 159, 174, 222, 254]. Current screening programs vary – anything between every 2–5 years. Given that some patients are more likely to progress to malignancy than others, various groups have attempted to identify a selective group of patients that would most benefit from routine screening, by stratifying risk factors for malignant transformation, e.g., increasing age, intestinal metaplasia [275], dysplasia [101, 209, 213, 258], and esophagitis [110]. Such attempts have so far been unsuccessful without compromising the sensitivity of the surveillance program [166].

In 1998, the American College of Gastroenterology provided guidelines for the surveillance intervals based on the grade of dysplasia identified [213] (Fig. 2).

The method of surveillance is as important as its frequency. The lack of standardized histological criteria for BE and inter and intraobserver variations in their interpretation [162, 178, 198] have left wide variations in results of screening programs. Furthermore, active inflammation at the time of biopsy can result in cellular atypia that may be misinterpreted as dysplasia. It is therefore essential that patients with GER should be treated for their gastritis/esophagitis to achieve mucosal healing, before surveillance biopsies are obtained. Multiple biopsies should be obtained due to the focal nature of dysplasia and cancer in patients with BE. These may be obtained using the technique of "four quadrant biopsies" taken every 2 cm of the Barrett's seg-

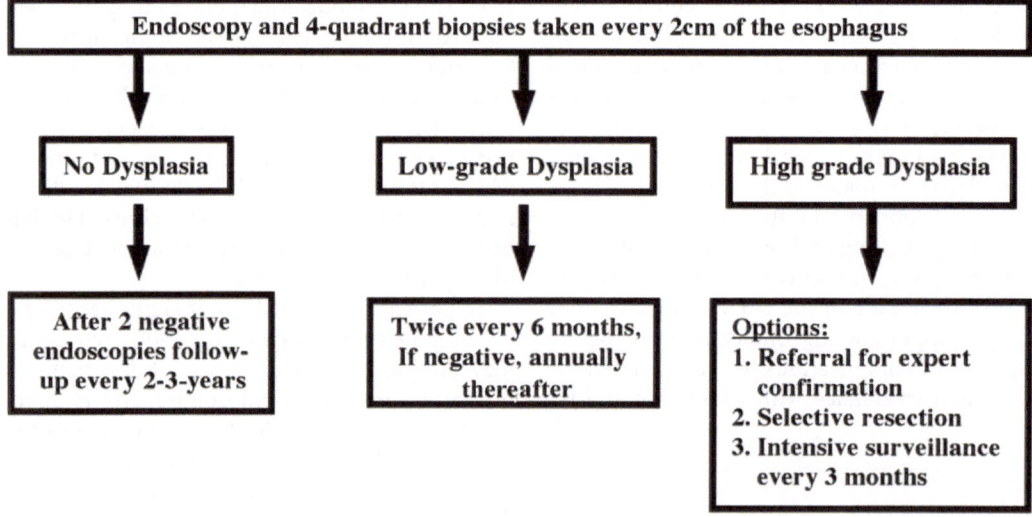

Fig. 2. The American College of Gastroenterology guidelines for surveillance intervals based on the grade of dysplasia (modified)

ment [142], including any mucosal abnormalities identified, e.g., ulcers, strictures. Given the differing risks of malignancy discussed between cardiac intestinal metaplasia and Barrett's intestinal metaplasia, the site of biopsy should also be recorded, e.g., at gastroesophageal junction.

9.5
Management of Barrett's Esophagus in Adults

The goals of treatment in patients with BE are to eliminate symptoms of GER, heal erosive esophagitis, and reverse the metaplastic mucosa, with the ultimate goal of reducing the incidence of esophageal adenocarcinoma.

9.5.1
Medical Therapy

The medical treatment for the symptoms of BE are the same as those for GER. Drugs that may promote GER, e.g., tricyclic antidepressants and calcium channel blockers, should be avoided. The suppression of acid is the backbone of treatment for GER, the main risk factor for BE, and may be achieved using antacids, Histamine H-2 receptor antagonists, and proton pump inhibitors. Proton pump inhibitors are more potent at healing inflammation [253] and ulceration [176], and in preventing strictures [231, 247], and freedom from symptoms can be achieved more effectively by using proton pump inhibitors than histamine H-2 receptor antagonists (77.4% versus 47.6%) [43]. Patients with BE have greater esophageal acid exposure than any other GER patients [242, 255], and control of symptoms may therefore require higher than usual doses of proton pump inhibitors [127]. Furthermore, Ortiz et al. demonstrated, using 24-h pH monitoring, that control of clinical symptoms of GER alone is not a reliable indicator of eradication of pathological reflux in patients with BE [179]. The authors concluded that 24-h pH monitoring should be performed to allow appropriate adjustment of the dose of medication in these patients. Abrupt discontinuation of these medications should be avoided, as recovery from acid inhibition may cause a "rebound hypersecretion" of acid, with a return of the symptoms of reflux. Prokinetic agents may be used, but with caution. Domperidone (motilium) and metoclopramide are generally safe prokinetics for short-term use, but the latter can cause drowsiness or restlessness, while the use of cisapride has generally lost favor due to its adverse cardiac effects. It should be noted that there is no data to suggest that medical treatment reverses metaplasia of BE or arrests the development of malignancy. Evidence suggests that even high dose proton pump inhibitor therapy to reduce esophageal acid exposure will not usually result

in the reversal of BE [51, 149, 225]. Long-term proton pump inhibitor therapy can lead to the development of squamous islands within the Barrett's mucosa, but biopsies of these squamous islands have revealed intestinal metaplasia underlying the squamous epithelium [224]. Thus, the appearance of macroscopic squamous islands may not equate with a reduction in the total surface area of BE. Medical treatment should therefore be reserved for symptom relief and is not warranted for asymptomatic patients.

In adults, in addition to drug therapy, certain lifestyle maneuvers such as avoidance of tobacco and excess alcohol, addressing any obesity, dietary changes (e.g., reducing fat, caffeine, and acid fluids) are important. Adjustment of resting positions, e.g., avoiding sleeping in supine position may also help symptoms of reflux.

9.5.2
Surgical Therapy

The surgical treatment of uncomplicated BE is also directed at symptom relief, i.e., symptoms of GER, as there is no evidence to suggest antireflux surgery decreases the risk of developing subsequent esophageal cancer [168]. The indications for surgery include failure of medical therapy to control symptoms of GER, poor compliance (particularly in children), and those with anatomic defects predisposing to ongoing GER, e.g., large hiatal hernia, a weak lower esophageal sphincter pressure.

Operative options available for treatment of GER are the Nissen's fundoplication [82, 173], Thal [82, 249], Toupet [82], Dor, Boerema, Boix-Ochoa, Collis-Belsey, Hill procedures, and Duodenal diversion. The Nissen's fundoplication is the most popular method, and involves a 360° wrap of the fundus of the stomach, brought round the posterior aspect of the esophagus. It controls GER by increasing the acuteness of the angle of His and lengthening the intra-abdominal esophagus, thereby increasing the high-pressure zone at the lower esophageal sphincter. The Thal procedure is an anterior fundoplication with a partial (180°–270°) wrap of the fundus of the stomach to the intra-abdominal esophagus. The benefit of the Thal procedure is that it allows the patient to belch and release any bloating, which is not feasible with the Nissen's fundoplication. Fundoplication for BE may be performed by the open or laparoscopic method [6, 22, 41, 56, 63, 78, 112, 155, 179, 184, 240, 265, 271]. We performed a meta-analysis of 1 randomised controlled trials comparing these 2 approaches in adults (unpublished). We found that both approaches reduced gastroesophageal acid reflux equally effectively open fundoplication is associated with shorter operative time and less dysphagia post-operatively but higher incidence of post-operative of an other complications, longer hospital stay and longer sick-leave. Reliable data comparing outcomes between the two approaches is, however, limited in children. In cases where esophageal shortening from long-term inflammation and fibrosis prevents a tension-free fundoplication from being done, a Collis gastroplasty may be performed [41, 200]. The addition of esophageal elongation by gastroplasty thus allows a tension-free Nissen's repair. Fundoplication can achieve resolution of reflux symptoms in up to 90% [6, 22, 41, 56, 63, 78, 112, 155, 179, 184, 240, 265, 271]. It should be noted, however, that while fundoplication aims to arrest the insult from acid reflux to the existing BE, cumulative evidence suggests that this has little effect on regression of the metaplastic epithelium [212] or prevention of the development of dysplasia and carcinoma [210, 212, 215]. Furthermore, some authors report that the failure rate of Nissen's fundoplication or Hill's posterior gastropexy in patients with BE to be significantly higher (up to 60%) than those with reflux esophagitis without BE [56, 58]. This may in part be due to the fact that the pathogenesis of BE involves a refluxate into the esophagus containing not only acid but also duodenal contents, with the classic antireflux procedures having little effect on the persistence of duodenal reflux into the esophagus. These groups instead advocate a more aggressive approach in these patients comprising "acid suppression" (vagotomy-partial gastrectomy) and "duodenal diversion" (Roux-en-Y anastomosis), particularly in patients who have either failed antireflux surgery or developed complications, e.g., stricture. The authors applied the technique in 65 patients with BE and reported a significant reduction of acid reflux from 24.8% to 4.8% on 24-h pH monitoring, complete abolition of duodenal reflux, resolution of associated dysplasia in three of seven patients, and morbidity associated with the procedure in 14% [55]. However, as with antireflux procedures, there is a lack of definite evidence of regression of the metaplastic epithelium, the technique is very aggressive, and its application in children remains unclear.

Recently, two further endoscopic techniques have been described for the treatment of GER, which may be applied in BE. The first is endoscopic radiofrequency energy delivery to the gastroesophageal junction around the lower esophageal sphincter. Early data suggests it can achieve resolution of symptoms of GER in 87% of patients [252], but is associated with significant mortality and morbidity, including aspiration, pleural effusion, and atrial fibrillation [126]. The second is endoscopic gastroplication [81], which involves internally plicating the stomach on itself approximately 1 cm below the gastroesophageal junction to alter the angle of His and thereby decrease reflux of gastric contents. Early results indicate poorer outcomes compared to fundoplications, with 75% still requiring adjuvant medical treatment and 6% undergoing fundoplication due to

therapeutic failure [208]. Furthermore, the data reported with both these two procedures have so far been limited to adult populations, and their application in pediatrics remains unclear.

9.5.3
Ablative Therapy

Patients in whom associated comorbidities preclude surgery may be treated with endoscopic ablative techniques, using either endoscopically applied energy delivery or mucosal resection. Although largely used for Barrett's dysplasia, the application of these techniques, described below, for BE without dysplasia is being investigated. All ablative therapies require subsequent acid suppression therapy either with drugs or antireflux surgery to prevent the recurrence of BE and allow the esophageal tissue to heal in an environment that is conducive to squamous mucosa.

9.5.4
Treatment of Barrett's Stricture

The two main complications of BE are malignant transformation or the development of a benign stricture from chronic reflux and fibrosis. The management of the former is discussed in Sect. 9.5.5; meanwhile, data relating to the optimum management of benign stricture in BE is limited. Therapeutic options described include medical treatment, esophageal bouginage, antireflux surgery, acid suppression, and duodenal diversion (described above), and esophageal resection. Esophageal bouginage remains the most popular initial treatment of a stricture. Surgical alternatives to serial bouginages include either resection of the affected segment or bouginage followed by acid suppression and duodenal diversion. In a study of 280 such patients with stricture following BE or following failed antireflux surgery, Csendes et al. reported that this approach eliminated excess acid, on 24-h pH monitoring, in 85% of patients, and completely eliminated duodenal reflux, with none of the patients demonstrating dysplasia after 6 years of followup [57]. In a separate study by the same group, the results of the different treatment modalities were compared following initial bouginage [23]. Among a total cohort of 185 patients with benign stricture from esophagitis and BE, recurrence rates in the groups treated by medical therapy, antireflux surgery, acid suppression and duodenal diversion, and esophageal resection were 73%, 41%, 4.4%, and 0%, respectively. The mortality rate in those undergoing acid suppression and duodenal diversion was 2.9% compared to one death among the seven patients undergoing esophageal resection [23].

9.5.5
Treatment of Barrett's Dysplasia and Adenocarcinoma

The treatment of Barrett's dysplasia is largely determined by the degree of dysplasia identified. "Low-grade dysplasia" and "indefinite dysplasias" are managed simply by continuing endoscopic biopsy surveillance. According to the guidelines of the American College of Gastroenterology [213], the followup interval for these patients is shortened from every 2–3 years (for BE without dysplasia) to every 6 months. Esophagectomy is not warranted for low-grade or indefinite dysplasia unless the patient develops high-grade dysplasia or cancer during the surveillance. Meanwhile, the presence of high-grade dysplasia may indicate that esophageal malignancy is already present. The initial approach to such cases should be to confirm the histology and assessment of the extent of the disease. For instance, computerized tomography scanning and more recently endoscopic ultrasound described above have proved useful in staging early cancers and dysplasia to determine the depth and amount of tissue involved. Thereafter, the management options available for high-grade dysplasia include continued surveillance, esophagectomy, mucosal resection, ablative therapy, and chemoprevention.

9.5.5.1
Esophagectomy

The *gold standard* for management of high-grade dysplasia and Barrett's adenocarcinoma has traditionally been esophagectomy [62, 133, 199, 235, 236], with or without a gastric or colonic transposition procedure. The advantage of surgery is that it allows dissection of involved lymph nodes and complete removal of the potentially malignant tissue that is otherwise often left in the residual Barrett's segment when endoscopic local treatment is used. The results of surgical treatment largely depend on the tumor stage, as demonstrated by Holsher, et al. [113]. In a study of 41 patients with early esophageal adenocarcinoma who underwent subtotal or total esophageal resection, the 5-year survival rate for all patients was 83%. However, all ten of the patients with mucosal tumors survived 5 years compared to 79% of the 31 patients with submucosal tumor invasion [113]. The benefits of resection surgery are, however, at the expense of a relatively high incidence of morbidity and mortality. Reported mortality rates were 3.3–4.8%, while complications occurred in 20–44% [108, 113]. Postoperative complications of esophagectomy include delayed gastric emptying, transient hoarseness, and strictures, while patients require several months to regain a quality of life similar to that which they had before surgery. Furthermore, its demolitive nature means

that it is not always amenable for patients who are physiologically unfit for major surgery, e.g., due to associated co-morbidities. In such groups, less invasive endoscopic techniques described recently, such as endoscopic mucosal resection or endoscopic ablative therapy, which are discussed below, are gaining popularity.

9.5.5.2
Surveillance, and Esophagectomy Reserved for Malignant Disease

Although there is little evidence to suggest that high-grade dysplasia may regress spontaneously without treatment [85, 108], it is also true that the majority of patients with high-grade dysplasia are unlikely to progress to esophageal adenocarcinoma. Some patients with this grade dysplasia therefore opt to simply have intensive endoscopic followup. According to the guidelines of the American College of Gastroenterology [213], in these individuals intensive endoscopic biopsy surveillance every 3 months should be done. The understanding is that surgery would be undertaken if carcinoma were found in the course of the follow-up. This has not been a universally popular approach as it requires a commitment on the part of the endoscopist to obtain meticulous surveillance biopsies frequently and also requires that the patient be content with the frequent followup and with the uncertainty of what the future holds.

9.5.5.3
Endoscopic Mucosal Resection

Endoscopic mucosal resection is a minimally invasive endoscopic technique that may be used both as a diagnostic tool for obtaining full-thickness biopsies, or for the therapeutic resection of patients with circumscribed mucosal dysplasia or carcinoma. Using the "suck-and-cut" technique, with or without prior ligation, large areas can be removed with inclusion of the submucosa. Compared to the other endoscopic ablative techniques, endoscopic mucosal resection has the advantage of allowing histological assessment of the resected specimen with respect to the depth of invasion of the wall layers and allows a complete resection within healthy margins. The limited reports of its use suggest complete resection with successful resolution of the dysplasia or early Barrett's adenocarcinoma can be achieved in 95–97% of cases, in most cases with a single session [72, 262]. The main complication reported is hemostasis, with Ell [72] and Wehrmann [252] reporting hemorrhage in 12% and 64%, respectively. Long term results are not yet available but recurrence rates at 12 months in both studies were 5–14%.

9.5.5.4
Endoscopic Mucosal Ablative Therapy

Endoscopic ablation was first used by Ertan et al. in patients with adenocarcinoma who were poor operative candidates [74]. Ablation techniques are now also being applied in patients with high-grade dysplasia and benign Barrett's mucosa, as a less interventional therapeutic modality to surgery. A number of techniques are available to ablate the affected area, including thermocoagulation procedures [argon plasma coagulation, titanyl phosphate (KTP) laser, and neodymium ± yttrium ± aluminum ± garnet (Nd:YAG) laser] and nonthermal procedures such as photodynamic therapy.

Photodynamic therapy is the most frequently used method of ablation in Barrett's dysplasia and early adenocarcinoma [15, 96, 139, 182]. The technique described earlier is useful not only to obtain targeted biopsies of porphyrin-sensitized dysplastic or neoplastic tissue cells, but also in the targeted destruction of these affected areas. Photodynamic ablation exploits the phenomenon that light can activate the photosensitized substances (e.g., sodium porfimer) stored in the tissue and destroy the tissue by means of oxidation processes. In contrast to conventional high-energy lasers, photodynamic therapy thus allows a selective, nonthermal destruction of the target tissue while to an extent protecting the healthy surroundings. Using a combination of photodynamic therapy and long-term acid suppression using a proton pump inhibitor, partial or complete regression of the Barrett's metaplasia with regeneration of normal squamous epithelium in more than 75% of patients has been achieved by various groups [95, 139, 181]. However, some BE remains behind and all ablations must be followed up by surveillance with additional biopsy and if necessary additional sessions of ablation. The advantage of photodynamic therapy is that the ablation is homogeneous and extensive, allowing long Barrett's segments to be completely treated in a few sessions. In comparison with other ablative techniques, this method requires the lowest number of sessions to achieve ablation of the Barrett's epithelium. Side-effects that have been observed include dysphagia and odynophagia, strictures, pleural effusion, and skin photosensitivity. Photosensitivity of the skin may persist for 6 - weeks or more, subjecting them to increased risk of sunburn. Patients therefore must remain out of the sunlight for this period. These side-effects have, however, occurred mainly with first generation photosensitizing agents (e.g., sodium porfimer). Photodynamic therapy using 5-aminolaevulinic acid, a new endogenous photosensitizer, has a reduced depth of penetration and thus a lower rate of stenosis [95, 96]. In addition, the agent possesses faster decay kinetics than other photosensitizers, so that the risk of phototoxic effects in the skin is present only for 48 h [131]. This markedly improves patients' quality of life since they do not have to remain in darkened rooms for several weeks.

Argon plasma coagulation is a noncontact thermocoagulation procedure with the advantage of a limited depth of penetration, thus minimizing the risk of perforation, and is substantially less expensive compared with laser ablation. Partial or complete regression of Barrett's metaplasia can be achieved [12, 31, 70, 97, 165, 257], but may require several sessions. The technique, however, is associated with a relatively high risk of leaving residual islands of metaplasia, and it is possible for dysplastic tissue to remain under the regenerated squamous epithelium. As a result, its use is limited to ablation of low-grade dysplasia and shorter segments of Barrett's dysplasia. Despite the limited depth of mucosal destruction, massive hemorrhage or perforation resulting in mortality have also been reported [31, 97]. The successful use of argon plasma coagulation in early Barrett's carcinoma has been documented only in a single case report including a total of three patients [153]. The malignancies were completely ablated in all cases, and complete re-epitheliazation occurred in two patients with additional omeprazole treatment. During a mean followup period of 24.3 months, a recurrence was observed in one case, which was in turn successfully treated using photodynamic therapy.

Laser therapy methods of ablating BE are rarely used, and include KTP and Nd:YAG laser ablation and monopolar or multipolar electrocoagulation.

1. The limited data reporting the use of *Nd:YAG laser* ablation have been encouraging, although several sessions have been required for complete ablation to be achieved. No severe complications were observed even when high power was used, but permanent high-dose acid suppression therapy was needed to prevent recurrence [24, 74, 147, 211, 216].

2. The *KTP laser* is a double-frequency Nd:YAG laser into which a KTP crystal has been incorporated to reduce the wavelength of the laser, thus allowing a surface temperature of more than 65°C in the esophageal mucosa, with an external temperature on the serosa of only 21°C. Complete ablation of Barrett's mucosa may be achieved, although it is possible for residual columnar epithelium to remain underneath the newly formed squamous epithelium [9, 15, 94].

3. *Multipolar electrocoagulation* has also been used. Reported data suggests that the success rate for complete ablation of the Barrett's epithelium correlates with the length of the Barrett's segment, with successful regression being achieved in only 25% of patients with segments longer than 4 cm. Other disadvantages of this technique are that the number of sessions required is higher than with any of the other methods, as well as the high rate of complications. Forty to fifty percent of patients have reportedly suffered complications including dysphagia, odynophagia, and gastrointestinal hemorrhage [135, 161, 214, 223].

9.5.5.5
Chemoprevention with Drugs

Given the association of Barrett's dysplasia with overexpression of the Cyclo-oxygenase (COX)-2 gene, a number of pharmacological COX-2 inhibiting agents are being investigated that attempt to downgrade or reverse Barrett's dysplasia. This was first achieved in vitro by Buttar et al. [29] using the inhibitor NS-398 and then in patients by Kaur, et al. [130] using the agent Rofecoxib. Both groups demonstrated that use of a COX-2 inhibitor not only normalizes proliferation in vitro and in vivo, but COX-2 overexpression is normalized as well. Perhaps most importantly, an animal model of Barrett's has recently been used by Buttlar et al. to demonstrate the ability of a specific COX-2 inhibitor to decrease cancer incidence by 55% and cancer volume [30]. The use of chemoprevention in BE is clearly still experimental, but these early findings suggest that COX-2 inhibition may play a critical role in the future management of esophageal adenocarcinoma.

In conclusion, the apparent growing incidence of BE in adults has become a challenging issue given that traditional medical and surgical treatments both have had little impact in reversing the metaplasia or development of esophageal adenocarcinoma. Greater emphasis has therefore been placed on surveillance to ensure early detection of dysplasia or malignant transformation. An optimum surveillance strategy that is both sensitive and cost-effective, however, remains elusive. A number of therapeutic modalities are now available for the treatment of BE, Barrett's dysplasia, and adenocarcinoma. Surgical resection of the affected esophagus is still regarded as the gold standard for the treatment of high-grade dysplasia and early Barrett's carcinoma. Given the measurable morbidity and mortality associated with invasive surgery, recent advances using endoscopic techniques also need consideration. These techniques have shown early promise, particularly in achieving regression of the metaplasia. Some, however, are still experimental while others require expertise, are not yet widely available, and data on their long-term effects remain sparse. What is most important is that the interplay between these various procedures should not be regarded as competitive but rather as complementary to achieve optimal management. We will now take a closer examination of aspects of BE and its management specific to the pediatric population.

9.6
Barrett's Esophagus in Children

The importance of BE in children, as in adults, relates to the recognition of a time-related increase in incidence and severity of dysplasia and subsequent risk of adeno-

carcinoma [101, 194]. Qualman identified goblet cell (intestinal) metaplasia in 50% of pediatric patients with BE compared to 84% of adults, and identified dysplasia, carcinoma in situ, or invasive carcinoma only in patients over the age of 41 years.[194] Hameeteman followed 50 patients with BE for a period of 1.5–14 years (mean 5.2 years) and identified a rising incidence of dysplasia from 14% at study entry to 26% at last follow-up. An additional 10% of patients had developed adenocarcinoma at this stage [101]. However, there are a number of differences between the features and management of this condition in adults and children that warrant specific consideration.

The true incidence of BE in children is difficult to ascertain as the number of cases seen by any one pediatric surgeon is likely to be limited. Over a 15-year period at Great Ormond Street Hospital, London, Beddow identified only 38 cases of BE.[11] Only 16 cases were seen by Cheu over a similar time period [42]. Despite the relatively common diagnosis of GER in children, BE has traditionally been considered an uncommon condition in this age group. However, a number of groups have challenged this preconception.[42, 60, 106] In a group of children who underwent endoscopy and esophageal biopsy for symptoms of GER, Dahms reported a prevalence of 13% with BE [60], while in a subgroup of children with esophageal strictures secondary to GER on endoscopic examination, the incidence of BE may be as high as 25% [106].

The reasons for this disparity are not immediately evident. It has been documented that the characteristic macroscopic appearances of BE seen in adults are not always seen in children [106] and that endoscopic appearances correlate poorly with histological findings [16]. Thus, a child with apparently normal endoscopic appearances may not have a biopsy taken of the esophageal mucosa when in fact BE may be present and identifiable only on histological section. Secondly, not all children with symptoms of GER or proven GER on the basis of a 24-h pH study undergo endoscopy and evaluation of the lower esophageal mucosa. Endoscopy is reserved for those with protracted or recurrent symptoms. It is possible that this conservative approach misses a number of cases of BE. Conversely, it may be that a figure of 13% represents an overestimation of the true incidence as this figure relates only to those children undergoing endoscopy and biopsy, not all those with GER.

The actual occurrence of esophageal adenocarcinoma in childhood appears to be extremely rare. Hoeffel [111] reported two children with a history of GER who developed esophageal adenocarcinoma, both of whom died, and a fatal case of esophageal adenocarcinoma has been reported in an 8-year-old boy [83]. Hassall reported a survivor of adenocarcinoma secondary to BE who underwent esophagectomy at the age of 17 years [103].

It is likely that in the majority of cases the timescale required for the development of adenocarcinoma secondary to GER or BE is beyond the realms of pediatric practice. Recently, a population-based study has attempted to estimate the risk of esophageal malignancy in a large cohort of patients with BE in a single country [166]. An overall incidence of 0.26 esophageal malignancies per 100 patient years was reported. Using this figure, 13 out of 100 children with BE followed for 50 - years would be expected to develop adenocarcinoma.

There are particular groups of children who may be at increased risk of BE and adenocarcinoma. In the early part of the twentieth century almost all infants born with esophageal atresia died, yet now survival rates in excess of 80% are reported [69]. Case reports of both adenocarcinoma and squamous cell carcinoma exist in patients born with esophageal atresia [2, 64]. Two series have examined the incidence of BE among patients born with esophageal atresia and identified an incidence of 7% at a median age of 14 years [220] and 13% at a mean followup of 7.6 years [144]. However, in this second series the diagnosis of BE was based on endoscopic appearance and metaplasia was only evident in 8% of cases on histological examination. It is possible that in the future this particular group of patients may have previously unrecognized complications relating to their now corrected congenital malformations and long-term followup may be indicated [144]. Children with cystic fibrosis also have a predisposition to develop GER and their potential to develop BE has also been reported [104].

9.6.1
Management of the Child with Barrett's Esophagus

Issues relating to the management of the child with BE are complex. Firstly, should the reflux itself be treated and if so how? Secondly, how should these children be followed up to identify those at risk of developing adenocarcinoma later in life? And finally, what should be done about the BE itself – will it regress, should it be excised, or are other treatment options available? These issues are further complicated by the lack of evidence in the pediatric literature concerning all aspects of the management of BE. Therefore, data from the adult population are extrapolated and applied to children.

9.6.1.1
Treatment of GER in Children with BE

GER in children is generally treated to relieve symptoms and other secondary complications of reflux. Whether control of reflux itself has any direct benefit over and above symptom control for patients with BE is poorly understood. It is generally considered that BE does not regress following control of reflux (see BE in adults). However, Conti-Nibali et al. have reported resolution of BE following antireflux surgery (itself preceded by failure of medical therapy) in an infant aged 4 months at diagnosis [49]. Hassell reported partial regression of BE in a 12-year-old boy following fundoplication [105]. These reports suggest that in some cases, perhaps limited to the pediatric population, BE itself can be eradicated by adequate antireflux treatment. Recently, data from a study comparing medical and surgical treatment of GER in adults with BE suggests that eradication of reflux into the esophagus may have a beneficial influence on the natural history of BE, reducing the development of dysplasia and adenocarcinoma [183]. Unfortunately, there are no studies in which this relationship is more clearly defined.

In general, as in adults, the treatment of reflux is approached by either medical or surgical treatment. Medical treatment involves the use of H_2 receptor antagonists or proton pump inhibitors or both. Surgical treatment is most commonly by Nissen fundoplication, performed either via the open or laparoscopic approach. Both medical and surgical approaches to GER in children with BE are reported [11, 42]. However, patients in neither series underwent post-treatment pH studies to ensure adequate eradication of reflux. It has been the authors' practice to perform a surgical antireflux procedure (Nissen fundoplication) on children with BE rather than submit them to a trial of medical treatment with monitoring. Whether this is the most satisfactory approach remains unclear. Perhaps what is most important is eradication of the reflux rather than the method by which this is done. While we may assume that a surgical procedure is superior to medical treatment in this respect, there is no evidence in support of this at present.

9.6.1.2
Surveillance of Children with BE

As previously described in adults, the aims of endoscopic surveillance are to identify those with dysplasia at increased risk of developing adenocarcinoma and those with adenocarcinoma requiring treatment. There is no doubt that surveillance of some description is indicated in children, but the frequency at which endoscopic examination should be performed is unclear. Essentially, the challenge, as in adults, is that of identifying those at risk of dysplastic or malignant change while minimizing the inconvenience, disruption to lifestyle, and costs involved with overzealous surveillance. Due to the low risk of adenocarcinoma in childhood, a more liberal policy of endoscopy and biopsy every 3–4 years has been recommended [11, 103] and this surveillance should be continued into adult life. Recently, however, Stepanov advocated a more aggressive surveillance policy of endoscopy and esophageal biopsy every 6–12 months [243].

9.6.1.3
Treatment of BE Itself

Although it has generally been considered that BE does not regress following antireflux treatment, there are cases in which resolution has been observed in both adult and pediatric [49, 105] patients. Thus, for a selective small group, antireflux treatment may in itself be sufficient treatment for BE. For the majority, however, it has been standard practice to observe those with BE for evidence of dysplasia or adenocarcinoma and offer definitive treatment only when present. Thus surveillance has been the preferred treatment regime in children.

The use of endoscopic laser ablation has been described in adults (see adults). Salo described 17 patients with BE that initially underwent successful antireflux surgery [211]. In eleven of these, the Barrett's epithelium was ablated using an endoscopic laser technique. The regenerated epithelium was squamous type in all but two, in whom intestinal metaplasia persisted. Garcia also reported a 13-year-old child with BE who had been treated with antireflux surgery and endoscopic bipolar coagulation, who subsequently was free from BE after 15 months of followup [84].

Stepanov et al. reported surgical excision of the BE segment when associated with esophageal stricture not responding to dilatation by bouginage [243]. Colonic interposition was performed to maintain esophageal length. While this approach is radical, it is also effective at removing the BE segment. Stepanov advises that in addition to BE with high-grade dysplasia or suspicion of adenocarcinoma, multiple failed antireflux surgical procedures be considered an absolute indication for surgical excision of BE. They further introduce the concept that these peptic strictures not responsive to antireflux surgery and bouginage and young patients with BE may be regarded as having relative indications for surgical excision. Evidence for this aggressive approach is, however, lacking. The potential risks and complications of a demolitive procedure must be balanced against the lifetime risk of adenocarcinoma, which as stated previously, is shown to be small.

Whether BE really requires treatment rather than surveillance alone remain controversial. It is unclear whether surveillance will be required following successful treatment and eradication of BE. This strategy may be particularly applicable to children who developed BE early in life.

9.6.1.4
Authors Recommended Strategy for Management of BE in Children

The paucity of reliable evidence makes the development of precise guidelines for the pediatric population hazardous. However, the strategy described below is based upon our current practice and recent published evidence.

Children identified as having BE are offered antireflux surgery in the form of Nissen fundoplication performed either via the open or laparoscopic approach. Following surgery, a pH study is performed to ensure adequate eradication of GER. A surveillance program is initiated comprising endoscopic examination with biopsies at 3–4 yearly intervals. Care is formally transferred to adult gastroenterologists at an appropriate age and surveillance continued according to adult guidelines. Aggressive therapy is reserved for children who show evidence of adenocarcinoma.

References

1. Achkar E, Carey W (1988) The cost of surveillance for adenocarcinoma complicating Barrett's esophagus. Am J Gastroenterol 83(3):291–294
2. Adzick NS, Fisher JH, Winter HS, Sandler RH, Hendren WH (1989) Esophageal adenocarcinoma 20 years after esophageal atresia repair. J Pediatr Surg 24(8):741–744
3. Allison PR (1948) Peptic ulcer of oesophagus. Thorax 3:20–42
4. Allison PR, Johnstone AS (1953) The esophagus lined with gastric mucous membrane. Thorax 8:87–91
5. Almasan A, Linke SP, Paulson TG, Huang LC, Wahl GM (1995) Genetic instability as a consequence of inappropriate entry into and progression through S-phase. Cancer Metastasis Rev 14(1):59–73
6. Attwood SE, Barlow AP, Norris TL, Watson A (1992) Barrett's oesophagus: effect of antireflux surgery on symptom control and development of complications. Br J Surg 79(10): 1050–1053
7. Attwood SE, DeMeester TR, Bremner CG, Barlow AP, Hinder RA (1989) Alkaline gastroesophageal reflux: implications in the development of complications in Barrett's columnar-lined lower esophagus. Surgery 106(4):764–770
8. Attwood SE, Smyrk TC, DeMeester TR, Mirvish SS, Stein HJ, Hinder RA (1992) Duodenoesophageal reflux and the development of esophageal adenocarcinoma in rats. Surgery 111(5):503–510
9. Barham CP, Jones RL, Biddlestone LR, Hardwick RH, Shepherd NA, Barr H (1997) Photothermal laser ablation of Barrett's oesophagus: endoscopic and histological evidence of squamous re-epithelialization. Gut 41(3):281–284
10. Barrett NR (1950) Chronic peptic ulcer of the oesophagus and "oesophagitis." Br J Surg 38:175–182
11. Beddow EC, Wilcox DT, Drake DP, Pierro A, Kiely EM, Spitz L (1999) Surveillance of Barrett's esophagus in children. J Pediatr Surg 34(1):88–90
12. Berenson MM, Johnson TD, Markowitz NR, Buchi KN, Samowitz WS (1993) Restoration of squamous mucosa after ablation of Barrett's esophageal epithelium. Gastroenterol 104(6):1686–1691
13. Berenson MM, Riddell RH, Skinner DB, Freston JW (1978) Malignant transformation of esophageal columnar epithelium. Cancer 41(2):554–561
14. Bersentes K, Fass R, Padda S, Johnson C, Sampliner RE (1998) Prevalence of Barrett's esophagus in Hispanics is similar to Caucasians. Dig Dis Sci 43(5):1038–1041
15. Biddlestone LR, Barham CP, Wilkinson SP, Barr H, Shepherd NA (1998) The histopathology of treated Barrett's esophagus: squamous reepithelialization after acid suppression and laser and photodynamic therapy. Am J Surg Pathol 22(2): 239–245
16. Biller JA, Winter HS, Grand RJ, Allred EN (1983) Are endoscopic changes predictive of histologic esophagitis in children? J Pediatr 103(2):215–218

17. Blot WJ, Devesa SS, Kneller RW, Fraumeni JF Jr (1991) Rising incidence of adenocarcinoma of the esophagus and gastric cardia. JAMA 265(10):1287–1289

18. Blount PL, Ramel S, Raskind WH, Haggitt RC, Sanchez CA, Dean PJ, et al. (1991) 17p allelic deletions and p53 protein overexpression in Barrett's adenocarcinoma. Cancer Res 51(20):5482–5486

19. Bonelli L (1993) Barrett's esophagus: results of a multicentric survey. G.O.S.P.E. (Gruppo Operativo per lo Studio delle Precancerosi Esofagee. Endoscopy 25(9):652–654

20. Borhan-Manesh F, Farnum JB (1993) Study of Helicobacter pylori colonization of patches of heterotopic gastric mucosa (HGM) at the upper esophagus. Dig Dis Sci 38(1):142–146

21. Borrie J, Goldwater L (1976) Columnar cell-lined esophagus: assessment of etiology and treatment. A 22 year experience. J Thorac Cardiovasc Surg 71(6):825–834

22. Bowers SP, Mattar SG, Smith CD, Waring JP, Hunter JG (2002) Clinical and histologic follow-up after antireflux surgery for Barrett's esophagus. J Gastrointest Surg 6(4):532–538

23. Braghetto I, Csendes A, Burdiles P, Korn O, Compan A, Guerra JF (2002) Barrett's esophagus complicated with stricture: correlation between classification and the results of the different therapeutic options. World J Surg 26(10):1228–1233

24. Brandt LJ, Kauvar DR (1992) Laser-induced transient regression of Barrett's epithelium. Gastrointest Endosc 38(5):619–622

25. Bremner CG (1982) Benign strictures of the esophagus. Curr Probl Surg 19(8):401–489

26. Brown LM, Silverman DT, Pottern LM, Schoenberg JB, Greenberg RS, Swanson GM, et al. (1994) Adenocarcinoma of the esophagus and esophagogastric junction in white men in the United States: alcohol, tobacco, and socioeconomic factors. Cancer Causes Control 5(4):333–340

27. Burbige EJ, Radigan JJ (1979) Characteristics of the columnar-cell lined (Barrett's) esophagus. Gastrointest Endosc 25(4):133–136

28. Burgess JN, Payne WS, Andersen HA, Weiland LH, Carlson HC (1971) Barrett esophagus: the columnar-epithelial-lined lower esophagus. Mayo Clin Proc 46(11):728–734

29. Buttar NS, Wang KK, Anderson MA, Dierkhising RA, Pacifico RJ, Krishnadath KK, et al. (2002) The effect of selective cyclooxygenase-2 inhibition in Barrett's esophagus epithelium: an in vitro study. J Natl Cancer Inst 94(6):422–429

30. Buttar NS, Wang KK, Leontovich O, Westcott JY, Pacifico RJ, Anderson MA, et al. (2002) Chemoprevention of esophageal adenocarcinoma by COX-2 inhibitors in an animal model of Barrett's esophagus. Gastroenterol 122(4):1101–1112

31. Byrne JP, Armstrong GR, Attwood SE (1998) Restoration of the normal squamous lining in Barrett's esophagus by argon beam plasma coagulation. Am J Gastroenterol 93(10):1810–1815

32. Bytzer P, Christensen PB, Damkier P, Vinding K, Seersholm N (1999) Adenocarcinoma of the esophagus and Barrett's esophagus: a population-based study. Am J Gastroenterol 94(1):86–91

33. Caldwell MT, Lawlor P, Byrne PJ, Walsh TN, Hennessy TP (1995) Ambulatory oesophageal bile reflux monitoring in Barrett's oesophagus. Br J Surg 82(5):657–660

34. Cameron AJ, Lomboy CT (1992) Barrett's esophagus: age, prevalence, and extent of columnar epithelium. Gastroenterol 103(4):1241–1245

35. Cameron AJ, Ott BJ, Payne WS (1985) The incidence of adenocarcinoma in columnar-lined (Barrett's) esophagus. N Engl J Med 313(14):857–859

36. Cameron AJ, Zinsmeister AR, Ballard DJ, Carney JA (1990) Prevalence of columnar-lined (Barrett's) esophagus. Comparison of population-based clinical and autopsy findings. Gastroenterol 99(4):918–922

37. Canto MI, Setrakian S, Petras RE, Blades E, Chak A, Sivak MV Jr (1996) Methylene blue selectively stains intestinal metaplasia in Barrett's esophagus. Gastrointest Endosc 44(1):1–7

38. Casson AG, Mukhopadhyay T, Cleary KR, Ro JY, Levin B, Roth JA (1991) p53 gene mutations in Barrett's epithelium and esophageal cancer. Cancer Res 51(16):4495–4499

39. Chak A, Lee T, Kinnard MF, Brock W, Faulx A, Willis J, et al. (2002) Familial aggregation of Barrett's oesophagus, oesophageal adenocarcinoma, and oesophagogastric junctional adenocarcinoma in Caucasian adults. Gut 51(3):323–328

40. Champion G, Richter JE, Vaezi MF, Singh S, Alexander R (1994) Duodenogastroesophageal reflux: relationship to pH and importance in Barrett's esophagus. Gastroenterol 107(3):747–754

41. Chen LQ, Nastos D, Hu CY, Chughtai TS, Taillefer R, Ferraro P, et al. (1999) Results of the Collis-Nissen gastroplasty in patients with Barrett's esophagus. Ann Thorac Surg 68(3):1014–1020

42. Cheu HW, Grosfeld JL, Heifetz SA, Fitzgerald J, Rescorla F, West K (1992) Persistence of Barrett's esophagus in children after antireflux surgery: influence on follow-up care. J Pediatr Surg 27(2):260–264

43. Chiba N, De Gara CJ, Wilkinson JM, Hunt RH (1997) Speed of healing and symptom relief in grade II to IV gastroesophageal reflux disease: a meta-analysis. Gastroenterol 112(6):1798–1810

44. Chobanian SJ, Cattau EL Jr, Winters C Jr, Johnson DA, Van Ness MM, Miremadi A, et al. (1987) In vivo staining with toluidine blue as an adjunct to the endoscopic detection of Barrett's esophagus. Gastrointest Endosc 33(2):99–101

45. Collins BJ, Abbott M, Thomas RJ, Morstyn G, St John DJ (1991) Clinical profile in Barrett's esophagus: who should be screened for cancer? Hepatogastroenterology 38(4):341–344

46. Collins JB, III, Georgeson KE, Vicente Y, Hardin WD Jr (1995) Comparison of open and laparoscopic gastrostomy and fundoplication in 120 patients. J Pediatr Surg 30(7):1065–1070

47. Conio M, Cameron AJ, Romero Y, Branch CD, Schleck CD, Burgart LJ, et al. (2001) Secular trends in the epidemiology and outcome of Barrett's oesophagus in Olmsted County, Minnesota. Gut 48(3):304–309

48. Conio M, Filiberti R, Blanchi S, Ferraris R, Marchi S, Ravelli P, et al. (2002) Risk factors for Barrett's esophagus: a case-control study. Int J Cancer 97(2):225–229

49. Conti NS, Barresi G, Tuccari G, Rivosecchi M, Magazzu G (1988) Barrett's esophagus in an infant: a long standing history with final postsurgical regression. J Pediatr Gastroenterol Nutr 7(4):602–607

50. Cooper BT, Barbezat GO (1987) Barrett's oesophagus: a clinical study of 52 patients. Q J Med 62(238):97–10851. Cooper BT, Neumann CS, Cox MA, Iqbal TH (1998) Continuous treatment with omeprazole 20 mg daily for up to 6 years in Barrett's oesophagus. Aliment Pharmacol Ther 12(9):893–897

52. Cooper JE, Spitz L, Wilkins BM (1987) Barrett's esophagus in children: a histologic and histochemical study of 11 cases. J Pediatr Surg 22(3):191–196

53. Corley DA, Levin TR, Habel LA, Weiss NS, Buffler PA (2002) Surveillance and survival in Barrett's adenocarcinomas: a population-based study. Gastroenterol 122(3):633–640

54. Crabb DW, Berk MA, Hall TR, Conneally PM, Biegel AA, Lehman GA (1985) Familial gastroesophageal reflux and development of Barrett's esophagus. Ann Intern Med 103(1):52–54

55. Csendes A, Braghetto I, Burdiles P, Diaz JC, Maluenda F, Korn O (1997) A new physiologic approach for the surgical treatment of patients with Barrett's esophagus: technical considerations and results in 65 patients. Ann Surg 226(2):123–133

56. Csendes A, Braghetto I, Burdiles P, Puente G, Korn O, Diaz JC, et al. (1998) Long-term results of classic antireflux surgery in 152 patients with Barrett's esophagus: clinical, radiologic, endoscopic, manometric, and acid reflux test analysis before and late after operation. Surgery 123(6):645–657

57. Csendes A, Burdiles P, Braghetto I, Korn O, Diaz JC, Rojas J (2002) Early and late results of the acid suppression and duodenal diversion operation in patients with Barrett's esophagus: analysis of 210 cases. World J Surg 26(5):566–576

58. Csendes A, Burdiles P, Korn O, Braghetto I, Huertas C, Rojas J (2000) Late results of a randomized clinical trial comparing total fundoplication versus calibration of the cardia with posterior gastropexy. Br J Surg 87(3):289–297

59. Dahms BB, Greco MA, Strandjord SE, Rothstein FC (1987) Barrett's esophagus in three children after antileukemia chemotherapy. Cancer 60(12):2896–2900

60. Dahms BB, Rothstein FC (1984) Barrett's esophagus in children: a consequence of chronic gastroesophageal reflux. Gastroenterol 86(2):318–323

61. Decarli A, Liati P, Negri E, Franceschi S, La Vecchia C (1987) Vitamin A and other dietary factors in the etiology of esophageal cancer. Nutr Cancer 10(1–2):29–37

62. DeMeester SR, DeMeester TR (1999) The diagnosis and management of Barrett's esophagus. Adv Surg 33:29–68

63. DeMeester TR, Attwood SE, Smyrk TC, Therkildsen DH, Hinder RA (1990) Surgical therapy in Barrett's esophagus. Ann Surg 212(4):528–540

64. Deurloo JA, van Lanschot JJ, Drillenburg P, Aronson DC (2001) Esophageal squamous cell carcinoma 38 years after primary repair of esophageal atresia. J Pediatr Surg 36(4):629–630

65. Devesa SS, Blot WJ, Fraumeni JF Jr (1998) Changing patterns in the incidence of esophageal and gastric carcinoma in the United States. Cancer 83(10):2049–2053

66. Donehower LA, Bradley A (1993) The tumor suppressor p53. Biochim Biophys Acta 1155(2):181–205

67. Dorsch ER, Graham DY, Lie JT, Estrada RG (1977) The columnar-cell-lined (Barrett's) esophagus: a premalignant condition? South Med J 70(4):505–507

68. Drewitz DJ, Sampliner RE, Garewal HS (1997) The incidence of adenocarcinoma in Barrett's esophagus: a prospective study of 170 patients followed 4.8 years. Am J Gastroenterol 92(2):212–215

69. Driver CP, Shankar KR, Jones MO, Lamont GA, Turnock RR, Lloyd DA, et al. (2001) Phenotypic presentation and outcome of esophageal atresia in the era of the Spitz classification. J Pediatr Surg 36(9):1419–1421

70. Dumoulin FL, Terjung B, Neubrand M, Scheurlen C, Fischer HP, Sauerbruch T (1997) Treatment of Barrett's esophagus by endoscopic argon plasma coagulation. Endoscopy 29(8):751–753

71. Eckardt VF, Kanzler G, Bernhard G (2001) Life expectancy and cancer risk in patients with Barrett's esophagus: a prospective controlled investigation. Am J Med 111(1):33–37

72. Ell C, May A, Gossner L, Pech O, Gunter E, Mayer G, et al. (2000) Endoscopic mucosal resection of early cancer and high-grade dysplasia in Barrett's esophagus. Gastroenterol 118(4):670–677

73. Eng C, Spechler SJ, Ruben R, Li FP (1993) Familial Barrett esophagus and adenocarcinoma of the gastroesophageal junction. Cancer Epidemiol Biomarkers Prev 2(4):397–399

74. Ertan A, Zimmerman M, Younes M (1995) Esophageal adenocarcinoma associated with Barrett's esophagus: long-term management with laser ablation. Am J Gastroenterol 90(12):2201–2203

75. Esposito C, Garipoli V, De Pasquale M, Russo S, Palazzo G, Cucchiara S (1997) Laparoscopic versus traditional fundoplication in the treatment of children with refractory gastro-oesophageal reflux. Ital J Gastroenterol Hepatol 29(5):399–402

76. Everhart CW Jr, Holtzapple PG, Humphries TJ (1983) Barrett's esophagus: inherited epithelium or inherited reflux? J Clin Gastroenterol 5(4):357–358

77. Fahmy N, King JF (1993) Barrett's esophagus: an acquired condition with genetic predisposition. Am J Gastroenterol 88(8):1262–1265

78. Farrell TM, Smith CD, Metreveli RE, Johnson AB, Galloway KD, Hunter JG (1999) Fundoplication provides effective and durable symptom relief in patients with Barrett's esophagus. Am J Surg 178(1):18–21

79. Fein M, Ireland AP, Ritter MP, Peters JH, Hagen JA, Bremner CG, et al. (1997) Duodenogastric reflux potentiates the injurious effects of gastroesophageal reflux. J Gastrointest Surg 1(1):27–33

80. Ferreres JC, Fernandez F, Rodriguez VA, Gonzalez-Rodilla I, Ursua I, Ramos R, et al. (1991) Helicobacter pylori in Barrett's esophagus. Histol Histopathol 6(3):403–408

81. Filipi CJ, Lehman GA, Rothstein RI, Raijman I, Stiegmann GV, Waring JP, et al. (2001) Transoral, flexible endoscopic suturing for treatment of GERD: a multicenter trial. Gastrointest Endosc 53(4):416–422

82. Fonkalsrud EW, Ashcraft KW, Coran AG, Ellis DG, Grosfeld JL, Tunell WP, et al. (1998) Surgical treatment of gastroesophageal reflux in children: a combined hospital study of 7,467 patients. Pediatrics 101(3 Pt 1):419–422

83. Gangopadhyay AN, Mohanty PK, Gopal SC, Gupta DK, Sahi UP, Aryya NC, et al. (1997) Adenocarcinoma of the esophagus in an 8-year-old boy. J Pediatr Surg 32(8):1259–1260

84. Garcia MC, Brandalise NA, Deliza R, Servidoni MF, Ferraz JG, Magalhaes AF (1998) Regression of childhood Barrett's esophageal mucosa by antireflux surgery and bipolar electrocoagulation. J Pediatr Surg 33(5):747–749

85. Garewal HS, Sampliner R, Gerner E, Steinbronn K, Alberts D, Kendall D (1988) Ornithine decarboxylase activity in Barrett's esophagus: a potential marker for dysplasia. Gastroenterol 94(3):819–821

86. Garewal HS, Sampliner R, Liu Y, Trent JM (1989) Chromosomal rearrangements in Barrett's esophagus. A premalignant lesion of esophageal adenocarcinoma. Cancer Genet Cytogenet 42(2):281–286

87. Gelfand MD (1983) Barrett esophagus in sexagenarian identical twins. J Clin Gastroenterol 5(3):251–253

88. Gerson LB, Shetler K, Triadafilopoulos G (2002) Prevalence of Barrett's esophagus in asymptomatic individuals. Gastroenterol 123(2):461–467

89. Gilchrist AM, Levine MS, Carr RF, Saul SH, Katzka DA, Herlinger H, et al. (1988) Barrett's esophagus: diagnosis by double-contrast esophagography. AJR Am J Roentgenol 150(1):97–102

90. Gillen P, Keeling P, Byrne PJ, Healy M, O'Moore RR, Hennessy TP (1988) Implication of duodenogastric reflux in the pathogenesis of Barrett's oesophagus. Br J Surg 75(6):540–543

91. Glickman JN, Wang H, Das KM, Goyal RK, Spechler SJ, Antonioli D, et al. (2001) Phenotype of Barrett's esophagus and intestinal metaplasia of the distal esophagus and gastroesophageal junction: an immunohistochemical study of cytokeratins 7 and 20, Das-1 and 45 MI. Am J Surg Pathol 25(1):87–94

92. Goldstein NS (2000) Gastric cardia intestinal metaplasia: biopsy follow-up of 85 patients. Mod Pathol 13(10):1072–1079

93. GOSPE (1991) Barrett's esophagus: epidemiological and clinical results of a multicentric survey. Gruppo Operativo per lo Studio delle Precancerosi dell'Esofago (GOSPE). Int J Cancer 48(3):364–368

94. Gossner L, May A, Stolte M, Seitz G, Hahn EG, Ell C (1999) KTP laser destruction of dysplasia and early cancer in columnar-lined Barrett's esophagus. Gastrointest Endosc 49(1):8–12

95. Gossner L, Sroka R, Hahn EG, Ell C (1995) Photodynamic therapy: successful destruction of gastrointestinal cancer after oral administration of aminolevulinic acid. Gastrointest Endosc 41(1):55–58

96. Gossner L, Stolte M, Sroka R, Rick K, May A, Hahn EG, et al. (1998) Photodynamic ablation of high-grade dysplasia and early cancer in Barrett's esophagus by means of 5-aminolevulinic acid. Gastroenterol 114(3):448–455

97. Grade AJ, Shah IA, Medlin SM, Ramirez FC (1999) The efficacy and safety of argon plasma coagulation therapy in Barrett's esophagus. Gastrointest Endosc 50(1):18–22

98. Graham S, Marshall J, Haughey B, Brasure J, Freudenheim J, Zielezny M, et al. (1990) Nutritional epidemiology of cancer of the esophagus. Am J Epidemiol 131(3):454–467

99. Gray MR, Donnelly RJ, Kingsnorth AN (1993) The role of smoking and alcohol in metaplasia and cancer risk in Barrett's columnar lined oesophagus. Gut 34(6):727–731

100. Haggitt RC, Tryzelaar J, Ellis FH, Colcher H (1978) Adenocarcinoma complicating columnar epithelium-lined (Barrett's) esophagus. Am J Clin Pathol 70(1):1–5

101. Hameeteman W, Tytgat GN, Houthoff HJ, van den Tweel JG (1989) Barrett's esophagus: development of dysplasia and adenocarcinoma. Gastroenterol 96(5 Pt 1):1249–1256

102. Harle IA, Finley RJ, Belsheim M, Bondy DC, Booth M, Lloyd D, et al. (1985) Management of adenocarcinoma in a columnar-lined esophagus. Ann Thorac Surg 40(4):330–336

103. Hassall E, Dimmick JE, Magee JF (1993) Adenocarcinoma in childhood Barrett's esophagus: case documentation and the need for surveillance in children. (Review, 35 refs). Am J Gastroenterol 88(2):282–288

104. Hassall E, Israel DM, Davidson AG, Wong LT (1993) Barrett's esophagus in children with cystic fibrosis: not a coincidental association. Am J Gastroenterol 88(11):1934–1938

105. Hassall E, Weinstein WM (1992) Partial regression of childhood Barrett's esophagus after fundoplication. Am J Gastroenterol 87(10):1506–1512

106. Hassall E, Weinstein WM, Ament ME (1985) Barrett's esophagus in childhood. Gastroenterol 89(6):1331–1337

107. Hawe A, Payne WS, Weiland LH, Fontana RS (1973) Adenocarcinima in the columnar epithelial lined lower (Barret) oesophagus. Thorax 28(4):511–514

108. Heitmiller RF, Redmond M, Hamilton SR (1996) Barrett's esophagus with high-grade dysplasia. An indication for prophylactic esophagectomy. Ann Surg 224(1):66–71

109. Herlihy KJ, Orlando RC, Bryson JC, Bozymski EM, Carney CN, Powell DW (1984) Barrett's esophagus: clinical, endoscopic, histologic, manometric, and electrical potential difference characteristics. Gastroenterol 86(3):436–443

110. Hillman LC, Chiragakis L, Clarke AC, Kaushik SP, Kaye GL (2003) Barrett's esophagus: Macroscopic markers and the prediction of dysplasia and adenocarcinoma. J Gastroenterol Hepatol 18(5):526–533

111. Hoeffel JC, Nihoul-Fekete C, Schmitt M (1989) Esophageal adenocarcinoma after gastroesophageal reflux in children.(erratum appears in J Pediatr 1989 Nov; 115(5 Pt 1): 836). J Pediatrics 115(2):259–261

112. Hofstetter WL, Peters JH, DeMeester TR, Hagen JA, DeMeester SR, Crookes PF, et al. (2001) Long-term outcome of antireflux surgery in patients with Barrett's esophagus. Ann Surg 234(4):532–538

113. Holscher AH, Bollschweiler E, Schneider PM, Siewert JR (1997) Early adenocarcinoma in Barrett's oesophagus. Br J Surg 84(10):1470–1473

114. Houck JA, Lucas JG (1989) Absence of Campylobacter-like organisms in Barrett's esophagus. Arch Pathol Lab Med 113(5):470–472

115. Hu FZ, Preston RA, Post JC, White GJ, Kikuchi LW, Wang X, et al. (2000) Mapping of a gene for severe pediatric gastroesophageal reflux to chromosome 13q14. JAMA 284(3): 325–334

116. Iftikhar SY, James PD, Steele RJ, Hardcastle JD, Atkinson M (1992) Length of Barrett's oesophagus: an important factor in the development of dysplasia and adenocarcinoma. Gut 33(9):1155–1158

117. Iftikhar SY, Ledingham S, Steele RJ, Evans DF, Lendrum K, Atkinson M, et al. (1993) Bile reflux in columnar-lined Barrett's oesophagus. Ann R Coll Surg Engl 75(6):411–416

118. Iftikhar SY, Steele RJ, Watson S, James PD, Dilks K, Hardcastle JD (1992) Assessment of proliferation of squamous, Barrett's and gastric mucosa in patients with columnar lined Barrett's oesophagus. Gut 33(6):733–737

119. Incarbone R, Bonavina L, Szachnowicz S, Saino G, Peracchia A (2000) Rising incidence of esophageal adenocarcinoma in Western countries: is it possible to identify a population at risk? Dis Esophagus 13(4):275–278

120. Jankowski J, McMenemin R, Yu C, Hopwood D, Wormsley KG (1992) Proliferating cell nuclear antigen in oesophageal diseases; correlation with transforming growth factor alpha expression. Gut 33(5):587–591

121. Jochem VJ, Fuerst PA, Fromkes JJ (1992) Familial Barrett's esophagus associated with adenocarcinoma. Gastroenterol 102(4 Pt 1):1400–1402

122. Johnston MH, Hammond AS, Laskin W, Jones DM (1996) The prevalence and clinical characteristics of short segments of specialized intestinal metaplasia in the distal esophagus on routine endoscopy. Am J Gastroenterol 91(8):1507–1511

123. Kabat GC, Ng SK, Wynder EL (1993) Tobacco, alcohol intake, and diet in relation to adenocarcinoma of the esophagus and gastric cardia. Cancer Causes Control 4(2):123–132

124. Kalogeropoulos NK, Whitehead R (1988) Campylobacter-like organisms and Candida in peptic ulcers and similar lesions of the upper gastrointestinal tract: a study of 247 cases. J Clin Pathol 41(10):1093–1098

125. Kastan MB, Canman CE, Leonard CJ (1995) P53, cell cycle control and apoptosis: implications for cancer. Cancer Metastasis Rev 14(1):3–15

126. Katz PO (2002) Gastroesophageal reflux disease: new treatments. Rev Gastroenterol Disord 2(2):66–74

127. Katzka DA, Castell DO (1994) Successful elimination of reflux symptoms does not insure adequate control of acid reflux in patients with Barrett's esophagus. Am J Gastroenterol 89(7):989–991

128. Kauer WK, Burdiles P, Ireland AP, Clark GW, Peters JH, Bremner CG, et al. (1995a) Does duodenal juice reflux into the esophagus of patients with complicated GERD? Evaluation of a fiberoptic sensor for bilirubin. Am J Surg 169(1): 98–103

129. Kauer WK, Peters JH, DeMeester TR, Ireland AP, Bremner CG, Hagen JA (1995b) Mixed reflux of gastric and duodenal juices is more harmful to the esophagus than gastric juice alone. The need for surgical therapy re-emphasized. Ann Surg 222(4):525–531

130. Kaur BS, Khamnehei N, Iravani M, Namburu SS, Lin O, Triadafilopoulos G (2002) Rofecoxib inhibits cyclooxygenase 2 expression and activity and reduces cell proliferation in Barrett's esophagus. Gastroenterol 123(1):60–67

131. Kennedy JC, Pottier RH (1992) Endogenous protoporphyrin IX, a clinically useful photosensitizer for photodynamic therapy. J Photochem Photobiol B 14(4):275–292

132. Kim R, Weissfeld JL, Reynolds JC, Kuller LH (1997) Etiology of Barrett's metaplasia and esophageal adenocarcinoma. Cancer Epidemiol Biomarkers Prev 6(5):369–377

133. Koop H (2000) Reflux disease and Barrett's esophagus. Endoscopy 32(2):101–107

134. Kouklakis GS, Kountouras J, Dokas SM, Molyvas EJ, Vourvoulakis GP, Minopoulos GI (2003) Methylene blue chromoendoscopy for the detection of Barrett's esophagus in a Greek cohort. Endoscopy 35(5):383–387

135. Kovacs BJ, Chen YK, Lewis TD, DeGuzman LJ, Thompson KS (1999) Successful reversal of Barrett's esophagus with multipolar electrocoagulation despite inadequate acid suppression. Gastrointest Endosc 49(5):547–553

136. Kuerbitz SJ, Plunkett BS, Walsh WV, Kastan MB (1992) Wildtype p53 is a cell cycle checkpoint determinant following irradiation. Proc Natl Acad Sci USA 89(16):7491–7495

137. Lagergren J, Bergstrom R, Lindgren A, Nyren O (1999) Symptomatic gastroesophageal reflux as a risk factor for esophageal adenocarcinoma. N Engl J Med 340(11):825–831

138. Lagergren J, Bergstrom R, Nyren O (1999) Association between body mass and adenocarcinoma of the esophagus and gastric cardia. Ann Intern Med 130(11):883–890

139. Laukka MA, Wang KK (1995) Initial results using low-dose photodynamic therapy in the treatment of Barrett's esophagus. Gastrointest Endosc 42(1):59–63

140. Lehman GA, Berke MA, Biegel AA (1979) Familial gastroesophageal reflux (GER) with Barrett's esophagus (abstract). Gastroenterol 76:1183

141. Levi F, Ollyo JB, La Vecchia C, Boyle P, Monnier P, Savary M (1990) The consumption of tobacco, alcohol and the risk of adenocarcinoma in Barrett's oesophagus. Int J Cancer 45(5): 852–854

142. Levine DS, Haggitt RC, Blount PL, Rabinovitch PS, Rusch VW, Reid BJ (1993) An endoscopic biopsy protocol can differentiate high-grade dysplasia from early adenocarcinoma in Barrett's esophagus. Gastroenterol 105(1):40–50

143. Lieberman DA, Oehlke M, Helfand M (1997) Risk factors for Barrett's esophagus in community-based practice. GORGE consortium. Gastroenterol Outcomes Research Group in Endoscopy. Am J Gastroenterol 92(8):1293–1297

144. Lindahl H, Rintala R, Sariola H (1993) Chronic esophagitis and gastric metaplasia are frequent late complications of esophageal atresia. J Pediatr Surg 28(9):1178–1180

145. Liron R, Parrilla P, Martinez de Haro LF, Ortiz A, Robles R, Lujan JA, et al. (1997) Quantification of duodenogastric reflux in Barrett's esophagus. Am J Gastroenterol 92(1):32–36

146. Loffeld RJ, Ten Tije BJ, Arends JW (1992) Prevalence and significance of Helicobacter pylori in patients with Barrett's esophagus. Am J Gastroenterol 87(11):1598–1600

147. Luman W, Lessels AM, Palmer KR (1996) Failure of Nd-YAG photocoagulation therapy as treatment for Barrett's oesophagus – a pilot study. Eur J Gastroenterol Hepatol 8(7):627–630

148. Macdonald CE, Wicks AC, Playford RJ (2000) Final results from 10 year cohort of patients undergoing surveillance for Barrett's oesophagus: observational study. BMJ 321(7271):1252–1255

149. Malesci A, Savarino V, Zentilin P, Belicchi M, Mela GS, Lapertosa G, et al. (1996) Partial regression of Barrett's esophagus by long-term therapy with high-dose omeprazole. Gastrointest Endosc 44(6):700–705

150. Mann NS, Tsai MF, Nair PK (1989) Barrett's esophagus in patients with symptomatic reflux esophagitis. Am J Gastroenterol 84(12):1494–1496

151. Martinez JM, Halverson A, Magnuson DK, Sackier JM (1997) Laparoscopic versus open Nissen fundoplication: outcome of surgery in monozygotic twins. J Laparoendosc Adv Surg Tech A 7(5):323–326

152. Mattioli G, Repetto P, Carlini C, Torre M, Pini PA, Mazzola C, et al. (2002) Laparoscopic vs open approach for the treatment of gastroesophageal reflux in children. Surg Endosc 16(5):750–752

153. May A, Gossner L, Gunter E, Stolte M, Ell C (1999) Local treatment of early cancer in short Barrett's esophagus by means of argon plasma coagulation: initial experience. Endoscopy 31(6):497–500

154. McDonald GB, Brand DL, Thorning DR (1977) Multiple adenomatous neoplasms arising in columnarlined (Barrett's) esophagus. Gastroenterol 72(6):1317–1321

155. McDonald ML, Trastek VF, Allen MS, Deschamps C, Pairolero PC, Pairolero PC (1996) Barrett's esophagus: does an antireflux procedure reduce the need for endoscopic surveillance? J Thorac Cardiovasc Surg 111(6):1135–1138

156. Menke-Pluymers MB, Hop WC, Dees J, van Blankenstein M, Tilanus HW (1993) Risk factors for the development of an adenocarcinoma in columnar-lined (Barrett) esophagus. The Rotterdam Esophageal Tumor Study Group. Cancer 72(4):1155–1158

157. Messian RA, Hermos JA, Robbins AH, Friedlander DM, Schimmel EM (1978) Barrett's esophagus. Clinical review of 26 cases. Am J Gastroenterol 69(4):458–466

158. Messmann H, Knuchel R, Endlicher E, Hauser T, Szeimies RM, Kullmann F, et al. (1998) (Photodynamic diagnosis of gastrointestinal precancerous lesions after sensitization with 5-aminolevulinic acid. A pilot study). Dtsch Med Wochenschr 123(17):515–521

159. Miros M, Kerlin P, Walker N (1991) Only patients with dysplasia progress to adenocarcinoma in Barrett's oesophagus. Gut 32(12):1441–1446

160. Moghissi K, Sharpe DA, Pender D (1993) Adenocarcinoma and Barrett's oesophagus. A clinico-pathological study. Eur J Cardiothorac Surg 7(3):126–131

161. Montes CG, Brandalise NA, Deliza R, Novais de Magalhaes AF, Ferraz JG (1999) Antireflux surgery followed by bipolar electrocoagulation in the treatment of Barrett's esophagus. Gastrointest Endosc 50(2):173–177

162. Montgomery E, Bronner MP, Goldblum JR, Greenson JK, Haber MM, Hart J, et al. (2001) Reproducibility of the diagnosis of dysplasia in Barrett esophagus: a reaffirmation. Hum Pathol 32(4):368–378

163. Morales TG, Camargo E, Bhattacharyya A, Sampliner RE (2000) Long-term follow-up of intestinal metaplasia of the gastric cardia. Am J Gastroenterol 95(7):1677–1680

164. Morales TG, Sampliner RE, Bhattacharyya A (1997) Intestinal metaplasia of the gastric cardia. Am J Gastroenterol 92(3):414–418

165. Mork H, Barth T, Kreipe HH, Kraus M, Al Taie O, Jakob F, et al. (1998) Reconstitution of squamous epithelium in Barrett's oesophagus with endoscopic argon plasma coagulation: a prospective study. Scand J Gastroenterol 33(11):1130–1134

166. Murray L, Watson P, Johnston B, Sloan J, Mainie IM, Gavin A (2003) Risk of adenocarcinoma in Barrett's oesophagus: population based study. BMJ 327(7414):534–535

167. Naef AP, Savary M (1972) Conservative operations for peptic esophagitis with stenosis in columnar-lined lower esophagus. Ann Thorac Surg 13(6):543–551

168. Naef AP, Savary M, Ozzello L (1975) Columnar-lined lower esophagus: an acquired lesion with malignant predisposition. Report on 140 cases of Barrett's esophagus with 12 adenocarcinomas. J Thorac Cardiovasc Surg 70(5):826–835

169. Nandurkar S, Talley NJ (1998) Surveillance in Barrett's oesophagus: a need for reassessment? J Gastroenterol Hepatol 13(10):990–996

170. Nehra D, Howell P, Pye JK, Beynon J (1998) Assessment of combined bile acid and pH profiles using an automated sampling device in gastro-oesophageal reflux disease. Br J Surg 85(1):134–137

171. Nehra D, Howell P, Williams CP, Pye JK, Beynon J (1999) Toxic bile acids in gastro-oesophageal reflux disease: influence of gastric acidity. Gut 44(5):598–602

172. Newton M, Bryan R, Burnham WR, Kamm MA (1997) Evaluation of Helicobacter pylori in reflux oesophagitis and Barrett's oesophagus. Gut 40(1):9–13

173. Nissen R (1961) Gastropexy and fundoplication in surgical treatment of hiatal hernia. Am J Dig Dis 6:959–961

174. O'Connor JB, Falk GW, Richter JE (1999) The incidence of adenocarcinoma and dysplasia in Barrett's esophagus: report on the Cleveland Clinic Barrett's Esophagus Registry. Am J Gastroenterol 94(8):2037–2042

175. Oberg S, Ritter MP, Crookes PF, Fein M, Mason RJ, Gadenstatter M, et al. (1998) Gastroesophageal reflux disease and mucosal injury with emphasis on short-segment Barrett's esophagus and duodenogastroesophageal reflux. J Gastrointest Surg 2(6):547–553

176. Ollyo JB, Monnier P, Fontolliet C, Birchler R, Fasel J, Levi F, et al. (1988) Savary's ulcer: a new complication of gastroesophageal reflux? Apropos of 32 endoscopically observed cases. Schweiz Med Wochenschr 118(21):823–827

177. Ormsby AH, Goldblum JR, Rice TW, Richter JE, Falk GW, Vaezi MF, et al. (1999) Cytokeratin subsets can reliably distinguish Barrett's esophagus from intestinal metaplasia of the stomach. Hum Pathol 30(3):288–294

178. Ormsby AH, Petras RE, Henricks WH, Rice TW, Rybicki LA, Richter JE, et al. (2002) Observer variation in the diagnosis of superficial oesophageal adenocarcinoma. Gut 51(5):671–676

179. Ortiz A, Martinez de Haro LF, Parrilla P, Morales G, Molina J, Bermejo J, et al. (1996) Conservative treatment versus antireflux surgery in Barrett's oesophagus: long-term results of a prospective study (comment). Br J Surg 83(2):274–278

180. Ovaska J, Miettinen M, Kivilaakso E (1989) Adenocarcinoma arising in Barrett's esophagus. Dig Dis Sci 34(9):1336–1339181. Overholt BF, Panjehpour M (1996) Photodynamic therapy for Barrett's esophagus: clinical update. Am J Gastroenterol 91(9):1719–1723

182. Overholt BF, Panjehpour M, Haydek JM (1999) Photodynamic therapy for Barrett's esophagus: follow-up in 100 patients. Gastrointest Endosc 49(1):1–7

183. Parrilla P, Martinez de Haro LF, Ortiz A, Munitiz V, Molina J, Bermejo J, et al. (2003) Long-term results of a randomized prospective study comparing medical and surgical treatment of Barrett's esophagus. Ann Surg 237(3):291–298

184. Patti MG, Arcerito M, Feo CV, Worth S, De Pinto M, Gibbs VC, et al. (1999) Barrett's esophagus: a surgical disease. J Gastrointest Surg 3(4):397–403

185. Paull A, Trier JS, Dalton MD, Camp RC, Loeb P, Goyal RK (1976) The histologic spectrum of Barrett's esophagus. N Engl J Med 295(9):476–480

186. Paull G, Yardley JH (1988) Gastric and esophageal Campylobacter pylori in patients with Barrett's esophagus. Gastroenterol 95(1):216–218

187. Pera M, Cameron AJ, Trastek VF, Carpenter HA, Zinsmeister AR (1993) Increasing incidence of adenocarcinoma of the esophagus and esophagogastric junction. Gastroenterol 104(2):510–513

188. Peters JH, Clark GW, Ireland AP, Chandrasoma P, Smyrk TC, DeMeester TR (1994) Outcome of adenocarcinoma arising in Barrett's esophagus in endoscopically surveyed and nonsurveyed patients. J Thorac Cardiovasc Surg 108(5):813–821

189. Phillips RW, Wong RK (1991) Barrett's esophagus. Natural history, incidence, etiology, and complications. Gastroenterol Clin North Am 20(4):791–816

190. Polkowski W, van Lanschot JJ, Ten Kate FJ, Baak JP, Tytgat GN, Obertop H, et al. (1995) The value of p53 and Ki67 as markers for tumor progression in the Barrett's dysplasia-carcinoma sequence. Surg Oncol 4(3):163–171

191. Pottern LM, Morris LE, Blot WJ, Ziegler RG, Fraumeni JF Jr (1981) Esophageal cancer among black men in Washington, D.C. I. Alcohol, tobacco, and other risk factors. J Natl Cancer Inst 67(4):777–783

192. Prach AT, MacDonald TA, Hopwood DA, Johnston DA (1997) Increasing incidence of Barrett's oesophagus: education, enthusiasm, or epidemiology? Lancet 350(9082):933

193. Prior A, Whorwell PJ (1986) Familial Barrett's oesophagus? Hepatogastroenterology 33(2):86–87

194. Qualman SJ, Murray RD, McClung HJ, Lucas J (1990) Intestinal metaplasia is age related in Barrett's esophagus. Arch Pathol Lab Med 114(12):1236–1240

195. Radigan LR, Glover JL, Shipley FE, Shoemaker RE (1977) Barrett esophagus. Arch Surg 112(4):486–491

196. Ramel S, Reid BJ, Sanchez CA, Blount PL, Levine DS, Neshat K, et al. (1992) Evaluation of p53 protein expression in Barrett's esophagus by two-parameter flow cytometry. Gastroenterol 102(4 Pt 1):1220–1228

197. Ransom JM, Patel GK, Clift SA, Womble NE, Read RC (1982) Extended and limited types of Barrett's esophagus in the adult. Ann Thorac Surg 33(1):19–27

198. Reid BJ, Haggitt RC, Rubin CE, Roth G, Surawicz CM, Van Belle G, et al. (1988) Observer variation in the diagnosis of dysplasia in Barrett's esophagus. Hum Pathol 19(2):166–178

199. Reynolds JC, Waronker M, Pacquing MS, Yassin RR (1999) Barrett's esophagus. Reducing the risk of progression to adenocarcinoma. Gastroenterol Clin North Am 28(4):917–945

200. Richardson JD, Richardson RL (1998) Collis-Nissen gastroplasty for shortened esophagus: long-term evaluation. Ann Surg 227(5):735–740

201. Riddell RH, Goldman H, Ransohoff DF, Appelman HD, Fenoglio CM, Haggitt RC, et al. (1983) Dysplasia in inflammatory bowel disease: standardized classification with provisional clinical applications. Hum Pathol 14(11):931–968

202. Robbins AH, Hermos JA, Schimmel EM, Friedlander DM, Messian RA (1977) The columnar-lined esophagus – analysis of 26 cases. Radiology 123(1):1–7

203. Robertson CS, Mayberry JF, Nicholson DA, James PD, Atkinson M (1988) Value of endoscopic surveillance in the detection of neoplastic change in Barrett's oesophagus. Br J Surg 75(8):760–763

204. Rodriguez E, Rao PH, Ladanyi M, Altorki N, Albino AP, Kelsen DP, et al. (1990) 11p13–15 is a specific region of chromosomal rearrangement in gastric and esophageal adenocarcinomas. Cancer Res 50(19):6410–6416

205. Rogers EL, Goldkind SF, Iseri OA, Bustin M, Goldkind L, Hamilton SR, et al. (1986) Adenocarcinoma of the lower esophagus. A disease primarily of white men with Barrett's esophagus. J Clin Gastroenterol 8(6):613–618

206. Romero Y, Cameron AJ, Schaid DJ, McDonnell SK, Burgart LJ, Hardtke CL, et al. (2002) Barrett's esophagus: prevalence in symptomatic relatives. Am J Gastroenterol 97(5):1127–1132

207. Rothery GA, Patterson JE, Stoddard CJ, Day DW (1986) Histological and histochemical changes in the columnar lined (-Barrett's) oesophagus. Gut 27(9):1062–1068

208. Rothstein RI, Pohl H, Rogan E, et al. (2001) Endoscopic gastric plication for the treatment of GERD; two-year follow up results (abstract). Am J Gastroenterol 96:53

209. Rusch VW, Levine DS, Haggitt R, Reid BJ (1994) The management of high grade dysplasia and early cancer in Barrett's esophagus. A multidisciplinary problem. Cancer 74(4):1225–1229

210. Sagar PM, Ackroyd R, Hosie KB, Patterson JE, Stoddard CJ, Kingsnorth AN (1995) Regression and progression of Barrett's oesophagus after antireflux surgery. Br J Surg 82(6):806–810

211. Salo JA, Salminen JT, Kiviluoto TA, Nemlander AT, Ramo OJ, Farkkila MA, et al. (1998) Treatment of Barrett's esophagus by endoscopic laser ablation and antireflux surgery. Ann Surg 227(1):40–44

212. Sampliner RE (1997) New treatments for Barrett's esophagus. Semin Gastrointest Dis 8(2):68–74

213. Sampliner RE (1998) Practice guidelines on the diagnosis, surveillance, and therapy of Barrett's esophagus. The Practice Parameters Committee of the American College of Gastroenterol. Am J Gastroenterol 93(7):1028–1032

214. Sampliner RE, Fennerty B, Garewal HS (1996) Reversal of Barrett's esophagus with acid suppression and multipolar electrocoagulation: preliminary results. Gastrointest Endosc 44(5):532–535

215. Sampliner RE, Garewal HS, Fennerty MB, Aickin M (1990) Lack of impact of therapy on extent of Barrett's esophagus in 67 patients. Dig Dis Sci 35(1):93–96

216. Sampliner RE, Hixson LJ, Fennerty MB, Garewal HS (1993) Regression of Barrett's esophagus by laser ablation in an anacid environment. Dig Dis Sci 38(2):365–368

217. Sarr MG, Hamilton SR, Marrone GC, Cameron JL (1985) Barrett's esophagus: its prevalence and association with adenocarcinoma in patients with symptoms of gastroesophageal reflux. Am J Surg 149(1):187–193

218. Sartori S, Nielsen I, Indelli M, Trevisani L, Pazzi P, Grandi E (1991) Barrett esophagus after chemotherapy with cyclophosphamide, methotrexate, and 5-fluorouracil (CMF): an iatrogenic injury? Ann Intern Med 114(3):210–211

219. Saubier EC, Gouillat C, Samaniego C, Guillaud M, Moulinier B (1985) Adenocarcinoma in columnar-lined Barrett's esophagus. Analysis of 13 esophagectomies. Am J Surg 150(3):365–369

220. Schier F, Korn S, Michel E (2001) Experiences of a parent support group with the long-term consequences of esophageal atresia. J Pediatr Surg 36(4):605–610

221. Scotiniotis IA, Kochman ML, Lewis JD, Furth EE, Rosato EF, Ginsberg GG (2001) Accuracy of EUS in the evaluation of Barrett's esophagus and high-grade dysplasia or intramucosal carcinoma. Gastrointest Endosc 54(6):689–696

222. Shaheen NJ, Crosby MA, Bozymski EM, Sandler RS (2000) Is there publication bias in the reporting of cancer risk in Barrett's esophagus? Gastroenterol 119(2):333–338

223. Sharma P, Bhattacharyya A, Garewal HS, Sampliner RE (1999) Durability of new squamous epithelium after endoscopic reversal of Barrett's esophagus. Gastrointest Endosc 50(2):159–164

224. Sharma P, Morales TG, Bhattacharyya A, Garewal HS, Sampliner RE (1998) Squamous islands in Barrett's esophagus: what lies underneath? Am J Gastroenterol 93(3):332–335

225. Sharma P, Sampliner RE, Camargo E (1997) Normalization of esophageal pH with high-dose proton pump inhibitor therapy does not result in regression of Barrett's esophagus. Am J Gastroenterol 92(4):582–585

226. Sharma P, Weston AP, Morales T, Topalovski M, Mayo MS, Sampliner RE (2000) Relative risk of dysplasia for patients with intestinal metaplasia in the distal oesophagus and in the gastric cardia. Gut 46(1):9–13

227. Shen B, Ormsby AH, Shen C, Dumot JA, Shao YW, Bevins CL, et al. (2002) Cytokeratin expression patterns in noncardia, intestinal metaplasia-associated gastric adenocarcinoma: implication for the evaluation of intestinal metaplasia and tumors at the esophagogastric junction. Cancer 94(3):820–831

228. Shirvani VN, Ouatu-Lascar R, Kaur BS, Omary MB, Triadafilopoulos G (2000) Cyclooxygenase 2 expression in Barrett's esophagus and adenocarcinoma: Ex vivo induction by bile salts and acid exposure. Gastroenterol 118(3):487–496

229. Skinner DB (1989) The incidence of cancer in Barrett's esophagus varies according to series. In: Giuli R, McCallum RW (eds) Benign lesions of the esophagus and cancer: answers to 210 questions. Springer, New York, pp 764–765

230. Skinner DB, Walther BC, Riddell RH, Schmidt H, Iascone C, DeMeester TR (1983) Barrett's esophagus. Comparison of benign and malignant cases. Ann Surg 198(4):554–565

231. Smith PM, Kerr GD, Cockel R, Ross BA, Bate CM, Brown P, et al. (1994) A comparison of omeprazole and ranitidine in the prevention of recurrence of benign esophageal stricture. Restore Investigator Group. Gastroenterol 107(5):1312–1318

232. Snyder JD, Goldman H (1990) Barrett's esophagus in children and young adults. Frequent association with mental retardation. Dig Dis Sci 35(10):1185–1189

233. Spechler SJ (1992) Comparison of medical and surgical therapy for complicated gastroesophageal reflux disease in veterans. The Department of Veterans Affairs Gastroesophageal Reflux Disease Study Group. N Engl J Med 326(12):786–792

234. Spechler SJ (2000) Barrett's esophagus: an overrated cancer risk factor. Gastroenterol 119(2):587–589

235. Spechler SJ (2000a) Barrett's oesophagus: diagnosis and management. Baillieres Best Pract Res Clin Gastroenterol 14(5):857–879

236. Spechler SJ (2000b) Medical treatment of Barrett's esophagus. J Gastrointest Surg 4(2):119–121

237. Spechler SJ, Robbins AH, Rubins HB, Vincent ME, Heeren T, Doos WG, et al. (1984) Adenocarcinoma and Barrett's esophagus. An overrated risk? Gastroenterol 87(4):927–933

238. Spechler SJ, Sperber H, Doos WG, Schimmel EM (1983) The prevalence of Barrett's esophagus in patients with chronic peptic esophageal strictures. Dig Dis Sci 28(9):769–774

239. Spechler SJ, Sperber H, Doos WG, Schimmel EM (1983) The prevalence of Barrett's esophagus in patients with chronic peptic esophageal strictures. Dig Dis Sci 28(9):769–774

240. Starnes VA, Adkins RB, Ballinger JF, Sawyers JL (1984) Barrett's esophagus. A surgical entity. Arch Surg 119(5):563–567

241. Stein HJ, Feussner H, Kauer W, DeMeester TR, Siewert JR (1994) Alkaline gastroesophageal reflux: assessment by ambulatory esophageal aspiration and pH monitoring. Am J Surg 167(1):163–168

242. Stein HJ, Hoeft S, DeMeester TR (1993) Functional foregut abnormalities in Barrett's esophagus. J Thorac Cardiovasc Surg 105(1):107–111

243. Stepanov EA, Razumovskii AI, Bataev SK, Alkhasov AB, Nurik VI, Mart'ianov AV, et al. (2002) Treatment policy for children with gastroesophageal reflux complicated by Barrett esophagus. (Russian). Khirurgiia (11):8–13

244. Stepp H, Sroka R, Baumgartner R (1998) Fluorescence endoscopy of gastrointestinal diseases: basic principles, techniques, and clinical experience. Endoscopy 30(4):379–386

245. Stevens PD, Lightdale CJ, Green PH, Siegel LM, Garcia-Carrasquillo RJ, Rotterdam H (1994) Combined magnification endoscopy with chromoendoscopy for the evaluation of Barrett's esophagus. Gastrointest Endosc 40(6):747–749

246. Streitz JM Jr, Andrews CW Jr, Ellis FH Jr (1993) Endoscopic surveillance of Barrett's esophagus. Does it help? J Thorac Cardiovasc Surg 105(3):383–387

247. Swarbrick ET, Gough AL, Foster CS, Christian J, Garrett AD, Langworthy CH (1996) Prevention of recurrence of oesophageal stricture, a comparison of lansoprazole and high-dose ranitidine. Eur J Gastroenterol Hepatol 8(5):431–438

248. Talley NJ, Cameron AJ, Shorter RG, Zinsmeister AR, Phillips SF (1988) Campylobacter pylori and Barrett's esophagus. Mayo Clin Proc 63(12):1176–1180

249. Thal AP (1968) A unified approach to surgical problems of the esophagogastric junction. Ann Surg 168(3):542–550

250. Thier JS (1970) Morphology of the epithelium of the distal esophagus in patients with midesophageal peptic strictures. Gastroenterol 58(4):444–461

251. Thompson JJ, Zinsser KR, Enterline HT (1983) Barrett's metaplasia and adenocarcinoma of the esophagus and gastroesophageal junction. Hum Pathol 14(1):42–61

252. Triadafilopoulos G, Dibaise JK, Nostrant TT, Stollman NH, Anderson PK, Edmundowicz SA, et al. (2001) Radiofrequency energy delivery to the gastroesophageal junction for the treatment of GERD. Gastrointest Endosc 53(4):407–415

253. Triadafilopoulos G, Sharma R (1997) Features of symptomatic gastroesophageal reflux disease in elderly patients. Am J Gastroenterol 92(11):2007–2011

254. Tytgat GN (1995) Does endoscopic surveillance in esophageal columnar metaplasia (Barrett's esophagus) have any real value? Endoscopy 27(1):19–26

255. Vaezi MF, Richter JE (1996) Role of acid and duodenogastroesophageal reflux in gastroesophageal reflux disease. Gastroenterol 111(5):1192–1199

256. van der Burgh, BA, Dees J, Hop WC, van Blankenstein M (1996) Oesophageal cancer is an uncommon cause of death in patients with Barrett's oesophagus. Gut 39(1):5–8

257. Van Laethem JL, Cremer M, Peny MO, Delhaye M, Deviere J (1998) Eradication of Barrett's mucosa with argon plasma coagulation and acid suppression: immediate and mid term results. Gut 43(6):747–751

258. van Sandick JW, van Lanschot JJ, Kuiken BW, Tytgat GN, Offerhaus GJ, Obertop H (1998) Impact of endoscopic biopsy surveillance of Barrett's oesophagus on pathological stage and clinical outcome of Barrett's carcinoma. Gut 43(2):216–222

259. Vaughan TL, Davis S, Kristal A, Thomas DB (1995) Obesity, alcohol, and tobacco as risk factors for cancers of the esophagus and gastric cardia: adenocarcinoma versus squamous cell carcinoma. Cancer Epidemiol Biomarkers Prev 4(2):85–92

260. Walker SJ, Birch PJ, Stewart M, Stoddard CJ, Hart CA, Day DW (1989) Patterns of colonization of Campylobacter pylori in the oesophagus, stomach and duodenum. Gut 30(10):1334–1338

261. Wallner B, Sylvan A, Janunger KG, Bozoky B, Stenling R (2001) Immunohistochemical markers for Barrett's esophagus and associations to esophageal Z-line appearance. Scand J Gastroenterol 36(9):910–915

262. Wehrmann T, Lange P, Nakamura M, Riphaus A, Stergiou N (2001) Endoscopic mucosal resection of premalignant lesions of the upper gastrointestinal tract. Z Gastroenterol 39(11):919–928

263. Weston AP, Banerjee SK, Sharma P, Tran TM, Richards R, Cherian R (2001) p53 protein overexpression in low grade dysplasia (LGD) in Barrett's esophagus: immunohistochemical marker predictive of progression. Am J Gastroenterol 96(5):1355–1362

264. Weston AP, Krmpotich P, Makdisi WF, Cherian R, Dixon A, McGregor DH, et al. (1996) Short segment Barrett's esophagus: clinical and histological features, associated endoscopic findings, and association with gastric intestinal metaplasia. Am J Gastroenterol 91(5):981–986

265. Williamson WA, Ellis FH Jr, Gibb SP, Shahian DM, Aretz HT (1990) Effect of antireflux operation on Barrett's mucosa. Ann Thorac Surg 49(4):537–541

266. Williamson WA, Ellis FH Jr, Gibb SP, Shahian DM, Aretz HT, Heatley GJ, et al. (1991) Barrett's esophagus. Prevalence and incidence of adenocarcinoma. Arch Intern Med 151(11):2212–2216

267. Wilson KT, Fu S, Ramanujam KS, Meltzer SJ (1998) Increased expression of inducible nitric oxide synthase and cyclooxygenase-2 in Barrett's esophagus and associated adenocarcinomas. Cancer Res 58(14):2929–2934

268. Winters C Jr, Spurling TJ, Chobanian SJ, Curtis DJ, Esposito RL, Hacker JF III, et al. (1987) Barrett's esophagus. A prevalent, occult complication of gastroesophageal reflux disease. Gastroenterol 92(1):118–124

269. Wong WM, Lam SK, Hui WM, Lai KC, Chan CK, Hu WH, et al. (2002) Long-term prospective follow-up of endoscopic oesophagitis in southern Chinese – prevalence and spectrum of the disease. Aliment Pharmacol Ther 16(12):2037–2042

270. Woolf GM, Riddell RH, Irvine EJ, Hunt RH (1989) A study to examine agreement between endoscopy and histology for the diagnosis of columnar lined (Barrett's) esophagus. Gastrointest Endosc 35(6):541–544

271. Yau P, Watson DI, Devitt PG, Game PA, Jamieson GG (2000) Laparoscopic antireflux surgery in the treatment of gastroesophageal reflux in patients with Barrett esophagus. Arch Surg 135(7):801–805

272. Yonish-Rouach E, Grunwald D, Wilder S, Kimchi A, May E, Lawrence JJ, et al. (1993) p53-mediated cell death: relationship to cell cycle control. Mol Cell Biol 13(3):1415–1423

273. Younes M, Lebovitz RM, Lechago LV, Lechago J (1993) p53 protein accumulation in Barrett's metaplasia, dysplasia, and carcinoma: a follow-up study. Gastroenterol 105(6):1637–1642

274. Yu MC, Garabrant DH, Peters JM, Mack TM (1988) Tobacco, alcohol, diet, occupation, and carcinoma of the esophagus. Cancer Res 48(13):3843–3848

275. Zaninotto G, Avellini C, Barbazza R, Baruchello G, Battaglia G, Benedetti E, et al. (2001) Prevalence of intestinal metaplasia in the distal oesophagus, oesophagogastric junction and gastric cardia in symptomatic patients in north-east Italy: a prospective, descriptive survey. The Italian Ulcer Study Group "GISU." Dig Liver Dis 33(4):316–321

Chapter 10

Genetics of Gastroesophageal Reflux Disease

10

Susan R. Orenstein

Contents

10.1 Introduction

A possible genetic basis for gastroesophageal reflux disease (GERD) has begun to be proposed. The various strands of evidence that support this proposal, as well as the evidence for specific chromosomal loci in children, will be reviewed in this chapter. Genetic heterogeneity is likely in this disorder, with extensive phenotypic heterogeneity.

The first reports of familial hiatal hernia were published nearly half a century ago, but specific chromosomal loci have not been sought until very recently. In the decades following the first reports, multiple publications identified familial segregation of hiatal hernia (HH), Barrett's esophagus (BE), adenocarcinoma, and symptomatic or endoscopic GERD. These reports will be reviewed in the following pages.

10.2 Hiatal Hernia

The prevalence of sliding hiatal hernia is estimated to be about 10% in adults in the western world, being considerably less common in Asia and Africa. GERD is similarly common, with prevalence depending on the definition used. Although both conditions have been considered in the past to be acquired, reports of families with multiply affected members have accumulated. In 1959, Burke noted three families with multiple members affected by childhood hiatal hernia, including a mother with two children, a pair of twin boys, and three brothers in a third family, among his 137 cases of "partial thoracic stomach," as hiatal hernia was termed at the time [3]. One of the earliest publications related to epidemiological aspects of HH appeared in 1964. In that "negative" epidemiological report, Kim cited a *lower* incidence of HH in Korea (1.4% of 1,000 fluoroscopies) than had been reported in the western literature (2.3–50%) [25]. The huge variability cited in the proportion of positive fluoroscopies in the western literature suggests that fluoroscopic technique and interpretation may play a large role in whether an HH is found, and thus weakens any conclusions about inherited predisposition to HH that one might be tempted to draw.

Carre published several works examining a familial tendency for HH ("partial thoracic stomach") in his large database of young children with GERD [4]. He utilized radiographic HH as a gold standard for diagnosis of GERD, and identified a much higher incidence of HH than we are currently accustomed to observing in children with GERD; these differences impact our interpretation of his studies. In Carre's first publication citing a familial incidence, he screened relatives of children in whom he had found an HH. Siblings and other relatives (parents, grandparents, uncles/aunts, and cousins) were examined fluoroscopically, the former regardless of presence of symptoms and the latter only if they acknowledged symptoms. In this way he found 31 families with multiple affected members.

In 1970, Carre's next publication on familial pediatric HH reported it in three generations of a single family, wherein eight individuals (including six siblings) were affected, and suggested an autosomal dominant inheritance [5].

More than two decades later, Thomas and Carre published an enormous experience: fluoroscopic findings in 406 younger siblings of 465 probands with HH [40]. The authors asked about GERD symptoms in all of the younger siblings and elicited definite symptoms in 7%

and suggestive symptoms in 8%; thus 15% of the younger siblings had at least suggestive symptoms of GERD. The authors advised fluoroscopic evaluation of all of these 61 symptomatic younger siblings, and all complied. Additionally, they offered fluoroscopic screening of the 345 younger siblings without *any* suggestive symptoms; 210 of them complied. The fluoroscopic protocol was fairly provocative for reflux: it specified manual compression of the abdomen during the barium meal, and rolling the child to the right side and supine multiple times. In addition, duplicate studies were performed in 11% of the siblings who were negative for HH on their initial fluoroscopy. By these means the authors detected HH in 9 (3%) of the 271 siblings tested, comparable to the 2.3–50% reported incidence of HH in fluoroscopic examinations of western adults [25]. Thirty-nine (14%) of the 271 siblings manifested any reflux fluoroscopically, perhaps surprising for its low frequency, considering the number times a normal child refluxes following a meal.

Other brief reports of familial HH have appeared. In 1966 Sidd et al. described in the *British Journal of Radiology* four siblings, a pair of them twins, who had sliding HHs, illustrating the report with four nearly identical images of their fluoroscopic studies [39]. Two years later in *Gastroenterology*, Chaiken described four families with multiple HHs [6]. The following year, in the *Journal of Heredity*, Goodman et al. reported a large kindred that had HHs in six members and diabetes in seven [18]. Similarly, in the otolaryngologic literature Gage-White reported cosegregation of HH with 42% of cases of Zenker's diverticulum [16]. Familial HH was cited by Leung in the English literature, and by Boissieu et al. in the French literature [27, 2]. In 1996, Chana et al. described a father, two sons, and a daughter with sliding HHs, symptomatic reflux from infancy, and eventual antireflux surgery [8]. Finally, Coelho et al. reported an affected father and eight of his ten children who had symptomatic GERD, usually beginning in middle age; their symptomatic GERD was associated with HHs variously described as large, huge, or between 5 and 10 cm [9].

10.3
Barrett's Esophagus and Adenocarcinoma

Endoscopic diagnosis of mucosal complications of GERD gradually superseded fluoroscopic diagnosis of anatomic complications of (or predispositions for) GERD. As a result of the recognition of the increased sensitivity and specificity of endoscopic diagnosis of GERD, and particularly of its complications, the literature on the familial manifestations of GERD began to focus on Barrett's esophagus (BE) and adenocarcinoma.

The first such citation was an abstract by Lehman et al. *in Gastroenterology* in 1979, describing BE and GERD

in five offspring of a father with BE and a mother with HH [26]. Soon thereafter, Everhart et al. described BE in a father and two teenage sons [12]. In the 1980s, two pairs of sisters (one a set of twins) presenting with BE in their sixties were reported [17, 34].

Four articles published in the decade beginning in 1985 presented pedigrees of BE families with multiple afflicted members; three of these articles described several-generation pedigrees with four to seven individuals with BE, including a number with adenocarcinoma [10, 24, 11], and the fourth article documented four separate families with a total of 10 affected individuals [13]. Romero and Locke of the Mayo Clinic combined and summarized these reports in an editorial in which they indicated that 28% of the 88 individuals in these families had BE documented endoscopically, and an additional 42% had endoscopic esophagitis or heartburn, giving 70% as the total affected individuals in these families [36]. A 1996 publication described three more families in which there were a total of six BEs and adenocarcinomas [33].

The weight of the accumulated retrospective evidence for a familial tendency in BE prompted the first prospective evaluation, in 1997. The Mayo Clinic group used a questionnaire to evaluate relatives of 55 probands with reflux esophagitis, 40 probands with BE, and 27 probands with adenocarcinoma [35]. They evaluated reflux symptoms in 243 parents and siblings of their 122 probands, contrasting the results with those from all 122 spouses of their probands, and from 230 of the probands' spouses' parents and siblings, used as unrelated controls for some possible confounding variables. For the 55 probands with reflux esophagitis, reflux symptoms were not significantly more common in the probands' first-degree relatives (33%) than in their spouses' relatives (29%). However, for the 40 BE probands, reflux symptoms were more prevalent in their own parents and siblings than in parents and siblings of their spouses (46% vs. 27%, $p=0.013$, adjusted odds ratio 2.23); similar differences were found for the 27 probands with adenocarcinoma (43% vs. 23%, $p=0.034$, adjusted odds ratio 2.80). (The authors found statistical influences on GERD not only by family history, but also by obesity, smoking, and gender, and adjusted for those factors in their analysis.)

Several years later, Chak et al. performed a similar questionnaire study, comparing relatives of 106 control subjects (with esophagitis) to relatives of 58 case subjects with BE, esophageal adenocarcinoma, or esophagogastric junctional carcinoma [7]. However, those authors' primary outcome variables sought in the relatives were not reflux symptoms as sought by the Mayo Clinic study, but rather BE, adenocarcinoma, and junctional carcinoma. They found these diseases, too, to be increased in relatives of their cases, compared to the controls (24% vs. 5%, $p<0.005$; adjusted odds ratio

12.23, 95% confidence interval 3.34–44.76). In addition to male sex, the other factors they found to be significantly increased in their cases were age, obesity 10 years prior, and alcohol consumption, implicating environmental factors as well as genetic ones.

10.4
Symptomatic GERD and Esophagitis

Several publications have focused on familial symptomatic GERD or reflux esophagitis, rather than on HH or BE. Two early articles described symptoms or esophagitis in sibling pairs or twins, the twin report being one of the few pediatric publications related to familial GERD [37, 23]. Two studies have investigated the epidemiology of these symptoms. In a sequel to their earlier work devoted to reflux symptoms in relatives of patients with BE and adenocarcinoma [35], Locke et al. of the Mayo Clinic performed a cross-sectional study that broadened their examination of risk factors associated with symptomatic reflux [28]. As in their prior study, they mailed a validated questionnaire to residents of Olmsted County, sending out 2,118 mailings. Of those, 1,524 (72%) were returned. Heartburn, or stomach or esophageal disease in immediate family members, were significantly associated with reflux symptoms at least once weekly among the questionnaire respondents, using odds ratios with 95% confidence intervals. (As in their prior study, obesity and smoking were risk factors for reflux symptoms; alcohol consumption more than seven times a week and increased psychosomatic symptom checklist scores were additional risk factors.)

The second epidemiological study, published the same year by Trudgill et al. in the *American Journal of Gastroenterology*, was a prospective, questionnaire-based examination of the prevalence of reflux symptoms and use of antireflux medications in first-degree relatives of six evenly sized groups (30 patients each) of their patients [41]. Relatives of patients with (a) no reflux symptoms; (b) reflux symptoms but no objective evidence of increased esophageal acid exposure; (c) reflux symptoms and abnormal pH probe study (esophageal acid exposure >5% of the time, but normal lower esophageal sphincter pressure); (d) reflux symptoms, abnormal pH probe study, and lower esophageal sphincter pressure <10 mmHg; (e) BE; and (f) esophageal strictures were compared. Interestingly, the 418 (78%) respondents among the first-degree relatives of these 180 probands reported significantly increased symptoms and medication use only in the groups with BE or objective evidence of GERD (groups c, d, and e). Relatives of those with symptomatic reflux (but without abnormal pH probe studies or endoscopies) and of those with strictures did not report significantly increased symptoms and medication use.

Associative studies that show increased incidence of GERD or its complications in families, however, have a difficult time controlling for the many potential environmental confounders, including diet, tobacco smoke, and alcohol. Also, studies that show an increase in esophageal adenocarcinoma in families may be confounded by genetic influences on carcinogenesis, rather than on GERD. But by suggesting a possible genetic component in the pathophysiology of GERD, these associative studies have begun to prompt molecular investigations.

10.5
"Severe Pediatric GERD" Phenotype: 13q14 Locus

As data suggesting a genetic determinant for GERD accumulated, Hu et al. published a study in 2000 identifying a chromosome 13 locus to be linked to a phenotype they designated "severe pediatric GERD" [21]. Querying more than 1,000 members of their parent support group based in Washington, D.C., and Los Angeles, and receiving return surveys from 80 families, they identified 20 families large enough to suggest a mode of inheritance. From these 20, they selected five families (three related by marriage) with 26 affected members for study. Via linkage analysis, they found a 21-centiMorgan (cM) region of chromosome 13 to be strongly linked to the phenotype–maximum 2-point LOD (logarithm of odds) score of 5.58, indicating a >100,000:1 likelihood of linkage between the phenotype and locus. Further, their 7.15 multipoint LOD score indicates a likelihood of >10,000,000:1 that the phenotype is linked to the chromosomal locus.

To test a possible candidate gene they had chosen, Hu et al. followed up their study with one focused on a small area in the 21 cM locus on 13q14, the location of a gene which codes for the 5-hydroxytryptamine receptor 2A (HTR2A), a developmentally regulated serotonin receptor that affects smooth muscle function and myogenesis [22]. That study, however, excluded the role of this candidate gene in their five families. Other candidate genes in this locus have not been reported.

The clinical importance of GERD, combined with the strength of the linkage these investigators reported, underline the importance of phenotypic precision. In the first Hu et al. study, many of the symptoms for the phenotype were otolaryngologic or respiratory. Of the 26 individuals designated affected, 19 were evaluated by endoscopy or pH-metry, but the techniques and the criteria for positive studies were not described and were likely varied; much of the phenotyping was apparently performed historically.

10.6
"Infantile GERD" Phenotype: Exclusion of 13q14

The strength of the association reported by Hu et al. led our group to evaluate the 13q14 locus in our extensive database of well characterized infants with GERD. To do so, we performed linkage analysis in a set of our multiply affected families with thoroughly evaluated probands [30].

This study examined five proband infants who presented to our center at 1–5 months of age. All five had esophageal histology quantitatively confirming reflux esophagitis by morphometric parameters [1], and excluding eosinophilic esophagitis [30]. In addition, all five probands had scores on a validated Infant Gastroesophageal Reflux Questionnaire (I-GERQ, developed by Susan R. Orenstein, MD, copyright 1992, 2002, University of Pittsburgh) that further supported their diagnosis of infantile GERD [29]. Finally, all probands had barium fluoroscopy that excluded anatomic abnormalities as potential causes for their symptoms.

The five probands had been identified because their parents had described some of their siblings as also suffering from symptoms of GERD. Five of these siblings had also had complete consultative evaluations at our center, demonstrating histologic esophagitis in all five; GERD by I-GERQs in all three of them who were evaluated by the questionnaire; and no anatomic abnormalities by barium fluoroscopy in all four examined radiographically. The five probands' three-generational pedigrees contained a total of 127 individuals who had consented to representation in the pedigrees. Included among the 127 in the pedigrees were 54 children in the proband generation (including the five probands and five affected siblings described above). The 49 siblings and cousins from the proband generation, as well as the five probands, were also phenotyped as affected or not via a shortened form of the I-GERQ, finding 39% to be affected. DNA from 45 individuals in the five families was examined by linkage analysis for the Hu study's four most closely linked markers, excluding linkage of the 13q14 locus to the infantile GERD phenotype. LOD scores were <-2 (odds more than 100:1 against linkage) for multipoint linkage to all four of the markers [22]. In contrast, in a subsequent preliminary study of two of these five families, we detected linkage to a chromosome 9 locus [32].

The answer to why the two pediatric GERD studies of the 13q14 locus [21, 30] produced opposite results may lie in phenotypic disparity between the studies, in genetic heterogeneity of pediatric GERD, or both.

10.7
Phenotypic Disparity

Although the Hu et al. [21] and Orenstein et al. [30] studies were similar in that each used linkage analysis to assess five families with multiple members affected by symptoms considered to suggest pediatric GERD, the studies' considerable differences are listed in Table 1. The age and presenting symptoms of the affected children are the most important of these differences. In our study, the phenotype was typical infantile GERD with esophagitis, whereas in the Hu et al. study no children with exclusively infantile GERD were included, and preponderant symptoms of GERD were otolaryngologic. It has even been suggested that the Hu et al. phenotype might be related to allergy, rather than to GERD [15, 14].

Table 1. Pediatric GERD and 13q14: Contrasts between studies

13q14 [21]	Not 13q14 [30]
Did not require GERD in infancy	*Required GERD in infancy*
Excluded probands resolved by 1 year old	Did not exclude those resolving
5 families (3 related by marriage)	5 unrelated families
26 affected (any generation)	21 affected (proband generation}
Identified by mass mailing to >1000 in national pediatric GERD support group	Identified at single center
Evaluated by different physicians	Evaluated by one physician
Emphasis: Otolaryngologic GERD	*Emphasis: Typical infant GERD*
Gold standard: Diagnosis by unspecified gastroenterologist or otolaryngologist	Gold standard: Validated tests (histology for probands, questionnaires for others)
pH probe: 10/26 "affected"; methods and results unspecified	I-GERQ[a]: positive in 21/21 "affected"
Es Bx[b]: 9/26 "affected"; methods and results unspecified	Es Bx[b]: positive in 10/21 "affected"

[a] I-GERQ: Infant Gastroesophageal Reflux Questionnaire (developed by Susan R. Orenstein, MD, copyright 1992, 2002, University of Pittsburgh)
[b] Es Bx: Esophageal biopsy

Table 2. Pathophysiologic determinants of GERD

Refluxate toxicity
  Gastric acid secretion
  Duodenogastric reflux

Intrinsic gastric volume and pressure
  Gastric compliance
  Gastric emptying [37]
  Gastric acid volume secretion

Extrinsic pressure on gastric contents
  Weight (obesity [28])
  Somatic motor tone (spasticity [38])
  Somatic and crural episodic contractions (cough, wheeze, etc. [19, 20])

Gastroesophageal barrier
  Lower esophageal sphincter tone
  Gastric fundic sensory thresholds (for transient lower esophageal sphincter relaxations)
  Crural diaphragm location (relative to sphincter location) and function [3–6, 8–10]

Esophageal defenses
  Salivary secretion
  Peristaltic motor function
  Esophageal cytoprotection

10.8
Genetic Heterogeneity

Because GERD is so phenotypically and pathophysiologically diverse, it is likely that it would be determined or modified by more than one genetic locus. Thus the 13q14 locus might represent one of several GERD phenotypes. Several different loci might control several different physiological processes, disturbances of each of which might contribute to GERD in different families. Combined abnormalities at more than one locus could collaborate to produce a more severe phenotype. These molecular abnormalities could include both direct ("primary") determinants of the pathophysiology of GERD (as shown in Table 2) and more indirect ("secondary") mechanisms. Thus, for example, molecular causes for gastric stasis might represent a direct mechanism underlying GERD in families with gastric stasis and GERD [37], whereas molecular causes for more indirect triggers of reflux, such as increased abdominal pressure, might occur in familial GERD associated with obesity [28] or spasticity [38], or cough [19, 20]. Finally, as noted above, familial GERD might be mimicked by other disorders with underlying molecular mechanisms, such as familial tendencies to allergy [14, 15], without actually being familial GERD.

The identification of the molecular mechanisms underlying familial pediatric GERD and familial GERD in adults will have important consequences for our understanding of the pathophysiology of this common and costly disorder, and thus for our ability to target treatments at those mechanisms more accurately.

References

1. Black DD, Haggitt RC, Orenstein SR, Whitington PF (1990) Esophagitis in infants: morphometric histologic diagnosis and correlation with measures of gastroesophageal reflux. Gastroenterology 98(6):1408–1414
2. Boissieu D, Montis G, Badoual J (1990) Formes familiales du reflux gastro-oesophagien. Ann Pediatr 37:221–225
3. Burke JB (1959) Partial thoracic stomach in childhood. Br Med J:787–792
4. Carre I (1965) Familial incidence of the partial thoracic stomach ("hiatus hernia") in children. International Congress of Pediatrics, 11th, University of Tokyo Press, Tokyo
5. Carre IJ, Froggatt P (1970) Oesophageal hiatus hernia in three generations of one family. Gut 11:51–54
6. Chaiken BH (1968) Familial occurrence of esophageal hiatus hernia (abstract). Gastroenterology 54(6):1224
7. Chak A, Lee T, Kinnard MF, Brock W, Faulx A, Willis J, Cooper GS, Sivak Jr MV (2002) Familial aggregation of Barrett's oesophagus, oesophageal adenocarcinoma, and oesophago-gastric junctional adenocarcinoma in Caucasian adults. Gut 51:323–328
8. Chana J, Crabbe DCG, Spitz L (1996) Familial hiatus hernia and gastro-oesophageal reflux. Eur J Pediatr Surg 6:175–176
9. Coelho J, Sousa GS, Vianna RMM (1999) Familial hiatal hernia and gastro-oesophageal reflux disease. Eur J Surg 165:392–394
10. Crabb DW, Berk MA, Hall TR, Conneally PM, Biegel AA, Lehman GA (1985) Familial gastroesophageal reflux and development of Barrett's esophagus. Ann Int Med 103:52–54
11. Eng C, Spechler SJ, Ruben R, Li FP (1993) Familial Barrett esophagus and adenocarcinoma of the gastroesophageal junction. Cancer Epidemiol Biomarkers Prev 2:397–399
12. Everhart CW, Holtzapple PG, Humphries TJ (1983) Barrett's esophagus: Inherited epithelium or inherited reflux? J Clin Gastroenterol 5:357–360
13. Fahmy N, King JF (1993) Barrett's esophagus: An acquired condition with genetic predisposition. Am J Gastroenterol 88(8):1262–1265
14. Furuta G, Badizadegan K (2001) Mapping of a gene for severe pediatric gastroesophageal reflux to chromosome 13q14 (Selected Summaries). J Pediatr Gastroenterol and Nutr 32:617
15. Furuta G, Nurko S, Bousvaros A, Antonioli D, Badizadegan K (2000) The spectrum of pediatric gastroesophageal reflux (letter). JAMA 284(24):3125–3126
16. Gage-White L (1988) Incidence of Zenker's diverticulum with hiatus hernia. Laryngoscope 98:527–534
17. Gelfand MD (1983) Barrett esophagus in sexagenarian identical twins. J Clin Gastroenterol 5:251–253
18. Goodman RM, Wooley CF, Rupert RD, Freimanis AK (1969) A possible genetic role in esophageal hiatus hernia. J Hered 60:71–74
19. Hassall E (1997) Co-morbidities in childhood Barrett's esophagus [invited review]. J Pediatr Gastroenterol Nutr 25(3):255–260
20. Hassall E, Israel D, Davidson A, Wong L (1993) Barrett's esophagus in children with cystic fibrosis: Not a coincidental association. Am J Gastroenterol 88(11):1934–1938
21. Hu FZ, Post JC, Johnson S, Ehrlich GD, Preston RA (2000) Refined localization of a gene for pediatric gastroesophageal reflux makes HTR2A an unlikely candidate gene. Hum Genet 107:519–525
22. Hu FZ, Preston RA, Post JC, White GJ, Kikuchi LW, Wang X, Leal SM, Levenstien MA, Ott J, Self TW, Allen G, Siffler RS, McGraw C, Pulsifer-Anderson EA, Ehrlich GD (2000) Mapping of a gene for severe pediatric gastroesophageal reflux to chromosome 13q14. JAMA 284(3):325–334
23. Iacono G, Carroccio A, Montalto G, Cavataio F, Balsamo V (1992) Gastroesophageal reflux: Clinical presentation in two pairs of twins. J Pediatr Gastroenterol Nutr 14(4):460–462
24. Jochem VJ, Fuerst PA, Fromkes JJ (1992) Familial Barrett's esophagus associated with adenocarcinoma. Gastroenterology 102:1400–1402
25. Kim E (1964) Hiatus hernia and diverticulum of the colon: Their low incidence in Korea. N Engl J Med 271(15):764–768

26. Lehman GA, Berke MA, Biegel AA, et al. (1979) Familial gastroesophageal reflux (GER) with Barrett's esophagus (abstract). Gastroenterology 76(5):1183

27. Leung AKC (1987) Familial hiatal hernia. Pediatrics 80:462

28. Locke GRI, Talley NJ, Fett SL, Zinsmeister AR, Melton LJI (1999) Risk factors associated with symptoms of gastroesophageal reflux. Am J Med 106:642–649

29. Orenstein SR, Shalaby TM, Cohn JF (1996) Reflux symptoms in 100 normal infants: Diagnostic validity of the Infant Gastroesophageal Reflux Questionnaire. Clin Pediatr 35(12):607–614

30. Orenstein SR, Shalaby TM, Di Lorenzo C, Putnam PE, Sigurdsson L, Mousa H, Kocoshis SA (2000) The spectrum of pediatric eosinophilic esophagitis beyond infancy: A clinical series of 30 children. Am J Gastroenterol 95(6):1422–1430

31. Orenstein SR, Shalaby TM, Finch R, Pfuetzer RH, DeVandry S, Chensny LJ, Barmada MM, Whitcomb DC (2002) Autosomal dominant infantile gastroesophageal reflux disease: Exclusion of a 13q14 locus in five well characterized families. Am J Gastroenterol 97(11):2725–2732

32. Orenstein SR, Suman A, Shalaby TM, Whitcomb DC, Barmada MM (2002) Infantile GERD maps to chromosome 9. J Pediatr Gastroenterol Nutr 35(3):440–441

33. Poynton AR, Walsh TN, O'Sullivan G, Hennessy TPJ (1996) Carcinoma arising in familial Barrett's esophagus. Am J Gastroenterol 91(9):1855–1856

34. Prior A, Whorwell PJ (1986) Familial Barrett's oesophagus? Hepato-gastroenterol 33:86–87

35. Romero Y, Cameron AJ, Locke GR III, Schaid DJ, Slezak JM, Branch CD, Melton LJ III (1997) Familial aggregation of gastroesophageal reflux in patients with Barrett's esophagus and esophageal adenocarcinoma. Gastroenterology 113:1449–1456

36. Romero Y, Locke GR III (1999) Is there a GERD gene? Am J Gastroenterol 94:1127–1129

37. Schulze-Delrieu K, Anuras S (1983) Chronic esophagitis in two sisters. Dig Dis Sci 28(12):1101–1105

38. Seri M, Cusano R, Forabosco P, Cinti R, Caroli F, Picco P, Bini R, Morra VB, De Michele G, Lerone M, Silengo M, Pela I, Borrone C, Romeo G, Devoto M (1999) Genetic mapping to 10q23.3-q24.2, in a large Italian pedigree, of a new syndrome showing bilateral cataracts, gastroesophageal reflux, and spastic paraparesis with amyotrophy. Am J Hum Genet 64:586–593

39. Sidd JJ, Gilliam JI, Bushueff BP (1966) Sliding hiatus hernias in identical twins. Br J Radiol 39:703–704

40. Thomas PS, Carre IJ (1991) Findings on barium swallow in younger siblings of children with hiatal hernia (partial thoracic stomach). J Pediatr Gastroenterol Nutr 12:174–177

41. Trudgill NJ, Kapur KC, Riley SA (1999) Familial clustering of reflux symptoms. Am J Gastroenterol 94(5):1172–1178

Part II
Pediatrics

Esophageal Manometry in the Diagnostic Evaluation of Infants and Children with GER

11

Salvatore Cucchiara · Osvaldo Borrelli

Contents

11.1 Introduction

Esophageal manometry is a diagnostic tool that provides both a qualitative and quantitative assessment of esophageal motor functions measuring intraluminal pressures and coordination of esophageal muscle pressure activity. Since the first manometric recordings obtained more than a century ago [30], methodological improvements have steadily occurred, and esophageal manometry has changed from a purely research technique to an investigative tool commonly performed in adults and in children for clinical purposes [22]. Substantial development of the recording equipment, which can now digitize on-line manometric recordings, has been implemented so that the latter can be easily analyzed by computer programs.

Nevertheless, the dichotomy between the use of manometry in clinical settings as a diagnostic tool and as an investigational technique for research purposes continues to exist.

11.2 Physiology of the Esophagus

The main purpose of the esophagus is the aborad transport of food to the stomach. It consists of three functional regions: the upper esophageal sphincter (UES), the esophageal body, and the lower esophageal sphincter (LES).

The UES is a physiologic region composed of striated muscles cells, defined as a zone of high intraluminal pressure localized between the pharynx and the esophagus [41]. It is present by at least 32 weeks of gestation and functional at birth, although incoordination between pharynx and esophagus may be present in the first weeks of life or in premature infants less than 1500 g [36]. At birth it measures ~0.5–1 cm in length and increases to ~3 cm in adults. There is a general agreement that the cricopharyngeal muscle is the main component of the UES but, since it is only about 1 cm wide, other muscles of the hypopharynx and the proximal esophagus also contribute to some of this high-pressure zone. However, at present time the precise anatomical identity of the UES is still undefined [41]. The UES is closed at rest and opens momentarily in response to a swallow. Radial and axial pressure asymmetry has been widely demonstrated [31]. Resting pressure is markedly asymmetric with anterior and posterior values being higher those laterally, and the highest anterior pressures are recorded near the pharynx, whereas the highest posterior pressures occur closer to the esophagus. Because of asymmetry and rapid pressure changes as well as brief axial movements, the manometric study of the UES has been hampered in the past by recording methodology. With modern systems allowing the recording of very rapid pressure change and with special catheter devices, accurate measurements of the UES pressure have become more feasible in both adults and children. In adults there is no consensus on the "normal values," and depending on the measuring method used, a wide range of UES pressure values has been reported in children, varying from 8 mmHg to 70 - mmHg [14, 40, 43, 44].

The esophageal body length in adults is 20–22 cm, whereas in children the length depends on the patient's age. It begins at the caudal edge of the cricopharyngeal and extends to the rostral limit of the LES. In adults, the proximal 5% of the esophagus is composed of striated muscle, and the middle 35–40% includes both striated and smooth muscle cells, with an increasing proportion of smooth muscle distally, whereas the caudal half of the esophageal body consists entirely of smooth muscle [39]. No equivalent information is available regarding children. At rest the musculature of the esophageal body appears to have no rhythmic or tonic contraction at all. Intraluminal pressure varies from –5 to –15 mmHg during normal inspiration to –2 to +5 mmHg during expiration, relative to atmospheric pressure [5].

Different types of esophageal contraction are recorded. *Primary peristalsis* is initiated by swallowing and is evident shortly after the pharyngeal contraction traverses the UES. It progresses down the esophagus and is initiated by central mechanisms. *Secondary peristalsis* can be elicited at any level of the esophagus in response to luminal distension by fluid and air. Usually it starts at the highest level reached by the refluxed materials into the esophagus. It also contributes to esophageal clearance of bolus not cleared up by a primary wave. *Tertiary contractions* occur spontaneously and randomly in the mid- and lower esophagus, unrelated to swallowing or reflux and with no peristaltic function. The efficacy of esophageal emptying is strongly related to the peristaltic amplitude, and it has been shown that emptying becomes progressively impaired when peristaltic amplitude becomes less than 35 mmHg [26, 38]. In children, the mean amplitude values of peristaltic contractions range between 40 to 89 mmHg, the duration of peristaltic contractions is between 2.5 and 5 s, and the propagation velocity is around 3.0 cm/s [10, 25, 32]. One interesting phenomenon of the peristaltic mechanism is "deglutitive inhibition" [7]. A second swallow, initiated while an earlier peristaltic contraction is still progressing, determines a complete inhibition of the contraction induced by the first swallow. With repeated swallows at very short intervals, the esophagus remains inhibited and a large "clearing wave" will occur after the last swallow in the series.

The LES is the high-pressure zone localized at the esophagogastric junction. It is tonically contracted at rest to produce a roughly concentrically symmetrical occlusion. However, the occlusion is not perfectly uniform, showing a radial asymmetry [5]. In adults, the LES is generally found to be 2–4 cm long, whereas in children its length increases with age, ranging from few millimeters in newborns to adult values in adolescents. LES pressure also varies with age and recording methods, ranging from ~7 mmHg in premature infants younger than 29 weeks of age to 18 mmHg in term infants [35] and from 10 to 40 mmHg in children [10, 25]. However,

it has been suggested that LES pressures of 5–10 mmHg above intragastric pressure are sufficient to maintain esophagogastric competence [13]. LES pressure is influenced by several factors. It is significantly variable during the interdigestive migrating motor complex (MMC) cycle. There is a pattern of LES contraction closely related to the phase of MMC in the stomach, showing a significantly higher LES pressure during MMC phase III than phase I [17]. The postprandial LES pressure is rather constant at a level comparable with that measured during phase I of the MMC [42]. LES pressure also shows inspiratory augmentation due to the contraction of the crural diaphragm encircling the sphincter [33]. LES pressure is usually modified by intra-abdominal pressure, gastric distension, peptides, hormones, various foods, and many drugs [43].

At the time of swallowing, the LES relaxes promptly in response to the initial neural discharge from the swallowing center in order to minimize resistance to flow across the esophagogastric junction [2]. This relaxation starts well after the peristaltic contraction has begun in the proximal esophagus and lasts 5–10 s, until the peristaltic wave reaches the distal esophagus. During relaxation, LES pressure falls to the level of gastric pressure. A complex phenomenon of the LES is represented by the so called transient relaxation, i.e., when relaxation is not triggered by swallowing. Although transient LES relaxations (TLESRs) are classically thought to be involved in the pathogenic mechanism of gastroesophageal reflux [11, 18, 28], it is now clear that they represent an essential component of belch reflex [45].

11.3
Technical Aspects

Manometry is by nature a highly technical evaluation. When knowledgeably used, manometric examination provides an accurate description of the esophageal contractile function, but only if physical principles and equipment characteristics are respected. In general, manometric data are reliable only if the methodology used to acquire them is accurate.

A manometric apparatus consists of a pressure sensor and transducer combination that detects the esophageal pressure complex and transduces it into an electrical signal, and a recording device to amplify, record, and store that electrical signal [6, 16]. The pressure sensor/transducer components of a manometric assembly function as a matched pair and are available in two general designs: either water-perfused catheters connected to a pneumohydraulic perfusion pump and to volume displacement transducers, or strain-gauge transducers with solid-state circuitry.

11.3.1
Low-Compliance Perfused Manometric System

The water infusion system includes a catheter composed of small capillary tubes, a low-compliance hydraulic capillary infusion pump, and external transducers [1]. In adults, the small capillary tubes usually have an internal diameter of approximately 0.8 mm and an opening or port at a known point along the length of the catheter. In adults, the most commonly used catheters have an overall diameter of 4.5 mm. In children, in order to reduce the diameter of the catheter, fewer recording ports (generally four) and smaller capillary tubes (with internal diameter of 0.35 mm) are utilized; a lower infusion rate is also used. The manometric probes are usually tailored to the child's size, with recording sites 1 cm apart in premature babies, 3 cm apart in toddlers and children, and 5 cm apart in adolescents [20] (Fig. 1). Each capillary tube is connected to an external transducer. The infusion pump, a simple and essential device for stationary manometry, perfuses the capillary tubes, providing a constant flow rate without increasing the compliance of the manometric system. When a catheter port is occluded (e.g. by a muscular contraction), there is a pressure rise in the water-filled tubes that is transmitted to the external transducers. High-fidelity recordings of intraluminal pressure are achieved by infusion rates from 0.1 to 0.4 mL min^{-1}, although these rates may provide an unacceptable amount of water to small babies or premature infants [20]. In order to overcome this problem, perfusion rates as low as 0.02 mL min^{-1} have been successfully used [9].

Mobility of the sphincteric region relative to a manometric probe of any type poses a special challenge. Both upper and lower sphincters have a zone of maximal pressure which is only a few millimeters wide, whereas the perfused manometric side holes are focal-pressure sensors. Thus, signaling of maximal sphincter pressure requires precise positioning of focal-pressure sensors within the sphincteric area. It is impossible to maintain such a position for more than few seconds, because of the movements of the sphincters due to the respiration cycle, swallowing, and body position changes [19]. Although pull-through of pressure sensors across the sphincters is used to sample the pressure values, this method is of limited diagnostic value. UES and LES pressures vary greatly over time, and repeated manipulation of the manometric assembly is also uncomfortable. To cope with these problems, the Dent sleeve manometry catheter was developed [15]. It is an infusion flexible catheter with a specially constructed tip. One side of a 2.5- to 5-cm-long segment (depending on patient's age) at the distal end is covered with a thin, flexible membrane under which a constant infusion rate of water occurs (Fig. 2). The membrane represents a pressure-sensitive area along its entire length. When pressure is applied

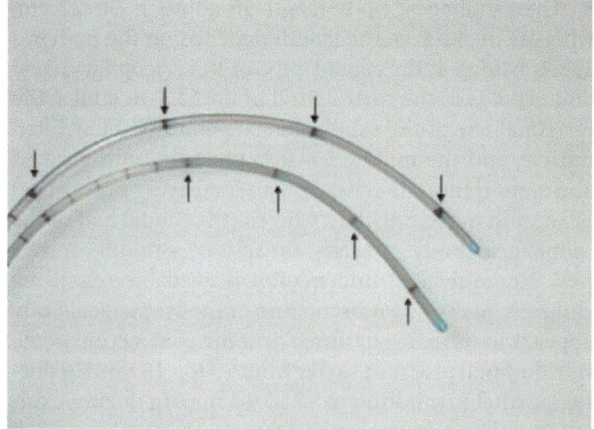

Fig. 1. Two manometric catheters with perfused side holes located at different distances apart (10 cm in the upper catheter, 5 cm in the lower catheter)

anywhere along the length of the membrane, the resistance to water flow beneath it increases, and pressure is registered on the corresponding manometric channel. Thus, this device is especially useful for long-term recording of the maximum resting pressure of esophageal sphincters, as it is not affected by small displacement of the sensor. It has been shown that a good correlation occurs between measurement of the resting LES pressure made with the side-hole sensors and the sphincteric sleeve measurement [15], whereas significant differences have been described in the measured duration of LES relaxation (shorter with the sleeve device) [8]. The disadvantages of a sleeve catheter include a limited frequency response, making it unsuitable for the recording of rapid changes in the contractile activity, recording from only one radial orientation, and the requirement of skilled personnel for its proper use [27].

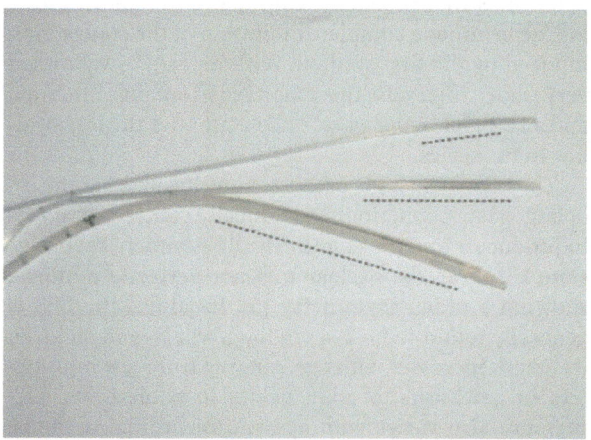

Fig. 2. Three manometric catheters incorporating a sleeve at the distal end. The *dotted lines* indicate sleeves of different size and length according to the age of the subjects investigated

A device activating the pressure transducers, storing their signals, and displaying the latter in such a way as to allow an immediate interpretation and analysis is needed. The personal computer has become the heart of the esophageal manometry system. It interfaces with purpose-designed electronic modules that activate and receive signals from pressure transducers, whereas commercially available software programs are essential for acquiring, displaying, and storing pressure recording data [16]. Actually, the technical adequacy of different commercially available device recording systems is quite comparable. Probably the dominant consideration that should determine the choice of a system is the level of technical assistance and the training locally available to support the user.

The required characteristics of a manometric recording apparatus are defined by the magnitude of the pressure to be recorded and the frequency content and waveform of esophageal contractile waves. It has been shown that the frequency response of a manometric system required to reproduce esophageal wave and sphincteric pressures with a 98% accuracy is 0–4 Hz (maximal recordable dP/dt: 300 mmHg/s) [37]. Most commercially available manometric systems can provide a pressure rise rate of 300–400 mmHg/s, which is adequate for faithful recordings in esophagus.

11.3.2
Solid-state Manometric System

The main alternative to the water-perfused manometric system is a manometric assembly incorporating strain-gauge sensors and solid-state electronic elements. In this system, the manometric probe contains miniature strain-gauge pressure transducers built into the catheter at a fixed location along its length, so that pressure changes directly influence the transducers to generate electrical output signals [7]. The probe plugs into a small box containing the electronics, which is then connected to the recording device. Such devices are blind and need to be connected to a personal computer with the appropriate software to display and analyze the recording. The main advantage of using solid-state catheters is that the pressures are recorded directly from the area and are unrelated to the relative position of the subject; therefore manometric studies may also be performed with the subject in the upright position. This, and the fact that it does not require water perfusion, make solid-state catheters suitable for long-term ambulatory monitoring of the intraluminal pressure. In addition, due to their vastly expanded frequency response, an accurate measurement of the cricopharyngeal region motor events is also possible. Limitations of the solid-state catheters include the high cost, the size, and fragility. It has been calculated that for a given number of

pressure recording points on a recording assembly, solid-state catheters are 10 to 20 times more expensive than a perfused manometric assembly [16]. Furthermore, the diameter of solid-state catheter with three microtransducers is comparable to that of the eight-lumen water infusion probe used in adults, too large to be used in small infants. Finally, there is very little experience in pediatric patients and controls.

11.4
Methodological Aspects

11.4.1
Preparation of the Patient

Before starting manometric recording, it is important to assess patient information regarding medical history, symptoms, medication, and allergies. Any drug with a known effect on gastrointestinal motility should be discontinued at least 72 h before the testing.

It is important to emphasize that esophageal manometry is performed in a different fashion in children and adults due to differences in esophageal size, cooperation, and neurological and developmental maturation. Performing manometry in children requires great patience from the physician. The parents should be present during the testing in order to tranquilize the child, and to provide the child with a model of cooperative behavior with the physician. The cooperation can also be improved by the use of age-appropriate relaxation techniques. For example, infants relax with swaddling and use of a pacifier. Having a favorite toy can comfort toddlers. School-age and older children benefit when equipment is examined and explained before starting the procedure. Esophageal manometry is best performed without sedation [20]. However, in many children sedation is necessary, and midazolam has been shown to be effective with minimal or no influence on pressure measurement [21]. It could be advisable to wait for a child's complete recovery from the drug effect before starting the motility tests. Finally, before starting the procedure it is important to verify signed informed consent, and it is necessary to check that infants have fasted for at least 3 h and children for at least 6 h, to avoid nausea, vomiting, and aspiration.

11.4.2
Study Procedure

The manometric catheter can be placed either nasally or orally, but there is a wide consensus that the studies are better tolerated when the catheter is introduced through the nose. The study should begin with all pressure sensors in the stomach. Normally, all channels at

~25 cm should be in the stomach in small babies as well as in the preterms, whereas in older children it occurs at ~35–40 cm. A relatively flat smooth tracing with small pressure rises during inspiration indicates gastric placement. This can be confirmed by asking the patient (if old enough) to take a deep breath, which is associated with a pressure rise in each channel. If some of the channels have not yet been introduced into the gastric cavity, the catheter should be pushed down 3–5 cm. Afterwards, it is necessary to establish a reference baseline at the average pressure in the stomach.

A complete motility study of the esophagus should include assessment of the LES, esophageal body, and UES. LES pressure can be assessed in adults by a rapid pull-through technique, a station pull-through technique, or a sleeve recording [27]. A rapid pull-through is performed by withdrawing the catheter across the sphincter at a rate of about 1 cm/s while the patient suspends respiration for 10–15 s. This method is obviously not suitable for infants and uncooperative children. Assessment of the LES in children is usually performed by a station pull-through technique. It involves a slow stepwise withdrawal of the catheter through the LES [4]. The catheter is moved in 0.5-cm increments and should remain at each position for 30–60 s. When the proximal channel reaches the lower border of the LES, an increase in the respiratory variation can be observed. As the catheter is withdrawn, a persistent rise above the end-expiratory baseline indicates that the channel has entered the LES (distal border; Fig. 3). It is at this point that LES relaxation can be assessed with 1 mL of water in infants and 3–5 mL in older children [20]. In small infants, water can be inserted in the mouth while they are using a pacifier, or a natural reflex swallow may be induced by gently blowing in the face or by moving the pacifier in the mouth [20]. Following a swallow, the LES

pressure should drop to about the level of the gastric baseline. As the catheter is advanced through the sphincter, the pressure tracing will pass a point where it will change from a positive deflection with inspiration to a negative one. This is known as the pressure inversion point (PIP): it marks the passage from the abdominal portion to the thoracic portion of the sphincter [23]. As the catheter is withdrawn, the pressure tracing will drop below the gastric baseline to the esophageal baseline. At this point the catheter has left the LES and has entered the esophagus. This procedure is performed until all channels pass through the LES.

An ideal method for assessing the LES is represented by sleeve recording. It is performed using a station pull-through technique by withdrawing the sleeve catheter across the sphincter until the sleeve device is positioned in the middle of the LES. The sleeve catheter is in a fixed position and does not require any movement during the recording time, increasing the comfort level of the patient and overcoming the single most difficult technical aspect of esophageal manometry, that is, a child's cooperation.

For complete evaluation of the esophageal body, measurements of both distal esophagus smooth muscle and proximal esophagus striated muscle should be included. In children the distal esophagus is evaluated by localizing the most distal recording port in the LES and the remaining ports in the esophageal body (Fig. 4). Ten wet swallows are given at 30-s intervals. During the catheter withdrawal, the proximal esophagus is evaluated in a similar manner with the proximal recording port being localized just below the UES.

In order to acquire a complete esophageal motility study, a manometric evaluation of the UES and pharynx should also be performed. Although the manometric evaluation of the UES and pharynx is the same as for the LES, it is of pivotal importance to increase the recording speed. After assessment of the proximal esophageal mo-

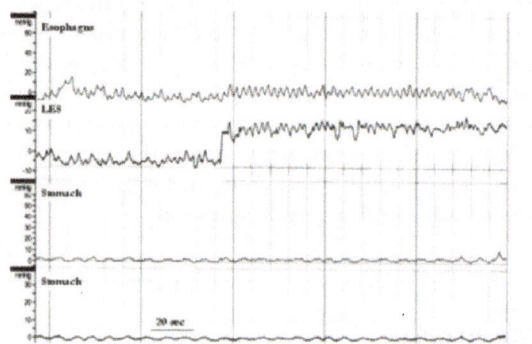

Fig. 3. Manometric tracing at the level of the distal esophagus and stomach. *From top to bottom*: distal esophagus (first channel), lower esophageal sphincter (second channel), stomach (third and fourth channels). At the level of the second channel, a sudden rise in the pressure profile is evident that corresponds to the entrance of the recording side hole of the manometric catheter into the lower esophageal sphincter region

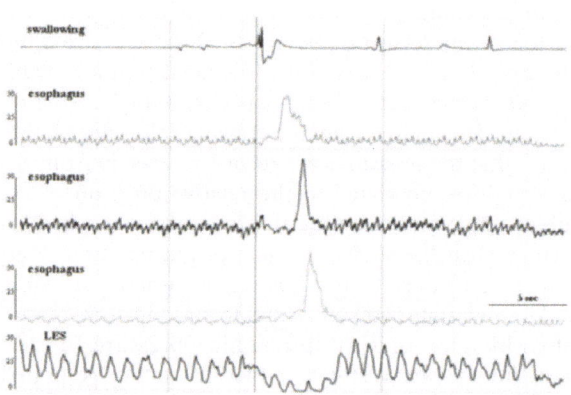

Fig. 4. Manometric recording of the esophageal peristalsis (second, third, and fourth channels) and relaxation of the lower esophageal sphincter (fifth channel). The first channel records the swallowing activity

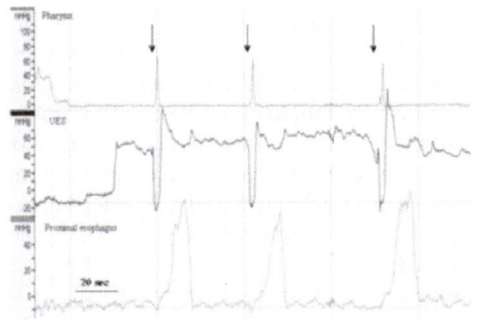

Fig. 5. Manometric recording at the level of the oropharyngeal region. The upper channel shows pharyngeal contractions, the middle channel records a profile of the upper esophageal sphincter that exhibits sequential relaxations in coincidence with pharyngeal contractions (oropharyngeal coordination), and the lower channel shows contractions at the level of the proximal esophagus

tility, as the catheter is slowly pulled back in 0.5-cm increments, a pressure rise in the proximal recording port above the esophageal baseline indicates that the channel has entered the UES. It is at this point that UES relaxation can be assessed. With continued the pull-back, the second recording port also enters the UES, and the proximal one is then localized in the pharynx. At this time, with a series of wet swallows the coordination between the sphincter relaxation and the pharyngeal contraction can also be evaluated (Fig. 5).

11.4.3
Analysis of Manometric Recording

The manometric assessment of the LES is performed in order to measure both LES resting pressure and swallow-related LES relaxation. The resting pressure of the LES is defined as the pressure rise measured from the gastric pressure, used as zero reference. The LES resting pressure measurement must take into account the influence of respiration. Several methods are used for the definition of LES pressure on a station pull-through technique. Some investigators define LES pressure at the point of end expiration; others emphasizing the important contribution of the diaphragmatic crura to the antireflux mechanism recommend end inspiration; still others advocate measurement at the mid-point of the respiratory oscillation. Although end-respiratory pressure corresponds most closely to true LES pressure, mid-expiratory measurements may prove better predictors of pathologic reflux [29]. The latter method is commonly used in the laboratory of the authors. Regarding studies of LES relaxation, the degree and the coordination of LES relaxation to swallowing need to be assessed. Normal LES should always relax to at least 4 - mmHg (residual pressure) of the gastric pressure with a wet swallow. LES relaxation in response to swallowing

can be expressed as the LES residual pressure, defined as the difference between the pressure at the nadir of the relaxation and gastric pressure, and as the percentage of LES relaxation, that is, the difference between the LES resting pressure and residual pressure, expressed as a percentage. A complete relaxation is defined as a 90% relaxation. Furthermore, LES relaxation needs to be coordinated for more than 90% of wet swallows.

The manometric assessment of the esophageal body is performed in order to evaluate the peristalsis, amplitude, duration, and velocity of the contractions, as well as the presence of abnormal contractions. The percentage of primary peristalsis is measured from at least 10 wet swallows, each separated by 30-s intervals. Amplitude defines the strength of the contraction and is expressed in mmHg. It is determined from the mean resting esophageal pressure to the peak of contraction. Peristaltic contractions where the overall mean amplitude is either very weak (≤30 mmHg) or very strong (≥180 - mmHg) are considered abnormal. Duration of the contraction is expressed in seconds and is measured from the onset of the major upstroke of the wave to its return to baseline. The velocity is the rate of progression of the contraction down the esophagus and is expressed in cm/s. It is measured by dividing the distance between the proximal and distal holes by the time required for the wave to transverse this distance. These measurements are also derived from the mean of 10 swallows. Esophageal contractions may also occur in simultaneous, retrograde, dropped, or interrupted sequences. In both normal adults and normal children, these abnormal motor responses with peristaltic failure can occur in less than 10% of all wet swallows [10, 38].

The manometric evaluation of the UES and pharynx includes the determination of the UES resting pressure, defined as the highest pressure in the sphincter above the esophageal baseline, the relaxation of the sphincter, defined as the pressure drop to baseline with swallowing, and the assessment of the coordination between the UES relaxation and pharyngeal contraction. However, the value of UES/pharyngeal measurements with standard catheters is as yet not well defined, and the clinical utility of such assessments in patients with GERD is not established [20].

11.4.4
Reference Values

Before interpreting the recorded data and deciding whether abnormalities of esophageal motility are present, it is of pivotal importance to define the limits of normality. Unfortunately, the lack of normal controls is an important limiting factor for the establishment of normal motility pattern, making the interpretation of manometric recording data difficult and subjective and leading to overinterpretation. However, some control data have been published. Although each center performing esophageal manometry should have its own set of normal values, it is suggested that "normal" ranges proposed by one group could be used by another if the investigation is performed and interpreted in the same way.

11.5
Esophageal Manometry and GERD

GERD is primarily a disorder of esophageal motility and is considered the common final pathway of a multifactorial pathophysiological process. Detected manometric abnormalities include impaired peristalsis, LES hypotension, and high rate of TLESRs (Fig. 6) [11–13]. Paradoxically, esophageal motility studies play a relatively small role in the diagnosis of GERD, because no single manometric defect discriminates between patients with GERD and controls. In theory, knowing the esophageal body and sphincter motor abnormalities leading to the development of GERD could help in the selection of the most appropriate treatment for correcting the defects underlying GERD. In recent years it has been shown that drugs targeting TLESRs, such as atropine, baclofen (GABA-B receptor agonist), L-NMMA (NO synthesis inhibitor), and loxiglumide (CCK_A receptor antagonist) reduce the rate of TLESRs and concomitantly the number of reflux episodes, suggesting their therapeutic implication [24]. Unfortunately, all data on these drugs derive from acute experiments; studies with their prolonged administration are still lacking. Furthermore, no similar data are available in children. Thus, at present, manometric assessment has no significant influence on the diagnosis, staging, and pharmacologic treatment of GERD [22].

Although at present there are no manometric findings that define an indication for antireflux surgery, it is widely agreed that all children being considered for antireflux surgery should be evaluated manometrically, mainly in those in whom there is uncertainty about the correct diagnosis of GERD, or when esophageal motility disorders, such as achalasia and scleroderma, are suspected [7, 27]. It has also been suggested that preoperative manometric assessment may aid in tailoring antireflux surgery, since it could identify patients at special risk for postsurgical dysphagia from defective peristalsis. Unfortunately, it has been shown in adults that preoperative manometric assessment does not predict surgical outcome, either in term of the development of postoperative dysphagia or the antireflux efficacy [34]. However, esophageal manometry is indicated for the evaluation of the effect of pharmacological or surgical treatment [3].

Finally, esophageal manometry is useful in defining the appropriate location of pH electrodes, in particular in patients with abnormal anatomy (i.e., hiatal hernia) [22].

11.6
Conclusions

Esophageal manometry has a small role in the diagnosis and management of patients with GERD. However, it is important to realize that symptoms arising from esophageal mucosal disease or abnormal esophageal motility can be very similar. So, even if it has few clinical indications, there are some situations in which esophageal manometry may be of value.

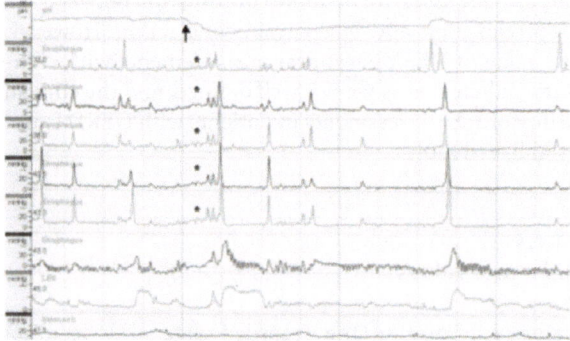

Fig. 6. Prolonged recording of the lower esophageal sphincter activity. *From top to bottom*: pH (first channel), esophageal body (second to seventh channels), lower esophageal sphincter (eighth channel), stomach (ninth channel). A transient lower esophageal sphincter relaxation is evident during the occurrence of a reflux episode (pH channel). During the reflux episode, a common cavity phenomenon is recorded along the esophageal body (*asterisks*)

References

1. Arndorfer RC, Stef JJ, Doods WJ et al (1977) Improved infusion system for intraluminal esophageal manometry. Gastroenterology 73:23–27
2. Biancani P, Harnett KM, Behar J (1999) Esophageal motor function. In: Yamada T (ed) Textbook of gastroenterology, 3rd edn. Lippincott Williams &Wilkins, Philadelphia, pp 157–187
3. Borrelli O, Mancini V, Bueno de Mesquita et al (2003) Long term esophageal function in children with severe gastroesophageal reflux disease after laparoscopic Nissen fundoplication. J Pediatr Gastroenterol Nutr 36:P106
4. Broag Dalton C (1987) The manometric study. In: Castell DO, Richter JE, Dalton CB (eds) Esophageal motility testing. Elsevier, New York, pp 35–60
5. Christensen J (1987) Motor function of the pharynx and esophagus. In: Johnson LR (ed) Physiology of the gastrointestinal tract, 2nd edn. Raven Press, New York, pp 595–612
6. Camilleri M (1993) Perfused tube manometry. In: Kumar D, Wingate D (eds) An illustrated guide to gastrointestinal motility. Churchill Livingstone, Cambridge, pp 183–199
7. Castell JA, Castell DO (1994) Stationary esophageal manometry. Functional investigation in esophageal disease. In: Modlin IR, Rozen P, Scarpignato C (eds) Frontiers of gastrointestinal research. Karger, Basel, pp 71–108

8. Castell JA, Dalton CB, Castell DO (1988) On-line computer analysis of human lower esophageal sphincter relaxation. Am J Physiol 255:G794–799
9. Chen WH, Omari TI, Holloway RH et al (1998) A comparison of micromanometric and standard manometric techniques for recording of oesophageal motility. Neurogastroenterol Motil 10:253–262
10. Cucchiara S, Staiano A, Di Lorenzo C et al (1986) Esophageal motor abnormalities in children with gastroesophageal reflux and peptic esophagitis. J Pediatr 108:907–910
11. Cucchiara, S, Staiano A, Di Lorenzo C et al (1988) Pathophysiology of gastroesophageal reflux and distal esophageal motility in children with gastroesophageal reflux disease. J Pediatr Gastroenterol Nutr 7:830–836
12. Cucchiara S, Bortolotti M, Minella R et al (1993) Fasting and postprandial mechanisms of gastroesophageal reflux in children with gastroesophageal reflux disease. Dig Dis Sci 38:86–92
13. Davidson GP, Omari TI (2001) Pathophysiological mechanisms of gastroesophageal reflux disease in children. Curr Gastroenterol Rep 3:257–262
14. Davidson GP, Dent J, Willing J et al (1991) Monitoring of upper oesophageal sphincter pressure in children. Gut 32:607–611
15. Dent J (1976) A new technique for continuous sphincter pressure measurement. Gastroenterology 71:263–267
16. Dent J, Holloway RH (1996) Esophageal motility testing and reflux testing. State of the art and clinical role in the twenty-first century. Gastroenterol Clin N Am 25:51–73
17. Dent J, Dodds WJ, Sekigushi T et al (1983) Interdigestive phasic contractions of the human lower esophageal sphincter. Gastroenterology 84:453–460
18. Dent J, Holloway RH, Toouli J et al (1988) Mechanisms of lower oesophageal sphincter incompetence in patients with symptomatic gastroesophageal reflux. Gut 29:1020–1028
19. Dodds WJ, Stewart ET, Hogan WJ (1974) Effect of esophageal movement on intraluminal esophageal pressure recording. Gastroenterology 67:592–600
20. Di Lorenzo C, Hillemeier C, Hyman P et al (2002) Manometry studies in children: minimum standards for procedures. Neurogastroenterol Mot 14:411–420
21. Fung KP, Math MV, Ho CO et al (1992) Midazolam as a sedative in esophageal manometry: a study of the effect on esophageal manometry. J Pediatr Gastroenterol Nutr 15:85–88
22. Gilger MA, Boyle JT, Sondhemeir JM et al (1997) Indications for pediatric esophageal manometry. J Pediatr Gastroenterol Nutr 24:616–618
23. Harris LD, Pope CE II (1966) The pressure inversion point: its genesis and variability. Gastroenterology 51:691–698
24. Hirsch DP, Tytgat GNJ, Boeckxstaens GEE (2002) Review article: transient lower oesophageal sphincter relaxations – a pharmacological target for gastro-oesophageal reflux disease. Aliment Pharmacol Ther 16:17–26
25. Hillemeier AC, Grill BB, McCallum R et al (1983) Esophageal and gastric motor abnormalities in infants with and without gastroesophageal reflux. Gastroenterology 84:741–746
26. Kahrilas PJ, Dodds WJ, Hogan WJ et al (1986) Peristaltic dysfunction in peptic esophagitis. Gastroenterology 91:897–904
27. Kahrilas PJ, Clouse RE, Hogan WJ (1994) American Gastroenterology Association technical review on the clinical use of esophageal manometry. Gastroenterology 107:1865–84
28. Kawahara H, Dent J, Davidson G (1997) Mechanism responsible for gastroesophageal reflux in children. Gastroenterology 113:399–408
29. Krauss BB, Wu WC, Castell DO (1990) Comparison of lower esophageal sphincter manometry and gastroesophageal reflux measured by 24-hour pH recording. Am J Gastroenterol 85:692–696
30. Kronecker H, Meltzer SJ (1883) Der Schluckmechanismus, seine Erregung und seine Hemmung. Arch Ges Anat Physiol 7(Suppl):328–332
31. Lang IM, Shaker R (2000) An overview of the upper esophageal sphincter. Curr Gastroenterol Rep 2:185–190
32. Mahony MJ, Migliavacca M, Spits L et al (1988) Motor disorders of the oesophagus in gastro-oesophageal reflux. Arch Dis Child 63:1333–1338
33. Mittal RK, Rochester DF, McCallum RW (1989) Sphincteric action of the diaphragm during a relaxed lower esophageal sphincter. Am J Physiol 256:9139–9144
34. Mughal MM, Bancewicz J, Maples M (1990) Oesophageal manometry and pH recording does not predict the bad results of Nissen fundoplication. Br J Surg 77:43–45
35. Newel SJ, Sarkar PK, Durbin GM et al (1988) Maturation of the lower esophageal sphincter in the preterm baby. Gut 95:52–62
36. Omari T, Snel A, Barnett C (1999) Measurement of upper esophageal sphincter tone and relaxation during swallowing in premature infants. Am J Physiol 277:G862–G866
37. Orlowski J, Dodds WJ, Linehan JH et al (1982) Requirement for accurate manometric recording of pharyngeal and esophageal peristaltic pressure waves. Invest Radiol 17:567–572
38. Richter JE, Wu WC, Johns DN et al (1987) Esophageal manometry in 95 healthy adult volunteers. Dig Dis Sci 32:583–592
39. Schofield GC (1968) Anatomy of muscular and neural tissues in the alimentary canal. In: Code CF (ed) Handbook of physiology. Section 6: Alimentary Canal. vol IV: Motility. American Physiological Society, Washington, DC, pp 1579–1627
40. Sondheimer JM (1983) Upper esophageal sphincter and pharingoesophageal motor function in infants with or without gastroesophageal reflux. Gastroenterology 85:301–305
41. Sivarao DV, Goyal RK (2000) Functional anatomy and physiology of the upper esophageal sphincter. Am J Med 108(4A):27S–37S
42. Smout AJPM, Bogaard JW, Grade AC et al (1985) Effects of cisapride, a new prokinetic substance, on interdigestive and postprandial motor activity of the distal esophagus in man. Gut 26:246–251
43. Willing J, Davidson GP, Dent J et al (1993) Effect of gastrooesophageal reflux on upper oesophageal sphincter motility in children. Gut 34:904–910
44. Willing J, Furukawa Y, Davidson GP et al (1994) Strain induced augmentation of upper oesophageal sphincter motility in children. Gut 35:159–164
45. Wyman JB, Dent J, Heddle R et al (1990) Control of belching by the lower oesophageal sphincter. Gut 31:639–646

Esophagogastric pH Monitoring in the Diagnostic Evaluation of Infants and Children with GER

12

Salvatore Cucchiara · Osvaldo Borrelli

Contents

measurement of their frequency and duration, has been regarded as the most sensitive and specific diagnostic tool for diagnosing reflux disease [11].

Spencer [52] first described the technique of using an indwelling glass electrode positioned above the LES for monitoring intraesophageal pH continuously; a landmark study was subsequently published by Johnson and DeMeester [29], who were the first to study both normal volunteers and symptomatic patients and to quantitatively analyze the results, introducing the concept of physiological reflux and defining the limits of pathological reflux in adults. Since its introduction, esophageal pH monitoring has rapidly gained a wide popularity. Furthermore, the development of small electrodes, the technology of portable compact recorders, and computer analysis programs have made this test the most common diagnostic tool for infants and children with suspected GERD. Despite the widespread acceptance of the test, however, it is not without limitations, and areas of disagreement about methodology, analysis, and interpretation are still present.

12.1
Introduction

Gastroesophageal reflux (GER), defined as the effortless retrograde passage of gastric contents into the lower esophagus, is a common physiological phenomenon occurring in both infants and children [8]. However, in a small percentage of cases it can be abnormal, leading to the development of disease, also called GER disease (GERD), characterized by a wide spectrum of intestinal and extraintestinal symptoms and signs.

Although different abnormalities in motility variables, such as lower esophageal sphincter (LES) function, esophageal peristalsis, and gastric motor activity can contribute to the development of GERD, the degree of esophageal acid exposure represents the key factor in the pathogenesis of GERD. Not surprisingly, esophageal pH monitoring, based on both the detection of acid reflux episodes (within the esophageal lumen) and the

12.2
Technical and Methodological Aspects

12.2.1
The Recording Device

The pH signals are digitized and stored in miniaturized, battery-powered dataloggers which can be worn by the patient himself on a waist belt or shoulder strap, permitting nearly normal activity during recording. These lightweight dataloggers may have up to four channels, although a single channel is usually sufficient for clinical purposes. Most recording devices work on rechargeable batteries and, with the use of a small internal backup power source, data are stored even when battery failure occurs. There is no continuous sampling, but a sampling rate of intraesophageal pH between 6 and 10 measurements/min is adequate for an accurate determination of median or threshold pH value [17]. A faster sampling rate would be needed to evaluate an intraesophageal pH decrease under the threshold lasting less than 15 s; however, these brief pH decreases are considered of no clinical relevance and may be ignored [37].

Dataloggers vary in the number and complexity of event markers allowing parents or older children to indicate the timing of symptoms and events, such as meals, recumbency (sleep), etc. Unfortunately, the experience of several authors is that many if not most people are unable to manage these buttons on a datalogger [15]. Therefore, it is preferable to use a detailed diary, in which all events and symptoms are written down by parents and/or nursery staff and subsequently correlated with the pH tracing [55].

12.2.2
pH Electrodes

Different types of pH electrodes are available for prolonged esophageal pH monitoring, such as antimony monocrystalline electrodes, glass electrodes, and ion-sensitive field effect transistor (ISFET) electrodes. Most of the electrodes currently in use are the antimony and glass electrodes; information regarding the ISFET type is not yet sufficient to allow adequate assessment.

The ideal pH probe should have certain features: it should have a small diameter so that it can be easily passed through the nose into the esophagus; it should be stable (with no drift during monitoring time) and minimally affected by temperature; it should have linear response (no hysteresis) and exhibit a short response time between pH 7 and pH 1 [23]. The probe should also be inexpensive, simple to calibrate, and disposable or easily sterilized. None of the currently available pH probes has all of these properties.

Glass electrodes have some technical advantages compared to antimony electrodes. They have a linear response over the pH range 1 to 12 occurring very rapidly after a pH change (usually more than 90% within 1 s) and are relatively drift-free, particularly when used with an internal reference in the form of a combination electrode [38]. From a practical point of view, they have the longest operational life (~50 studies with optimal care), and can be chemically sterilized. Unfortunately, their main disadvantages are that they are very expensive and fragile, with the possibility of being damaged during insertion. They are also larger in diameter (1–3.0 mm), stiffer and bulkier at their tip than antimony electrodes, thus making the intubation procedure difficult and/or less tolerable by children.

On the other hand, antimony monocrystalline electrodes are less expensive, smaller (<1–2.3 mm), more flexible, more comfortable and resistant to mechanical shock compared to the other types of electrodes. However, they are inferior to glass electrodes in terms of stability, temperature sensitivity, and response time;

moreover, they exhibit a nonlinear response even over the physiologic pH range of 1 to 7, showing a hysteresis phenomenon [38]. The pH-dependent function shown by antimony monocrystalline electrodes is due to a process of oxidation of the antimony crystal surface during the recording time. Thus, the pH probe properties change over time, resulting in somewhat greater drift (less stability) and a limited life span. Antimony monocrystalline electrodes are also not chemically resistant and, because they are degraded by glutaraldehyde, the frequent cleaning processes reduce their life span and impair their performance.

Considering all the characteristics of glass and antimony electrodes, it has been suggested that either can be used satisfactorily in the clinical setting for esophageal pH monitoring [23, 37, 58]. However, because antimony pH probes are less stiff and better tolerated than glass electrodes, the use of the former is suggested for infants and older children.

12.2.3
Reference Electrodes

pH electrodes require a reference electrode. Monopolar and combination electrodes suitable for intraesophageal use are commercially available; while the former requires an external cutaneous reference electrode [usually a silver/silver-chloride (Ag/AgCl) electrode], the latter has a built-in reference. Disadvantages of external cutaneous references are skin electrode dislodgment, poor skin contact due to drying out of the electrode gel, and skin changes in the composition of ions because of perspiration and skin-enteric potential difference (which introduces an error of up to 0.6 pH units) [38, 17]. Although careful attention to every detail can avoid most of the common problems occurring with cutaneous reference, the pH recordings with intraluminal references are usually more accurate. Until some years ago there was no reliable antimony electrode with an internal reference, and only combined glass electrodes were commercially available; nowadays, antimony pH probes with a built-in reference are also available.

Although pH probes with an internal reference have a relatively larger diameter and are slightly more expensive than those with external references, their use is usually recommended because of both technical advantages and recording accuracy.

12.2.4
Software

At completion of the pH recordings, data stored in the datalogger are downloaded into a computer and usually stored in a solid-state memory system (hard disk, floppy, or compact disks). Software from various manufacturers offer similar capabilities with regard to automated analysis, graphic display, and printing. The software should be able to display both a numerical summary and a time course of esophageal pH with indicators for specific time periods (such as meals, recumbency, etc.) and symptom events. Most programs are also able to calculate various reflux indices and create derivative graphs (such as circadian plot and frequency curve). It is of value (especially for research purposes) that the software is modifiable by users. Variables that may need to be changed include the pH threshold for the onset and end of reflux events, the minimum time below the pH threshold for defining a reflux event, and the time interval around the reflux episode for assessment of symptom association. The availability of after-sales service is also an important consideration.

12.2.5
Calibration

Whatever the type of pH probe used, it is of pivotal importance to carry out an accurate calibration, because even small errors in the procedure can lead to erroneous results. The probes are usually calibrated at room temperature, using both acidic (pH 1 or 4) and neutral buffer solution (pH 7), compatible with the type of electrode used. The calibration fluids for antimony electrodes should be those provided by the manufacturer. The pH buffer solution can change with increasing temperature, and a correction factor should be taken into account and incorporated into either the datalogger itself or the software analysis program.

The calibration should be repeated at the end of the monitoring period in order to rule out pH electrode failure and to ensure that no important drift has occurred during the recording time. For the diagnosis of GERD, a drift of less than 0.5 pH units over 24 h is considered acceptable (Emde et al. 1987). If antimony probes are used, sometimes it may be possible to restore proper electrode function by removing surface oxides with gentle abrasion of the crystal surface by means of an ultrafine abrasive paper.

12.2.6
Preparation of the Patient

Before starting pH monitoring, it is important to assess patient's information regarding medical history, symptoms, medication, and allergies. Histamine H_2 receptor antagonist and prokinetics should be stopped for at least 48 h before the study, whereas a washout period must be prolonged to at least 72 h for proton pump inhibitors. If pH monitoring is performed to evaluate the efficacy of treatment on esophageal acid exposure, the drug should be continued. Although various medications can alter LES function and esophageal pH (such as barbiturates, diazepam, smooth muscle relaxants, antiasthmatic drugs, etc.), their cessation is not usually essential.

It is also important to verify signed informed consent and explain the procedure to the child (if the child is old enough) and parents in order to obtain patient cooperation and increase his or her comfort level. Finally, before starting the procedure it is necessary to check that infants have fasted for at least 3 h and children for 6 h, to avoid nausea, vomiting, and aspiration.

12.2.7
Positioning the pH Probe

The pH probe is introduced through the nose and the tip is positioned in the lower esophagus at 87% of the esophageal length. Correct anatomic placement of the electrode is crucial for obtaining clinically useful esophageal pH measurements. Variation from the correct position directly affects the amount of acid reflux detected. Therefore, if the position of the gastroesophageal junction (GEJ) reference point is imprecise, the true distance between the GEJ and the probe tip will not be known. Thus, the distance could vary from patient to patient, producing results that are difficult to interpret, unreliable, and probably not reproducible. Patients with excessive acid exposure whose probe is positioned proximally to the correct position may appear to have normal acid reflux, and those with normal acid exposure may be considered abnormal if the probe is placed distally to the correct position above the LES [1].

Several methods exist for the correct placement of pH electrodes: manometry, fluoroscopy, endoscopy, and calculation of esophageal length. Manometry is the most accurate method for localizing the LES and defining pH probe placement [34], but because it is invasive, time-consuming, and not available in each center, its use is very limited. Fluoroscopy is the method recommended by the European Society for Pediatric Gastroenterology, Hepatology and Nutrition (ESPGHAN) working group on GER [55], since it can be applied in each center. The pH-sensitive point (localized at the tip of the glass electrodes and ~5 mm above the tip of the antimony electrodes) should be positioned so that it overlies the third vertebral body, above the diaphragm throughout the respiratory cycle. The disadvantage of the fluoroscopic method is that it can be inaccurate in the presence of severe thoracic malformation, previous esophageal or thoracic surgery, and in the presence of hiatal hernia. Endoscopy routinely assesses the GEJ but does not evaluate the nasopharynx and therefore cannot accurately provide the distance between the anterior nares and the GEJ. However, its invasiveness severely limits its use in children, and there is wide agreement that endoscopy is not an acceptable method for localizing the LES in children. In infants and in preterm newborns, different formulas have been used to calculate the approximate length of the esophagus from the nares to the LES [31, 51, 53]. In these patients, Strobel's formula ($5 + 0.252 \times$ length of the child) seems to be the noninvasive method of choice for pH probe placement [18], whereas in children over 1 m in height it may result in a placement too close to the GEJ [55].

12.2.8
Monitoring Conditions

A number of patient-dependent variables such as the type and amount of food ingested, the body position, and the degree of physical activity have been shown to affect the duration and the extent of esophageal acid exposure [47]. The acidity and the buffer capacity of meals and beverages consumed during the pH monitoring are variable: acid and liquid meals can increase the number of reflux episodes recorded, while feeding at short intervals buffers gastric contents and reduces the amount of reflux [14]. Body position, especially in infants, has profound effects on the frequency of reflux: in the prone position reflux episodes occur less frequently than in the supine position, and more acid reflux is recorded when infants are in a sitting position than when in a lying position, due to increased intraabdominal pressure [54]. Despite these considerations it is difficult to make a rigid set of guidelines for infants and children; this would reduce the ability of the pH test to detect a significant association between daily habits and reflux episodes, and pH patterns unrepresentative of the individual patient's situation would be obtained [19].

Therefore, it is commonly recommended that the monitoring conditions should be as unrestricted as possible, with emphasis placed on allowing daily habits that replicate the patient symptoms [55]. However, an accurate diary is essential to recognize and control the effects of all variables (feeding, position, activities, etc.) during the recording period in order to avoid erroneous interpretation of results.

Traditionally, ambulatory pH recording is performed over a 24-h period, although a 18-h period, including a daily and nightly recording, was also suggested by the ESPGHAN working group on GER [55]. Although shorter recording times such as 3 h postprandially and 12 h or 16 h overnight have been proposed [3, 20, 32], the appropriateness of these reduced monitoring periods is questionable [5, 30].

Several reasons support the use of prolonged recordings (18 or 24 h): longer recordings optimize diagnostic

sensitivity, specificity, and reproducibility, without deterioration of acceptability and compliance [6]; with the modern dataloggers there is no additional requirement of a hospital stay; finally, in some conditions it is of crucial importance to document the temporal relationship between symptoms (particularly atypical symptoms) and reflux events.

12.2.9
Dual pH Monitoring

Current technology allows pH recording at multiple sites into the esophagus using single probes. These probes are similar in design to those with a single channel, offering similar comfort levels and patient tolerance. The most common multichannel pH recording probes are those with two separate monitoring sites at different distances (5, 10, 15 cm; Fig. 1).

Some authors suggest that *dual esophageal pH monitoring* is particularly useful in patients with atypical symptoms, such as otolaryngologic and pulmonary features, in which it is desirable to assess the propensity of the patients to aspirate [44, 50] (Fig. 2). However, most commonly, reflux events result in distal esophageal acidification without affecting the proximal pH, suggesting that the atypical symptoms can be elicited more by a reflex mechanism than by aspiration of the gastric contents into the upper respiratory tract [27]. Furthermore, the reproducibility of proximal pH monitoring is very low (~55%). Finally, some unclear phenomena referred to as "pseudo-reflux" (i.e. proximal acidification without concomitant distal acid exposure) are not satisfactorily explained [61]. It is commonly agreed that this type of recording is mainly confined to the research area and should not be recommended as a routine clinical

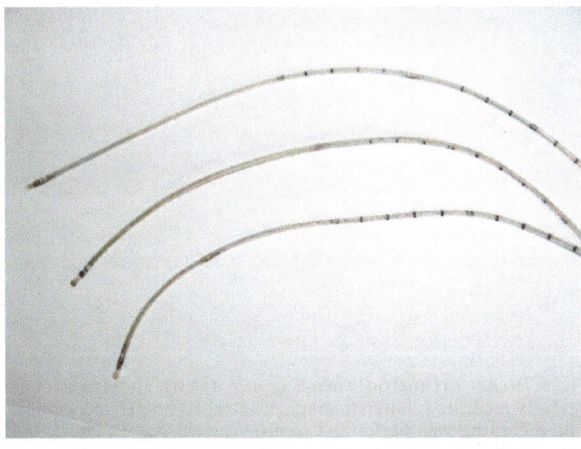

Fig. 1. Three thin (OD: 1.0 mm) flexible antimonial electrodes with recording electrodes spaced at variable distances (*from bottom to top*: 5 cm, 10 cm, and 15 cm apart)

Fig. 2.
Double pH-metric tracings.
The probe is positioned so that
the distal electrode records the
esophageal pH in the distal
esophagus above the lower
esophageal sphincter region,
whereas the proximal electrode records the intraesophageal proximal pH (at a site
10 cm proximally to the distal
electrode). The distal tracing
shows several clusters of GER
episodes; the proximal tracing
shows less frequent episodes of
GER. It is evident that a proportion of GER episodes occurring in the distal esophagus
are also recorded at the proximal site

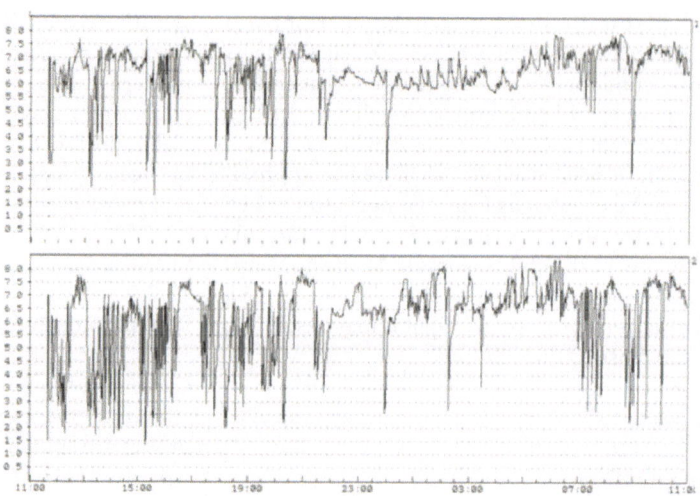

procedure without a strong validation through large trials [13, 23].

Combined gastric and esophageal pH monitoring has been proposed as the method of choice for investigating patients with GERD [21]. *Esophagogastric pH monitoring* provides a simultaneous assessment of esophageal and gastric pH profiles (Fig. 3). Some authors have emphasized its value in the diagnosis of the so called "non-acid" reflux, defined as an increase of at least 0.5 units in esophageal pH with simultaneous occurrence of a non-acid pH gastric profile [2]. "Non-acid" reflux is differentiated as "mixed reflux" and "alkaline reflux": the former is defined as the recording of both esophageal and gastric pH values between 4.0 and 7.0, with a difference between them equal to or lower than 0.5 pH units. The "alkaline reflux" is defined as the simultaneous recording of both esophageal and gastric pH above 7.0 [2]. Nevertheless, the significance of these findings obtained with the combined pH monitoring is unclear, and there is as yet no evidence that what is identified as "duodenogastric reflux" by the pH probe (i.e. an abrupt alkalinization of the stomach) truly corresponds to the reflux of intestinal juice into the stomach [36]. Thus, it is thought that pH monitoring cannot be reliably used for the diagnosis of alkaline reflux, because pH is a very poor indicator of the concentration of bile salts in the gastric content [26, 42]. However esophagogastric pH monitoring may be useful for interpreting negative esophageal pH monitoring (e.g. when it shows gastric anacidity) or for assessing the efficacy of a drug on gastric acid secretion. [24, 22]

12.3
Analysis

There are two major considerations in the analysis of pH recording: measurement of the degree of reflux, and the relationship between reflux episodes and patient symptoms.

12.3.1
Definition of Reflux Episodes

It is generally agreed that an episode of reflux starts whenever the distal esophageal pH falls below 4.0, generally accepted as the cutoff limit, for at least 15 s, and ends when the pH is restored to a value above 4.0 [55] (Fig. 4). There is no convincing evidence to suggest that any other cutoff limit is better than pH 4.0 [30]. If the pH drop under 4.0 occurs within 30 s after the previous episode has ended, it is not considered a reflux episode

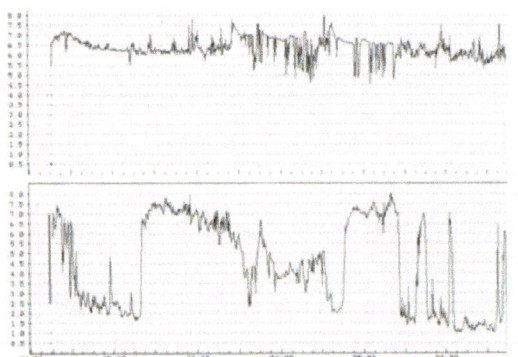

Fig. 3. Double pH-metric tracings (*upper* tracing, an intraesophageal pH recording; *lower* tracing, an intragastric pH recording). The recording was performed in a 6-year-old boy to check the antisecretory efficacy of a PPI drug. The intraesophageal tracing shows absence of significant GER episodes, whereas the intragastric tracing shows prolonged periods of an alkaline intragastric pH

Fig. 4.
The pH tracing shows an episode of gastroesophageal reflux as defined by pH-metric criteria. The reflux starts when the pH profile crosses the line of pH 4.0 (*black line* corresponding to the *left arrow*) and ends when the pH profile rises and crosses again the line of the pH 4.0 (*black line* corresponding to the *right arrow*). A short period of recording that is magnified by means of the analysis software is shown

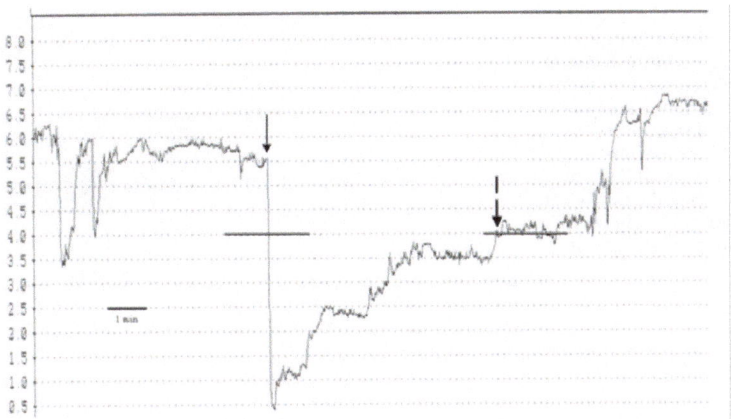

but a continuation of the previous one [4]. Some authors also define a reflux as any additional decrease of at least 1 pH unit or more during periods in which pH is less than 4.0.

12.3.2
Quantification of Degree of Reflux

With the development of computer facilities, excellent software packages are now available and most automated analysis systems are able to perform a large number of calculations, even though not all of these are necessary for the interpretation of the test.

The following parameters are usually analyzed:

1. Percentage of time during which pH is less than 4.0 (esophageal acid exposure time or reflux index);
2. Mean duration of reflux episodes (calculated by dividing reflux time by the number of reflux episodes);
3. Number of reflux episodes per 24 h;
4. Number of reflux episodes lasting more than 5 min per 24 h;
5. Longest episodes of reflux in minutes.

These values can be calculated for the total recording time, the time in the recumbent position, and the time in the upright position [16] (Figs. 5, 6).

There is a wide consensus to consider esophageal acid exposure as the best single determinant to discriminate normal subjects from patients with GERD [28, 48]. However, although this discriminant ability increases with the increasing degree of esophagitis, there is considerable overlap among subgroups of patients with reflux disease, particularly in those presenting with atypical symptoms and in those without endoscopic evidence of esophagitis [60]. The other variables usually measured (mean duration of reflux episodes, number of reflux episodes lasting more than 5 min, and total number of reflux episodes) are less reproducible; however, they give an estimate of the efficacy of the esophageal acid clearance [16].

The computed parameters previously considered do not take into account the degree of reflux episode acidity. Therefore, new parameters have been suggested, such as the area under pH 4.0 and the oscillatory index. The former evaluates the acidity of each reflux episode during its whole duration, and not only the minimal pH

Fig. 5.
pH tracing of a 24-h recording period. Clusters of numerous episodes of GER are evident in the postprandial period (*black vertical lines* indicate feeding time). A long-lasting episode of GER is also recorded during the nocturnal period (recording between 1:00 a.m. and 5: 00 a.m.)

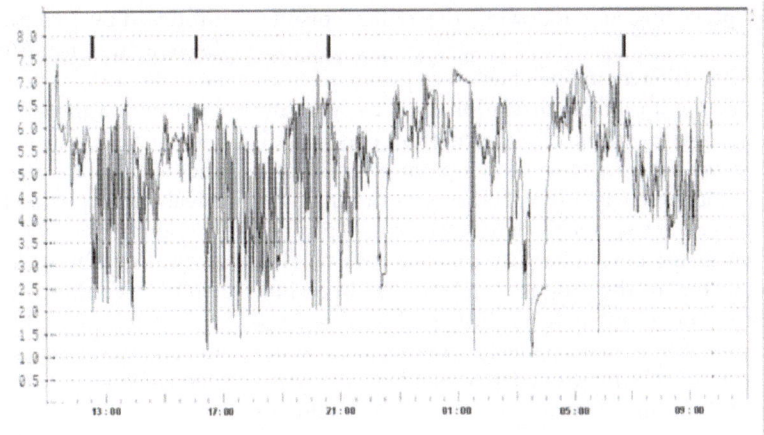

Fig. 6.
pH tracing showing a 24-h recording period. Clusters of numerous episodes of GER are evident in the postprandial period (*black vertical lines* indicate feeding time). No episodes of GER are recorded during the nocturnal period (recording between after 9:00 p.m. and shortly after 5:00 a.m.)

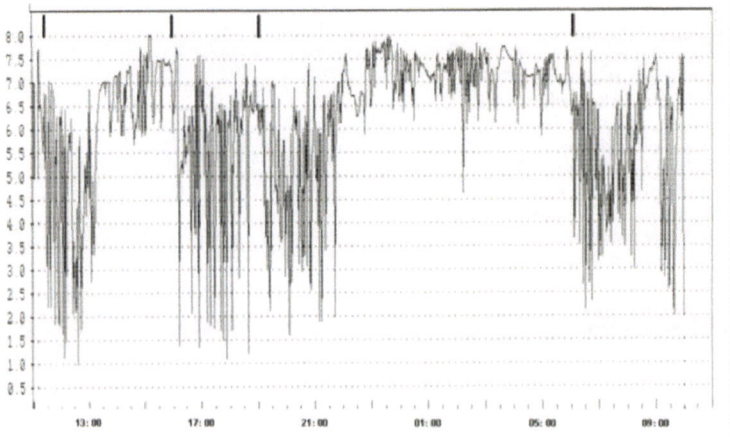

value obtained during that episode. The area under pH 4.0 could represent the real acid exposure of the distal esophagus and provide additional information on the severity of the disease [56]. The oscillatory index is a parameter which calculates the percentage of time in which the pH oscillates between the values of pH 4.25 and 3.75: it gives some idea of errors resulting from a fixed pH cutoff, and seems of great value in the "all-or-none" interpretation of the data, classified by computer with regard to a cutoff limit [57]. However, the general application of these parameters needs to be confirmed by further studies.

12.3.3
Symptom Analysis

Prolonged esophageal pH monitoring records not only the quantity of GER but also the temporal relationship between symptoms and reflux episodes. Symptom-reflux correlation is particularly important in patients presenting with atypical GER symptoms. Although strict criteria have not yet been defined, a symptom or event may be considered to be associated with GER if it occurs during the reflux episodes or within the 2-min periods preceding and following the reflux episodes [23].

In adults, different indexes have been proposed to assess the symptom-reflux correlation, such as symptom index (number of reflux-related symptom episodes divided by the total number of symptom episodes, expressed as a percentage) [60], and symptom sensitivity index (percentage symptom-associated reflux episodes, which evaluates the probability of relationship) [10]. However, none of the proposed indexes has been universally accepted, and none has been evaluated in a pediatric population. Most patients with atypical symptoms have a considerable overlap of esophageal acid exposure with healthy controls: in this group of patients

the quantitative results are probably less important than the evaluation of a relationship between pH changes and symptoms, obtained by a visual and qualitative assessment of the pH recording.

12.3.4
Reference Value

Before interpreting the recorded data and deciding whether a pathological reflux is present, it is of pivotal importance to define the upper limits of normality. The appropriate determination of normal values is essential for the sensitivity and specificity of the pH test and is the basis for determining whether a patient has an abnormal amount of acid reflux into the distal esophagus. Defining the upper limits of normal values as mean±SD is inappropriate, because pH data are typically skewed. Thus, a nonparametric method, such as the 95th percentile of the normal range or receiver operator curves, is more appropriate for choosing an optimal threshold that would discriminate between controls and patients [30, 45, 48]. Ideally, each center performing 24-h esophageal pH monitoring should use its own set of normal values. This is obviously difficult, and "normal" ranges proposed by one group could be used by another if the investigation is performed and interpreted in the same way. We suggest that those laboratories which have not determined their own normal range use the following cut-off points as acceptable upper "normal" limits for the routine diagnosis of GERD: (1) percentage of esophageal acid exposure time: 10% in infants, 5% thereafter; (2) number of reflux episodes: 80 in infants, 50 thereafter; (3) number of reflux episodes >5 min: eight in infants, three thereafter. These values represent the 95th percentiles (S. Cucchiara, personal data). The probe and the recording device which we routinely use have been described [9, 22].

12.4
Indications

In the diagnostic approach to GERD, esophageal pH monitoring is of value if the results will lead to a clinically important change in the management of patients [11]. The test is not necessary in all infants and children with suspected GERD. Generally, there is no indication for pH monitoring in children who regurgitate and/or vomit, and in whom the diagnosis can be made by combining of careful history and physical examination. After excluding other causes mimicking GERD, such as food allergy or infections, the children must be treated by choosing a therapy with the fewest side effects [46]. For most of these patients, esophageal pH monitoring would not change the therapeutic approach, whatever the pH analysis results are. If the child shows other symptoms suggesting a reflux esophagitis, endoscopic examination of the upper gastrointestinal tract is indicated [46]. Prolonged esophageal pH monitoring is not indicated in those patients with diagnosis of GERD through endoscopy and/or histology [11].

Thus, actually, the indications for prolonged pH monitoring are:

1. *Patients with unusual presentation of GERD.* Several studies provide evidence supporting the concept that acid reflux can induce extraintestinal clinical features, such as laryngeal symptoms, atypical chest pain, reactive airways disease, food refusal, dystonia, and recurrent chronic aspiration [40, 41, 49]. It has been shown that reflux may be the underlying cause in up to 20% of cases of apneic infants with no history of regurgitation [33], and in 2% of infants referred to an emergency room for acute, unexplained crying [43]. These conditions have other potential etiologies and may well coexist with GERD in an individual, without a causal relationship. Because it is of great clinical usefulness to establish such a causal relationship, the 24-h pH monitoring of the esophagus is of inestimable value in these conditions.

2. *Evaluation of GERD treatment.* Esophagogastric pH monitoring can be performed in order to assess the efficacy of a pharmacologic treatment of GER. In particular, the test may help in directing the optimal dose of antisecretory drugs [24].

3. *Pre- and postantireflux surgery.* Although esophageal pH monitoring should not be the sole indicator for surgery, it is one of the ways to document unresponsiveness of reflux to medical therapy. Prolonged pH recording could be a useful procedure in patient candidates for antireflux surgery [11]. The etiological role of GER and medical intractability should be reliably defined in order to avoid an unnecessary procedure. Prolonged pH monitoring is also indicated for the evaluation of patients with persistent or recurrent symptoms and suspected of having an ongoing abnormal reflux [34].

12.5
Limitations

One end of the GER spectrum is represented by physiological GER, occurring in healthy infants, and the other end is represented by pathological GER, occurring in children with endoscopic evidence of severe esophagitis. Between these two extremes, there is a variable degree of GER with or without associated esophagitis. In children with endoscopically and histologically documented reflux esophagitis, esophageal pH monitoring has been reported to have a diagnostic sensitivity of more than 90% [7]. This small discrepancy supports the view that a negative test might not exclude GER as the cause of the patient symptomatology [12]. Several mechanisms have been advocated: first, episodes of alkaline or "hypoacid" GER might be missed [23]; the increased flow of saliva that occurs after probe positioning can neutralize the acidity of the refluxed content, with a decrease in the esophageal exposure acid time [25]; in the first months of life a great intake of milk might neutralize gastric acidity [39]; finally, it is now well established that there is a substantial variability from day to day in the esophageal exposure to acid, determining a reproducibility rate of pH monitoring which varies from 70% to 95% [35]. Unfortunately, reproducibility is lowest in those patients with endoscopy negative GERD and in those with atypical symptoms, i.e. the groups in which esophageal pH monitoring is most applicable [44].

12.6
Conclusions

Prolonged pH monitoring may not be a true "gold" standard for identifying GERD. However, it is reasonably reliable as a diagnostic test once its limitations are understood. Although it has few clinical indications, prolonged pH monitoring remains the technique of choice whenever it is important to obtain objective evidence of both the amount of acid reflux and the relationship between symptoms and reflux episodes.

References

1. Anggiansah A, Sumboonnanonda K, Wang J et al (1993) Significantly reduced acid detection at 10 centimeters compared to 5 centimeters above lower esophageal sphincter in patients with acid reflux. Am J Gastroenterol 88:842–846
2. Baldi F, Longanesi A, Ferrarini F (1994). Combined gastric and esophageal pH-metry. Functional evaluation in esophageal disease. In: Modlin IR, Rozen P, Scarpignato C (eds) Frontiers of gastrointestinal research. Karger, Basel, pp 152–163
3. Barabino A, Costantini M, Ciccone MO et al (1995) Reliability of short-term esophageal pH monitoring versus 24-hour study. J Pediatr Gastroenterol Nutr 21:87–90
4. Bennett JR (1987) pH measurement in the oesophagus. Bailliere's Clin Gastroenterol 1:727–745

5. Bianchi Porro G, Pace F (1988) Comparison of three methods of intraesophageal pH recording in the diagnosis of gastroesophageal reflux. Scand J Gastroenterol 23:743–750

6. Bianchi Porro G, Pace F (1991) The role of continuous oesophageal pH monitoring in the diagnosis of gastro-oesophageal reflux. Eur J Gastroenterol Hepatol 3:501–509

7. Black DD, Haggitt RC, Orenstein SR et al (1990) Esophagitis in infants. Morphometric histological diagnosis and correlation with measures of gastroesophageal reflux. Gastroenterology 98:1408–1414

8. Boyle JT (1989) Gastroesophageal reflux in pediatric patient. Gastroenterol Clin North Am 18:315–338

9. Borrelli O, Cucchiara S, D'Armiento F et al (2003) Inflammation of the gastric cardia in children with symptoms of acid peptic disease. J Pediatr 143:520–524

10. Breumelhof R, Smout JPM (1991) The symptom sensitivity index: a valuable additional parameter in 24-hour esophageal pH monitoring. Am J Gastroenterol 86:160–164

11. Colletti RB, Christie DL, Orenstein SR (1995) Indications for pediatric esophageal pH monitoring: a medical position statement of North American Society for Pediatric Gastroenterology and Nutrition (NASPGN). J Pediatr Gastroenterol Nutr 21:253–262

12. Cucchiara S, Staiano A, Gobio Casali L et al (1990) Value of the 24 hour intraoesophageal pH monitoring in children. Gut 31:129–133

13. Cucchiara S, Santamaria F, Minella R et al (1995) Simultaneous prolonged recording of proximal and distal intraesophageal pH in children with gastroesophageal reflux disease and respiratory symptoms. Am J Gastroenterol 90:1791–1796

14. DeCaestecker JS, Blackwell JN, Pryde A et al (1987) Day-time gastro-oesophageal reflux is important in oesophagitis. Gut 28:519–526

15. Dent J, Holloway RH (1996) Esophageal motility testing and reflux testing. State of the art and clinical role in the twenty-first century. Gastroenterol Clin N Am 25:51–73

16. Dhiman RK, Saraswat VA, Naik SR (2002) Ambulatory esophageal pH monitoring. Technique, interpretations, and clinical indications. Dig Dis Sci 47:241–250

17. Emde C, Garner A, Blum AL (1987) Technical aspects of intraluminal pH metry in man: current status and recommendations. Gut 28:1177–1188

18. Emmerson AJB, Chant T, May J et al (2002) Assessment of three methods of pH probe positioning in preterm infants. J Pediatr Gastroenterol 35:69–72

19. Fass R, Hell R, Sampliner RE et al (1999) Effect of 24-hour esophageal pH monitoring on reflux-provoking activities. Dig Dis Sci 44:2263–2269

20. Fink SM, McCallum RW (1984) The role of prolonged esophageal pH monitoring in the diagnosis of gastroesophageal reflux. JAMA 252:1160–1164

21. Fiorucci S, Santucci L, Chiucchiu S et al (1992) Gastric acidity and gastroesophageal reflux patterns in patients with esophagitis. Gastroenterology 103:855–861

22. Franco MT, Salvia G, Terrin G et al (2000) Lansoprazole in the treatment of gastro-oesophageal reflux disease in children. Dig Dis Liv 32:660–666

23. Galmiche JP, Scarpignato C (1994) Esophageal pH monitoring. Functional evaluation in esophageal disease. In: Modlin IR, Rozen P and Scarpignato C (eds): Front Gastrointest Res. Karger, Basel, 71–108

24. Hassall E, Israel D, Shepherd R et al (2000) Omeprazole for treatment of chronic erosive esophagitis in children: a multicenter study of efficacy, safety, tolerability and dose requirements. J Pediatr 137:800–807

25. Helm JF, Dodds W, Hogan W et al (1982) Acid neutralizing capacity of human saliva. Gastroenterology 83:69–74

26. Hostein J, Bost R (1991) Intragastric pH monitoring is unsuitable for diagnosis of duodenogastric reflux. Dig Dis Sci 36:1341–1343

27. Jacob P, Kahrilas PJ, Herzon G (1991) Proximal esophageal pH-metry in patients with "reflux laryngitis." Gastroenterology 100:305–310

28. Jamieson JR, Stein HJ, DeMeester TR et al (1992) Ambulatory 24-h esophageal pH monitoring. Normal values, optima thresholds, specificity, sensitivity and reproducibility. Am J Gastroenterol 87:1102–1011

29. Johnson LF, DeMeester TF (1974) Twenty-four hour pH monitoring of the distal esophagus. A quantitative measure of gastroesophageal reflux. Am J Gastroenterol 62:325–332

30. Johnsson F, Joelsson B, Isberg PE (1987) Ambulatory 24-hour intra-esophageal pH monitoring in the diagnosis of gastroesophageal reflux disease. Gut 28:1145–1150

31. Jolley SG, Tunel WP, Carson JA et al (1984) The accuracy of abbreviated pH monitoring in children. J Pediatr Surg 19:848–853

32. Jorgensen F, Elsborg L, Hesse B (1988) The diagnostic value of computerized short-term esophageal pH monitoring in suspected gastroesophageal reflux. Scand J Gastroenterol 23:363–368

33. Kahn A, Rebuffat E, Franco P et al (1992) Apparent life-threatening events and apnea of infancy. In: Beckerman R, Brouilette R, Hunt C (eds) Respiratory control disorders in infants and children. William & Wilkins, Baltimore, pp 178–189

34. Kahrilas PJ, Quigley EMM (1996) Clinical esophageal pH recording: a technical review for practice guideline development. Gastroenterology 110:1982–1996

35. Mahajan L, Willie R, Oliva L et al (1998) Reproducibility of 24-hour intraesophageal pH monitoring in pediatric patients. Pediatrics 101:260–263

36. Mattioli S, Pilotti V, Felice V et al (1990) Ambulatory 24-hour pH monitoring of esophagus, fundus and antrum. A new technique for simultaneous study of gastroesophageal and duodenogastric reflux. Dig Dis Sci 35:929–938

37. Mattox HE, Richter JE (1990) Prolonged ambulatory esophageal pH monitoring in the evaluation of gastroesophageal reflux disease. Am J Med 89:345–356

38. McLauchlan G, Rawling JM, Lucas ML et al (1987) Electrodes for 24 hour pH monitoring – a comparative study. Gut 28:935–939

39. Mitchell DJ, McClure BG, Tubman TR (2001) Simultaneous monitoring of gastric and oesophageal pH reveal limitations of conventional oesophageal pH monitoring in milk fed infants. Arch Dis Child 84:273–276

40. Orenstein SR, Orenstein DM (1988) Gastroesophageal reflux and respiratory disease in children. J Pediatr 112:847–858

41. Orenstein SR, Kocoshis SA, Orenstein DM et al (1987) Stridor and gastroesophageal reflux: diagnostic use of intraluminal esophageal acid perfusion (Bernstein test). Pediatr Pulmonol 3:420–424

42. Penagini R, Yuen H, Misiewicz JJ et al (1988) Alkaline intraoesophageal pH and gastro-oesophageal reflux in patients with peptic oesophagitis. Scand J Gastroenterol 23:675–678

43. Poole S (1991) The infant with acute, unexplained and excessive crying. Pediatrics 88:450–455

44. Richter JE (1997) Ambulatory esophageal pH monitoring. Am J Med 103(5A):130S–134S

45. Richter JE, Bradley LA, DeMeester TR et al (1992) Normal 24-hour pH values. Influence of study center, pH electrodes, age and gender. Dig Dis Sci 37:849–856

46. Rudolph CD and the GER Guideline Committee of the North American Society for Pediatric Gastroenterology and Nutrition (NASPGN) (2001) Pediatric gastroesophageal reflux clinical practice guidelines. J Pediatr Gastroenterol Nutr 32(S2):1–31

47. Schofield PM, Bennett DH, Whornell PJ et al (1987) Exertional gastro-oesophageal reflux: a mechanism for symptoms in patients with angina pectoris and normal coronary angiograms. Br Med J 294:1459–1461

48. Schindlbeck NE, Heinrich C, Konig A et al (1987) Optimal threshold, sensitivity, and specificity of long term pH-metry for the detection of gastroesophageal reflux disease. Gastroenterology 93:85–90

49. Schmidt-Sommerfeld E (1994) Gastro-osesophageal reflux: presentation, evaluation and management. Bailliere's Clin Paediatr 2(4):767–785

50. Shaker R, Milbreath M, Ren J et al (1995) Esophagopharyngeal distribution of refluxed gastric acid in patients with reflux laryngitis. Gastroenterology 109:1575–1582

51. Song TJ, Kim YH, Ryu HS et al (1991) Correlation of esophageal lengths with measurable external parameters. Korean J Int Med 6:16–20
52. Spencer J (1969) Prolonged pH recording in the study of gastrooesophageal reflux. Br J Surg 56:9–12
53. Strobel CT, Bryne WJ, Ament M et al (1979) Correlation of esophageal length in children with height: application to the Tuttle test without prior esophageal manometry. J Pediatr 94:81–84
54. Vandenplas Y, Sacre-Smiths L (1985) Seventeen hour continuous esophageal monitoring in the newborns: evaluation of the influence of position in asymptomatic and symptomatic babies. J Pediatr Gastroenterol Nutr 4:356–361
55. Vandenplas and the working group of the ESPGAN (1992) A standardized protocol for the methodology of the esophageal pH monitoring and interpretation of the data for the diagnosis of gastroesophageal reflux. J Pediatr Gastroenterol Nutr 14:467–471
56. Vandenplas Y, Franckx-Goossens A, Pipeleers-Marichal M et al (1989) Area under pH 4: advantages of a new parameter in the interpretation of esophageal pH monitoring data in infants. J Pediatr Gastroenterol Nutr 8:31–36
57. Vandenplas Y, Lepoudre R, Helven R (1990) Dependability of esophageal pH monitoring data in infants on cut-off limits: the oscillatory index. J Pediatr Gastroenterol Nutr 11:304–309
58. Vandenplas Y, Helven R, Goyvaerts H (1991) A comparative study between glass and antimony electrodes for continuous oesophageal pH monitoring. Gut 32:708–712
59. Wiener GJ, Morgan TM, Cooper JB et al (1988) Ambulatory 24-hour esophageal pH monitoring. Reproducibility and variability of pH parameters. Dig Dis Sci 33:1127–1133
60. Wiener GJ, Richter JE, Cooper JB et al (1988) The symptom index: a clinically important parameter of ambulatory 24-hour esophageal pH monitoring. Am J Gastroenterol 83:358–361
61. Wiener GJ, Koufman JA, Wu WC, et al (1989) Chronic hoarseness secondary to gastroesophageal reflux disease. Documentation with 24-hour ambulatory pH monitoring. Am J Gastroenterol 84:1503–1508

Chapter 13

Gastroesophageal Endoscopy for the Diagnostic Evaluation of Infants with GER

13

Michèle Scaillon · Patrick Bontems · Samy Cadranel

Contents

In the pre-endoscopic era, evaluation of gastroesophageal reflux (GER) depended almost solely on black-and-white radiological imaging. Even without all the recent immense progress in medical imaging, radiology was able to deliver important information to the clinician such as the topographic situation of the gastroesophageal junction, hiatus hernia, gastric emptying, pyloric stenosis or intestinal malrotation. However, many borderline conditions could not be entirely and accurately assessed, and the clinician often remained frustrated, lacking the correct information about the mucosal involvement.

The introduction of fiberoptic endoscopes in pediatrics some thirty years ago [1–5] progressively but radically changed the evaluation of GER investigation in many conditions, especially in cases where gastrointestinal bleeding is present, which implies that a mucosal lesion will always be better detected by endoscopy than by any other "indirect visualization" means. In addition, biopsies for further study of microscopic lesions and endoscopic treatment have become possible.

Since GER is a very frequent (physiologic?) symptom in infants, it is obvious that not all infants presenting with GER need to undergo an endoscopic evaluation. Endoscopy and histology studies of biopsies have become some of the key tools used to distinguish between the vast majority of infants with GER from those at risk

of a gastroesophageal reflux disease (GERD). Considerable progress has been achieved in the miniaturization of endoscopes, handiness, optical qualities, and remote recording, and also in the field of sedation and anesthesia. The availability of instruments that can be used at any age, ranging from the slimmest 6-mm outer diameter "neonatoscope" to the standard 9-mm standard gastroscopes, has enabled pediatric gastroenterology to deal more easily with the diagnosis of any kind of disease involving the mucosa. An endoscopic investigation should be, whenever possible, completed by systematic biopsies, even when the mucosa looks apparently normal: microscopic lesions can be present without gross macroscopic changes, and many diagnoses can be missed if a comprehensive histology study is not performed. In addition, modern video-endoscopes greatly facilitate teamwork and training and have probably played an important role in allowing exchange and communication and setting of common criteria.

The remarkable progress in sedation and anesthesiology has made the investigation easier than in the early days of endoscopy. The endoscopist is therefore able to perform a safer procedure with less stressful conditions and less discomfort and risk of complications and side effects for the patient.

13.1
Indications

In 1994, a statement by a working group on gastroesophageal reflux disease of the European Society of Paediatric Gastroenterology and Nutrition recommended upper gastrointestinal (GI) endoscopy as the technique of choice in infants and children presenting with symptoms suggestive of reflux esophagitis [6] In 1996, the North American Society for Pediatric Gastroenterology and Nutrition issued a similar medical position. Indications for GI endoscopy include persistent refusal to eat, suspected esophageal or other pain during feeds, and follow-up of mucosal abnormalities. Endoscopy is recognized as the most sensible tool to discover mucosal abnormalities and to offer tissue diagnosis. It is not indicated for uncomplicated GER or X-ray findings of uncomplicated GER [7].

13.1.1
Symptoms of Overt GER

13.1.1.1
GI Bleeding

Frank bleeding such as hematemesis or nasogastric aspiration of fresh or old blood is indicative of an upper origin of gastrointestinal bleeding. In infants, melena or a hematochesia, despite a negative gastric aspirate, can also be linked to upper GI bleeding. Unless a clear clinical or biological explanation is evident, such alarm symptoms are strong indications for an upper GI endoscopy. In the newborn, suspected GI bleeding can be due to swallowed maternal blood and should be ruled out by the Apt test. It is based on the denaturation, in an alkaline milieu, of adult hemoglobin to a yellow-brown solution of alkaline globin hematin, whereas fetal hemoglobin resists and is colored pink.

The routine aspiration with a nasogastric tube may cause traumatic lesions and consequently moderate and self-limited bleeding. Hypovitaminosis K-related hemorrhage should be promptly ruled out before any endoscopy. In infants, it is important to be ready to perform the endoscopy using only specific equipment adapted to the size of the patient, whose hemodynamic conditions have been correctly stabilized.

Feeding tubes could produce two kinds of esophageal damage in very young infants: traumatic damage, and increased risk of reflux and consequently of esophagitis [8]. However, peptic esophagitis is not the only cause of GI bleeding. The development of safe endoscopy in neonates led to the identification of the occurrence of severe esophageal and gastric lesions in the first days of life even in asymptomatic newborns [9]. In a series of 5,180 full-term infants, 1.23% had upper GI bleeding within 26±20 h of life, and 24/53 who underwent an endoscopy presented with esophagitis; the origin of this esophagitis remains unclear [10].

13.1.1.2
Typical Symptoms

In infants, regurgitations are, in most cases, almost physiologic: several epidemiological studies insist on the frequency of this manifestation of overflow in the first year of life and that, in the vast majority of cases, it has a favorable outcome. In 50% of 0- to 3-month-old infants, at least one regurgitation is observed daily, and this frequency peaks at 67% of the 4-month-old infants and decreases dramatically to only 5% of those 12 months old

[11] (Fig. 1). Infants who vomit once a day outgrow the problem without treatment by 18 to 24 months [12].

The symptom "regurgitation" becomes even more rare after the first year of life and tends to be replaced by other symptoms such as pain or respiratory diseases, and can occur in older infants with or without a history of regurgitation. The long-term outcome is less benign, and some of these patients present with an undoubted chronic disease needing a careful follow-up [13].

The highest prevalence of "distressing" regurgitations in infants prompting the parents to seek advice occurs around the sixth month of life. The parents' anxiety is due to the frequency, the volume, and symptoms of discomfort or pain. Vomiting carries a more severe prognosis: once evident causes such as infections, obstructions, intracranial hypertension, and even metabolic diseases have been ruled out, cardial incompetence but also gastric outlet obstruction need a thorough work-up, in which endoscopy plays an important role.

A questionnaire based on the frequency and severity of certain symptoms such as regurgitations, refusal to eat, ceasing eating even when hungry, excessive crying or fussing, hiccups, arching back and also breathing difficulties and turning blue was recently validated and proposed to diagnose GERD without any complementary investigations [14]. A score of 16 on this questionnaire is consistent with the diagnosis of GERD and indicates the need for medication treatment after unsuccessful dietetic measures: it seems obvious that, in these circumstances, there is no need to demonstrate a GER that is clearly seen clinically [15]. However, a careful follow-up is needed, as some conditions could mimic

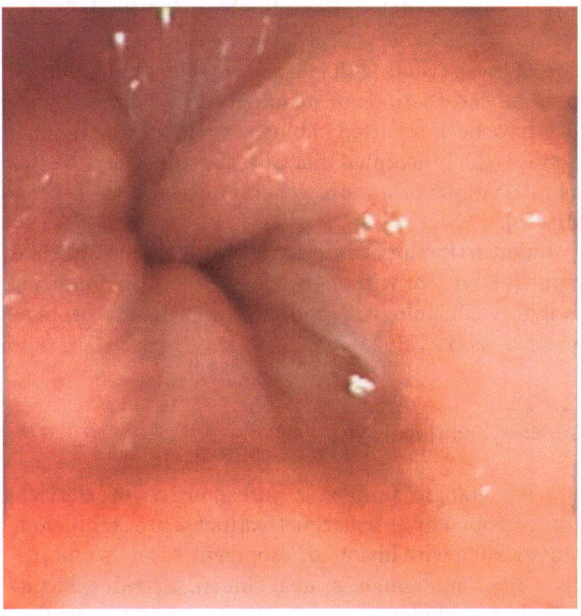

Fig. 1. Normal esophagus with a well-delineated Z-line

GERD and will not respond to the treatments prescribed currently. In our opinion, endoscopy can be particularly helpful in investigating a nonesophageal cause of reflux, showing a morphologic anomaly or a nonpeptic inflammation caused by allergy, infection, or any other reason, for instance eosinophilic esophagitis.

Anti-H2 receptor blockers and PPIs are increasingly being prescribed as primary treatments. This policy, very common for adult patients, needs careful systematic clinical evaluation and early investigation of the etiology in case of failure. Caution is needed whenever these treatments are prolonged, because little is known about the long-term effects in children [16–17].

On the other hand, esophagitis can be the cause of other symptoms such as iron-deficiency anemia, and endoscopy is the only reliable investigation explaining the underlying mechanism. Since early measures of prevention have been implemented for GER, peptic esophageal stenosis has become rare. It is still observed in children from socioeconomically depressed migrant families and in mentally retarded neurologically impaired children. Endoscopy is obviously the most suitable technique to explore and treat such lesions.

13.1.2
Atypical Symptoms Possibly Related To GER

Several symptoms are qualified as "atypical" or described in association with silent GERD. Among them are atypical loss of dental enamel, which is beyond the scope of this chapter devoted to infant GERD.

Numerous studies on the possible relation between GER and other major events such as ALTEs (acute-life-threatening-events), apneas, bradycardia, fussing, and crying are controversial in proving a straight correlation of these events with episodes of GER, and although in some cases lesions of histologically proven esophagitis have been reported in biopsy or autopsy material, it is more widely accepted that GER and apnea may be two manifestations of a more general developmental delay [18–20].

Infant irritability or discomfort has been associated with GER with or without esophagitis and an abnormal esophageal histology, sometimes with a normal esophageal pH-metry [21, 22].

13.1.2.1
Ear, Nose, and Throat Symptoms

Otolaryngologic problems unresponsive to classical antimicrobial or antiallergic treatments are significantly associated with histologic esophagitis and asthma, recurrent croup, cough, apnea, sinusitis, stridor, laryngomalacia, subglottic stenosis, posterior glottic erythema, and edema [23].

13.1.2.2
Bronchopulmonary Diseases

GER occurs more frequently in asthmatic children than in the general population. The issues regarding GER increasing bronchial obstruction and GER being a parallel phenomenon remain controversial. The different hypotheses are that acid micro-aspirations produce either bronchospasms or vagally transmitted reflex or, more probably, are coexisting phenomena. Refluxed gastric material aspirated into the lungs is an important cause of acute and chronic pulmonary disease. Currently, pulmonary contamination is rarely seen during esophageal scintigraphy, and the presence of fat-laden macrophages in tracheobronchial secretions of children, a conventional marker for reflux aspiration, is limited by its apparent lack of specificity [24].

Much remains to be learned about the developmental aspects of these supraesophageal manifestations of GER; further knowledge will provide a greater understanding of developmental pathophysiology, and will improve the clinical care of many infants [25].

In most studies, diagnosis of GER is based essentially on prolonged pH monitoring, where a negative result cannot completely and reliably rule out the responsibility of GER in the symptoms observed. Criteria of pH-metry are based on detecting an acid aggression and do not take into account the mechanical, physical, or chemical (other than acidity) effect of the refluxate. The rare studies using impedancemetry, a promising new technique not yet entirely available for routine clinical practice, show that GER seems much more frequent than is detected by pH-metry, although the results do not answer all of our questions [26]. In addition, in the expectation of more data from impedancemetry, aero-digestive tract endoscopy remains a valuable and reliable technique for infants [27].

In the end, in the face of a sufficient body of evidence, it is the effectiveness of the antireflux treatment which will make it possible to establish a link between GER and the supraesophageal manifestations observed [28]. We believe that these many unanswered questions about the relationship between some supraesophageal symptoms and GER could usefully promote prospective studies based on systematic endoscopy and histology. These extra data could enable a better understanding of the role of GER and consequently improve the therapeutic management of these atypical symptoms.

13.1.3
Followup of Therapeutic Medical or Surgical Measures

Pathological reflux in children is often associated with the presence of only mild esophageal inflammation that seems unlikely to deteriorate. Therefore, an endoscopic check-up could be limited to cases with severe esophagitis [29]. In contrast, systematic and more frequent surveillance should be applied to children with severe respiratory diseases such as bronchodysplasia and mucoviscidosis, even before the development of severe respiratory problems, because pathologically increased reflux can be present before radiological lung disease is established and, most frequently, no useful clinical predictors of pathological reflux are to be found [30–31].

13.1.3.1
Neurological Symptoms

Findings of esophagitis due to GER are frequent in children with brain damage and are related to significant complications, including fatal course. Children with brain damage and other neuromuscular diseases should be systematically investigated (including endoscopically) in view of detecting GER that may cause anorexia, pain, anemia, and bronchial inhalation of reflux material. These complications aggravate and deteriorate the poor quality of life of these patients [32].

13.1.3.2
Fundoplicature

After surgical antireflux operations, a systematic regular check-up, at least one year after operation, is recommended for the evaluation of long-term results. Even in the absence of symptoms, endoscopy can show a defective wrap or esophagitis, indicating starting of early treatment [33–34].

13.1.3.3
Esophageal Atresia

Infants undergoing an esophageal atresia repair frequently suffer from esophageal dismotility and GER as well as lung dysplasia complicated by several long-term respiratory complications during infancy, and they are at high risk of severe GERD esophagitis and stenosis. A systematic endoscopic followup during childhood is necessary [35–36].

13.2
Diagnosis

In adults, the role of diagnostic testing in reflux disease is in evolution. There is little question that patients with dysphagia, bleeding, or other "alarm" symptoms should undergo early endoscopy. A substantial proportion of patients presenting with reflux symptoms have endoscopy-negative reflux disease. pH testing lacks the sensitivity and specificity required for a "gold standard," and

empirical trials of therapy using PPIs have shown that this "therapeutic trial" approach may be the most cost-effective strategy [37].

However, such a strategy is most inconvenient in children and even more so in infants: is a life-long treatment advisable? A motion that "all patients with GERD should be offered endoscopy once in a lifetime" was recently discussed, including its pros and cons [38–39]. Those authors debated the relative importance of endoscopy in adult patients, concerning Barrett's esophagus (BE) and its severe complications. Although BE does not occur infancy and although many so-called cases of BE lack a convincing histologic demonstration, the pediatrician should be aware of the possibility of later development of such a consequence of GERD [16, 29, 42].

13.2.1
Endoscopic Findings

The endoscopic characteristics of reflux esophagitis in children are graded on a scale from 0 to 5, in which grade 0 represents the normal appearance of esophageal mucosa, grades 1 and 2 are subjective mucosal changes such as patchy or linear erythema, edema, and vertical lines, Grade 3 corresponds to the presence of erosions, grade 4 to that of ulcerations, and grade 5 to that of stricture [40].

This classification clearly shows the limitations of endoscopy alone, because of its low sensitivity and specificity for the diagnosis of reflux esophagitis in children, particularly regarding grades 0 to 2. Unusual but classic lesions, such as an inflammatory polyp fold complex at the junction often in continuity with a prominent gastric fold, are associated with reflux esophagitis.

However, biopsy alone can be misleading, since the tiny samples are not always easy to process and to interpret. Performing an upper GI endoscopy in infants is always a delicate procedure, whether the child is heavily sedated or under general anesthesia: only adapted slim endoscopes should be used, and this has become easier since all manufacturers now have such instruments available in their catalog. The advantage of endoscopy resides in the fact that it can provide information concerning not only the extension of the possible lesions but also the movements of the distal esophagus in relation to the diaphragm. It is important to determine whether there are no obstacles in the upper part of the esophagus, and then concentrate on its distal part. The topography of the diaphragmatic ring and the Z-line should be evaluated (a few forceful respiratory movements imposed by the anesthetist can help in locating correctly the diaphragmatic ring) (Fig. 1). Severe hiatus hernia is not difficult to recognize, whereas cardial incompetence requires a good evaluation of the adaptation of the cardial "sphincter" muscle to the shaft of the endoscope. This is better assessed in the U-turn position when the cardial orifice is seen from the gastric cavity (Figs. 2, 3). This position also allows identification of the His angle, which is usually weakly marked in infants in the first months of life but grows progressively during the first year.

A stricture due to reflux esophagitis appears as a white annular infundibular narrowing with a central lumen surrounded by actively inflamed or pale mucosa

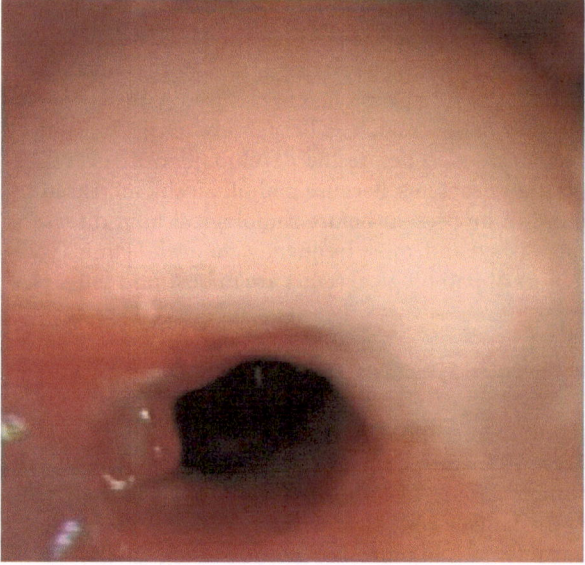

Fig. 4. Stenosis complicating a peptic esophagitis

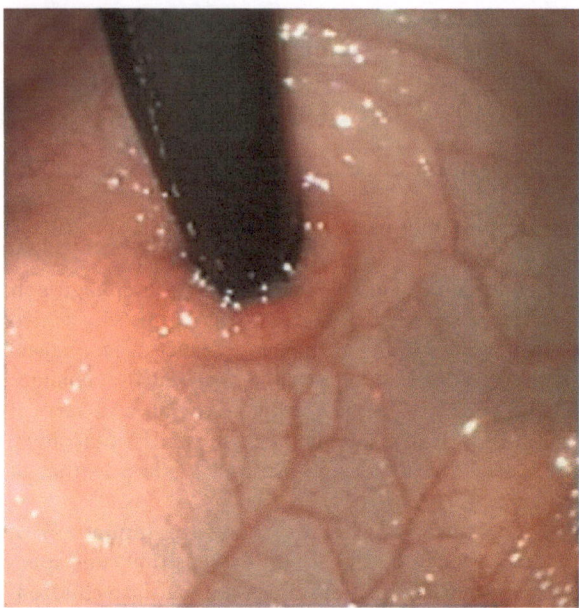

Fig. 2. Retrovision of the cardia from the gastric cavity: normal continence

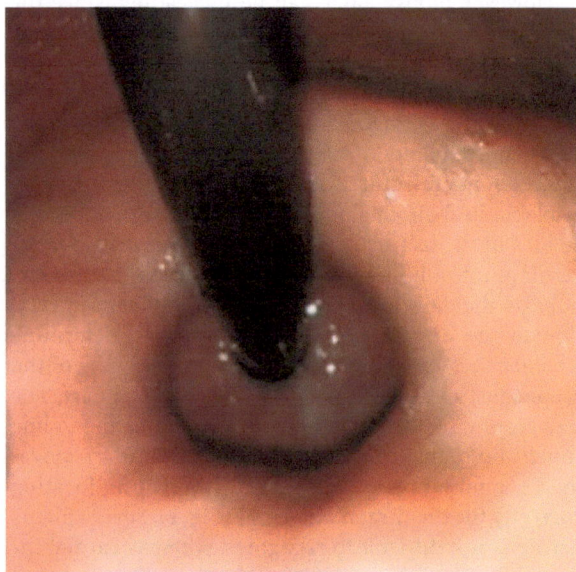

Fig. 3. Hiatus hernia

(Fig. 4). It is usually short and located in the distal esophagus, except in repaired esophageal atresia. Currently the development of such peptic strictures has become very rare, at least in the industrialized world, where much attention has been put on the prevention such complications of untreated GERD. Currently infants with GER are precociously treated with dietetic or postural measures, and recourse to medical treatments such as prokinetics and, more recently, anti-H2 receptor blockers or PPIs is recommended as soon as the former measures prove ineffective. In our routine medical practice we insist on performing a comprehensive investigation, including an endoscopy, before introducing any of these potent drugs, which need further evaluation before being used on a long-term basis in children [16].

13.2.2
Biopsies

13.2.2.1
Technique and Grading

One of the main goals and benefits of endoscopy is the opportunity to take target biopsies for histological confirmation of esophagitis or other esophageal involvement.

Grasp biopsies offer the advantage of being endoscopically guided. However proper material can sometimes be difficult to obtain from strongly adherent inflamed mucosa, and the samples are usually minute and tangential. Suction biopsies are deeper and more suitable for morphometric studies, but lack the endoscopic

Table 1. Grading of esophagitis according to histologic changes

Grade	Histologic criteria	Diagnosis
0	Normal	Normal
1a	Basal zone hyperplasia	Reflux
1b	Elongation stromal papillae	
1c	Vascular ingrowth	
2	Polymorphonuclear cells (epithelium and/or lamina propria)	Esophagitis
3	Polymorphs with epithelial defect	
4	Ulceration	
5	Aberrant columnar epithelium	

advantage of a reliable, comprehensive investigation and the possibility of targeting the right areas.

Endoscopic grading is based on the description of lesions; it may be difficult to be objective in this grading. Classification based on mixed endoscopic aspect and pathological findings drawn from classical criteria but adapted to the particular needs of infants and children has been proposed [6] (Table 1).

13.2.2.2
Interpretation

There has been some controversy in the literature about the usefulness of biopsies during esophageal endoscopies whether with a normal aspect, suspicion of esophagitis, and even frank erosive lesions [41] (Fig. 5).

Histology studies on biopsy material are recognized as useful for supporting the diagnosis of GERD but not for grading the severity of esophagitis or diagnosing

nonreflux disease entities [42]. Thickness of epithelium, basal zone thickness, and papillary length show increased epithelial cell turnover. Eosinophils, neutrophils, and "balloon cells" were observed only in patients with GER, thus serving as specific markers of this disease [43]. Cells with irregular nuclear contours and with the immunohistochemical profile of T-lymphocytes have been observed in significantly higher numbers in adults and young children patients with GERD [44–45].

Esophageal grasp biopsies taken at the time of endoscopy are of value in the assessment of patients with suspected reflux esophagitis. In a study of 113 infants aged 2–18 months with clinically significant GER, endoscopy was found to be highly specific (93%) for histological esophagitis but lacked sensitivity (25%). Intraepithelial lymphocytes were the earliest of the histological features noted and were present before 4 months of age. The numbers of intraepithelial eosinophils and lymphocytes and the presence of papillary elongation all increased with age [46].

Since 1982, intraepithelial eosinophilic infiltration has been considered to be due to a peptic aggression, and intraepithelial eosinophils are the most common and useful histologic criterion [47]. Eosinophils are easily identified, even in poorly oriented grasp biopsies. Recent studies of patients with symptoms of vomiting, regurgitation, or pain who do not respond to antireflux therapy, only to amino-acid based diets or steroids, suggest immunologic or allergic mechanisms [48]. In these patients, the eosinophilic infiltration is more severe than in patients with GER, and a count of more than seven eosinophils per field is predictive of an unsuccessful outcome of antireflux therapy in 86% of the cases [49].

Culture of biopsy samples for germs can yield an etiologic infectious diagnosis in otherwise endoscopically unspecific esophagitis, and subsequently guide the treatment. These conditions are mainly found in immunodepressed or oncologic patients [50].

Immunohistochemical studies based on the number of intraepithelial CD3+, CD25+, IL2 receptor, ICAM+, HLA-DR+, and mucosal mast cells appear useful in supporting the histological diagnosis of gastroesophageal reflux disease [51].

13.2.3
Alternative Techniques

Radiographic imaging of the upper GI tract is useful to diagnose anatomic abnormalities that cause symptoms similar to those observed in GERD such as obstacles (esophageal or antral webs, pyloric stenosis) and outlet total or partial obstructions such as in malrotation [52–53].

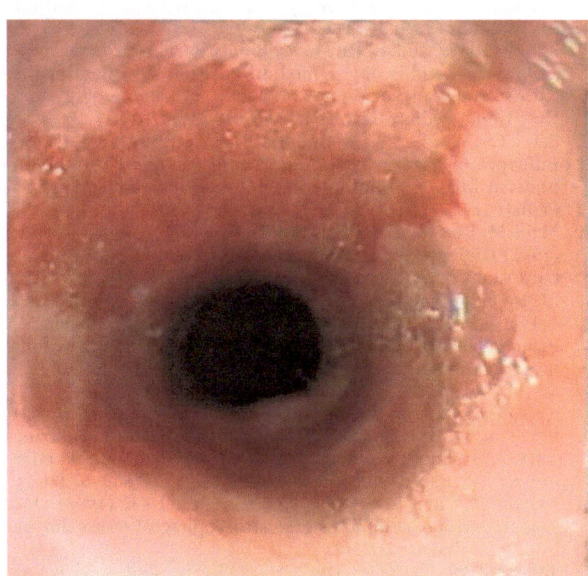

Fig. 5. Extensive esophagitis

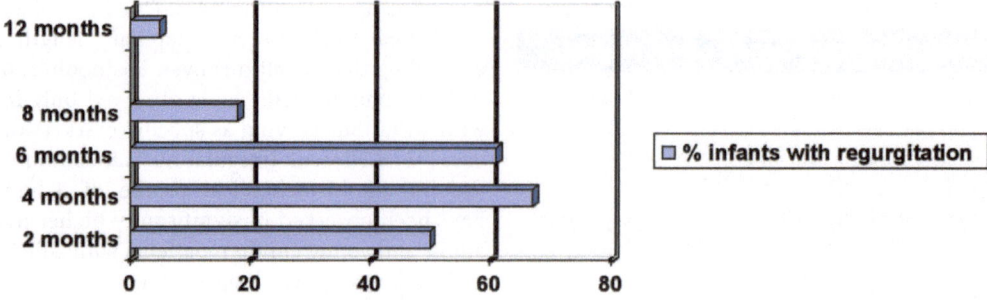

Fig. 6. Frequency of infants presenting with daily regurgitation according to age

Continuous 24-h esophageal pH monitoring has become a popular technique in pediatrics. Its role in GERD is, in our opinion, limited since it is unnecessary in overt GER. Its usefulness is mainly due to the detection of otherwise unsuspected GER in atypical symptoms, but it lacks sensitivity for the prediction of esophagitis. However, it remains a valuable tool for the assessment of the efficacy of an ongoing medical treatment.

Nuclear scintigraphy is based on the monitoring, up to 1 h, of episodes of GER following a normal feeding with an isotope-labeled formula. Less invasive than any of the other techniques of detection of GER, it has the important disadvantage of evaluating a period of time in which GER may occur in normal individuals [54].

Another noninvasive technique, ultrasonography of the gastroesophageal junction, also performed after a normal feeding, can show episodes of reflux. However, this elegant but time-consuming technique is extremely dependent on the motivation and skill of the echographist and does not answer many of the questions needed to distinguish between GER and GERD.

13.3
Conclusion

The role of gastroesophageal endoscopy in the diagnostic evaluation of infants with GER is an important one, as long as some rigorous guidelines are followed:
- Use of adapted miniaturized equipment
- Experienced, well-trained endoscopist
- Proper sedation or general anesthesia
- Careful monitoring of the gastric gas distension
- Comprehensive upper GI tract examination
- Proper checking of clotting factors
- Systematic biopsies at different levels
- Reliable pathology studies

It should be available in all pediatric gastroenterology units that deal with GERD or serve as referral centers for pediatricians confronted with the sometimes difficult decision to distinguish between GER and GERD. Fi-

nally, in many conditions, gastroesophageal endoscopy allows the clinician to go straight to the heart of the matter and avoid many other unnecessary and useless investigations of the patient.

References

1. Cremer M, Peeters JP, Emonts P, Rodesch P, Cadranel S (1974) Fiberendoscopy of the GI tract in children. Experience with newly designed fiberscopes. Endoscopy 6:18–19
2. Mougenot JF, Montagne JP, Faure C (1976) GI fibro-endoscopy in infants and children: radio-fibroscopic correlations. Ann Radiol 19:23–34
3. Cadranel S, Rodesch P, Peeters JP, Cremer M (1977) Fiberendoscopy of the GI tract in children. A series of 100 examinations. Amer J Dis Child 131:41-45
4. Ament ME, Christie DL (1977) Upper GI fiberoptic endoscopy in pediatric patients. Gastroenterology 72:1244–1248
5. Liebman WM (1977) Fiberoptic endoscopy of GI tract in infants and children. Amer J Gastroenterol 68:362–366
6. Vandenplas Y (1994) Reflux esophagitis in infants and children: a report from the Working Group on Gastro-Oesophageal Reflux Disease of the European Society of Paediatric Gastroenterology and Nutrition. J Pediatr Gastroenterol Nutr 18:413–422
7. Squires RH Jr, Colletti RB (1996) Indications for pediatric gastrointestinal endoscopy: a medical position statement of the North American Society for Pediatric Gastroenterology and Nutrition. J Pediatr Gastroenterol Nutr 23:107–110
8. Peter CS, Wiechers C, Bohnhorst B, Silny J, Poets CF (2002) Influence of nasogastric tubes on gastroesophageal reflux in preterm infants: a multiple intraluminal impedance study. J Pediatr 141:277–279
9. Maki M, Ruuska T, Kuusela AL, Karikoski-Leo R, Ikonen RS (1993) High prevalence of asymptomatic esophageal and gastric lesions in preterm infants in intensive care. Crit Care Med 21:1863–1867
10. Lazzaroni M, Petrillo M, Tornaghi R, Massironi E, Sainaghi M, Principi N, Porro GB (2002) Upper GI bleeding in healthy full-term infants: a case-control study. Am J Gastroenterol 97: 89–94
11. Nelson SP, Chen EH, Syniar GM, Christoffel KK (1997) Prevalence of symptoms of gastroesophageal reflux during infancy. A pediatric practice-based survey. Pediatric Practice Research Group. Arch Pediatr Adolesc Med 151:569–572
12. Nelson SP, Chen EH, Syniar GM, Christoffel KK (1998) One year followup of symptoms of gastroesophageal reflux during infancy. Pediatrics 102:E67
13. Tolaymat N, Chapman DM (1998) Gastroesophageal reflux disease in children older than two years of age. W V Med J 94: 22–25

14. Orenstein SR, Cohn JF, Shalaby TM, Kartan R (1993) Reliability and validity of an infant gastroesophageal reflux questionnaire. Clin Pediatr (Phila) 32:472–484
15. Kleinman L, Revicki D, Rothman ML (2003). Final report: infant gastroesophageal reflux questionnaire revised (I-GERD-R). Validation study final report. MEDTAP International, Bethesda, MD
16. Scaillon M, Cadranel S (2002) Safety data required for proton-pump inhibitor use in children. J Pediatr Gastroenterol Nutr 35:113–118
17. Laine L, Ahnen D, McClain C, Solcia E, Walsh JH (2000) Potential gastrointestinal effects of long-term acid suppression with proton pump inhibitors. Aliment Pharmacol Ther 14:651–668
18. Heine RG, Jaquiery A, Lubitz L, Cameron DJ, Catto-Smith AG (1995) Role of gastro-oesophageal reflux in infant irritability. Arch Dis Child 73:121–125
19. Suys B, De Wolf D, Hauser B, Blecker U, Vandenplas Y (1994) Role of gastro-esophageal reflux in infant irritability. J Pediatr Gastroenterol Nutr 19:187–190
20. Laukka MA, Cameron AJ, Schei AJ (1994) Gastroesophageal reflux and chronic cough: which comes first? J Clin Gastroenterol 19:100–104
21. Feranchak AP, Orenstein SR, Cohn JF (1994) Behaviors associated with onset of gastroesophageal reflux episodes in infants. Prospective study using split-screen video and pH probe. Clin Pediatr (Phila) 33:654–662
22. Heine RG, Cameron DJ, Chow CW, Hill DJ, Catto-Smith AG (2002) Esophagitis in distressed infants: poor diagnostic agreement between esophageal pH monitoring and histopathologic findings. J Pediatr 140:14–19
23. Yellon R, Coticchia J, Dixit S (2000) Esophageal biopsy for the diagnosis of gastroesophageal reflux associated otolaryngologic problems in children. Am J Med 180(Suppl 4a):S131–S138
24. Krishnan U, Mitchell JD, Tobias V, Day AS, Bohane TD (2002) Fat laden macrophages in tracheal aspirates as a marker of reflux aspiration: a negative report. J Pediatr Gastroenterol Nutr 35:309–313
25. Orenstein SR (2001) An overview of reflux-associated disorders in infants: apnea, laryngospasm, and aspiration. Am J Med 111(Suppl 8A):S60–S63
26. Wenzl TG, Schenke S, Peschgens T, Silny J, Heimann G, Skopnik H (2001) Association of apnea and nonacid gastroesophageal reflux in infants: investigations with the intraluminal impedance technique. Pediatr Pulmonol 31:144–149
27. Ungkanont K, Friedman EM, Sulek M (1998) A retrospective analysis of airway endoscopy in patients less than 1-month old. Laryngoscope 108(11 Pt 1):1724–1728
28. Sondheimer J (2002) Expanding the definition of GE reflux. J Ped Gastroenterol Nutr 34:511–512
29. Ashorn M, Ruuska T, Karikoski R, Laippala P (2002) The natural course of gastro-esophageal reflux disease in children. Scand J Gastroenterol 37:638–641
30. Heine RG, Button BM, Olinsky A, Phelan PD, Ctto-Smith AG (1998) Gastro-oesophageal reflux in infants under 6 months with cystic fibrosis. Arch Dis Child 78:44–48
31. Vic P, Tassin E, Turck D, Gottrand F, Launay V, Farriaux JP (1995) Frequency of gastro-esophageal reflux in infants and in young children with cystic fibrosis. Arch Pediatr 2:742–746
32. Gustafsson PM, Tibbling L (1994) Gastro-oesophageal reflux and oesophageal dysfunction in children and adolescents with brain damage. Acta Paediatr 83:1081–1085
33. Waag KL, Heller K, Eberhard R (1998) Long-term outcome after surgical treatment of gastro-esophageal reflux in infancy and childhood. Langenbecks Arch Chir Suppl Kongressbd 115:212–214
34. Guarino N, Ceriati E, Zaccara A, La Sala E, De Peppo F, Dall'Oglio L, Rivosecchi M (2002) Is endoscopic follow-up needed in pediatric patients who undergo surgery for GERD? Gastrointest Endosc 55:387–389
35. Somppi E, Tammela O, Ruuska T, Rahnasto J, Laitinen J, Turjanmaa V, Jarnberg J (1998) Outcome of patients operated on for esophageal atresia: 30 years' experience. J Pediatr Surg 33:1341–1346
36. Soto MC, Rivilla F, Dorado MJ, Rueda S, Balboa F, Casillas JG (2000) Pneumopathy in patients surgically treated for type 3 esophageal atresia. Cir Pediatr 13:136–140
37. Vakil N (2003) Review article: test and treat or treat and test in reflux disease? Aliment Pharmacol Ther 17(Suppl 2):57–59
38. Armstrong D (2002) Motion–all patients with GERD should be offered once in a lifetime endoscopy: arguments for the motion. Can J Gastroenterol 16:549–551
39. Freston JW (2002) Motion–all patients with GERD should be offered once in a lifetime endoscopy: arguments against the motion Can J Gastroenterol 16:555–558
40. Boyle JT (1989) Gastroesophageal reflux in the pediatric patients. Gastroenterol Clin North Am 18:315–337
41. Vandenplas Y (1996) Reflux esophagitis: biopsy or not? J Pediatr Gastroenterol Nutr 22:326–327
42. Hassall E (1996) Macroscopic versus microscopic diagnosis of reflux esophagitis: erosions or eosinophils? J Pediatr Gastroenterol Nutr 22:321–325
43. Mader AM, Alves MT, Kawakami E, Patricio FR (2002) Reflux esophagitis in children: histological and morphometric study. Arq Gastroenterol 39:126–131
44. Cucchiara S, D'Armiento F, Alfieri E, Insabato L, Minella R, De Magistris TM, Scoppa A (1995) Intraepithelial cells with irregular nuclear contours as a marker of esophagitis in children with gastroesophageal reflux disease. Dig Dis Sci 40:2305–2311
45. Wang HH, Mangano MM, Antonioli DA (1994) Evaluation of T-lymphocytes in esophageal mucosal biopsies. Mod Pathol 7:55–58
46. Chadwick LM, Kurinczuk JJ, Hallam LA, Brennan BA, Forbes D (1997) Clinical and endoscopic predictors of histological oesophagitis in infants. J Paediatr Child Health 33:388–393
47. Winter HS, Madara JL, Stafford RJ, Grand RJ, Quinlan JE, Goldman H (1982) Intraepithelial eosinophils: a new diagnostic criterion for reflux esophagitis. Gastroenterology 83:818–823
48. Teitelbaum JE, Fox VL, Twarog FJ, Nurko S, Antonioli D, Gleich G, Badizadegan K, Furuta GT (2002) Eosinophilic esophagitis in children: immunopathological analysis and response to fluticasone propionate. Gastroenterology 122:1216–1225
49. Ruchelli E, Wenner W, Voytek T, Brown K, Liacouras C (1999) Severity of esophageal eosinophilia predicts response to conventional gastroesophageal reflux therapy. Pediatr Dev Pathol 2:15–18
50. Isaac DW, Parham DM, Patrick CC (1997) The role of esophagoscopy in diagnosis and management of esophagitis in children with cancer. Med Pediatr Oncol 28:299–303
51. Tozzi A, Staiano A, Paparo F, Miele E, Maglio M, Di Meo M, Simeone D, Troncone R (2001) Characterization of the inflammatory infiltrate in peptic oesophagitis. Dig Liver Dis 33:452–458
52. Mehall JR, Chandler JC, Mehall RL, Jackson RJ, Wagner CW, Smith SD (2002) Management of typical and atypical intestinal malrotation. J Pediatr Surg 37:1169–1172
53. Cohen Z, Kleiner O, Finaly R, Mordehai J, Newman N, Kurtzbart E, Mares AJ (2003) How much of a misnomer is "asymptomatic" intestinal malrotation? Isr Med Assoc J 5:172–174
54. Fawcett H, Hayden C, Adams J, Swischuck L (1988) How useful is GER scintigraphy in suspected childhood aspiration? Pediatr Radiol 18:311–313

Chapter 14

Barium Swallow: An Useful Exam to Diagnose GER in Children

14

Biagio Zuccarello · Carmelo Romeo

Contents

Different diagnostic modalities have been used to confirm the clinical suspect of gastroesophageal reflux (GER). Each modality has a specific target and none can be used alone. The barium esophagogram is probably one of the most used and also one of the oldest techniques for making the diagnosis of GER. This technique was, in fact, described at the end of 1970s for the performance of the barium swallow in infants and children becoming a standardized approach for the diagnosis of GER. A morphologic classification was derived and still used.

A contrast study of the upper gastrointestinal tract should aim to characterize and determine not only simple gastroesophageal reflux but also any anomalies of deglutition, presence of nasopharyngeal reflux, anomalies of esophageal motility, presence of esophageal ulcer or stenosis, hiatal hernia, barium aspiration and gastric emptying.

14.1
Anatomic Details

The esophagus is a muscular canal extending from the pharynx to the stomach. It begins in the neck at the lower border of the cricoid cartilage, opposite the sixth cervical vertebra, descends along the front of the vertebral column, through the superior and posterior mediastinum, passes through the diaphragm, and, entering the abdomen, ends at the cardiac orifice of the stomach, opposite the eleventh thoracic vertebra.

From a functional point of view the esophagus can be divided into two segments: a superior segment, *tubular* or esophageal body, with merely peristaltic activity

ending just above the diaphragm; and a second part, *vestibular* with functional properties. The vestibular part can be divided into a supradiaphragmatic segment, or *epiphrenic ampulla* delimited in its lower part by the lower esophageal sphincter, an intrahiatal portion, and a subdiaphragmatic segment that terminates in the stomach.

From a topographical point of view the esophagus can be divided into one cervical segment; three thoracic segments: superior, mid- and lower esophagus and one abdominal segment.

14.2
Methods

A standard radiographic study of the esophagus should start with a plain x-ray of the thorax and the study should continue with the use of a contrast agent and in some instances with a double contrast, i.e., barium/air.

The ideal projection for an anatomic and functional study of the esophagogastric junction is the right lateral view. With this the hiatus is projected above, at the level or just below the diaphragm, depending on the acuity of the lateral position (Fig. 1).

In an infant, the presence of physiologic aerophagia allows the identification in some instances of the lumen of the esophagus as an air column behind the trachea in the lateral projections [14].

For a detailed examination of the region, focusing on the mechanism of continence, the examination should be performed dynamically, recording the entire examination with roentgen cineradiography. This will allow the clinician to review the examination several times without exposing infant patients to excess radiation.

One of the most frequent mistakes in administering a barium swallow is the use of an inadequate amount of barium given to an infant. For an adequate examination, the amount of barium introduced in the stomach should be equal to a normal meal [15]. Indeed, a not well distended stomach can significantly reduce the episodes of reflux. If the infant is unable to drink the barium, a soft nasogastric tube is introduced through the

Fig. 1.
Schematic draw showing the different projections of the esophageal hiatus according to the acuity of the lateral projection

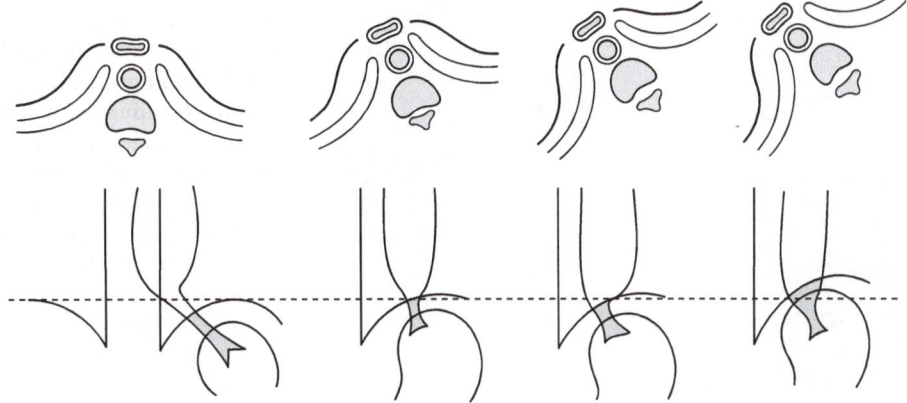

mouth into the stomach; then the appropriate volume of barium is infused and the tube is removed. Another important point is the examination time; an infant should be examined for at least 5 min, without continuous fluoroscopy but with intermittent spots for observation.

During the barium study the infant should be kept warm. Crying reduces reflux, and thus the infant should also be kept calm and comfortable. Deglutition and peristalsis are studied from the right lateral view. Then the infant should be placed in a supine position to look for reflux episodes and then turned in the right lateral position to empty the stomach and take a lateral view of the duodenal sweep. Once the contrast enters the last part of duodenum, the patient should be turned supine again to view the position of ligament of Treitz. Several movements of the baby from right to left should be attempted to induce reflux, but without using external abdominal pressure. In some circumstances a water siphon test can be necessary and is obtained with water, at small sips, after barium ingestion. A delayed image should be taken about 30 min after all the barium has been ingested, to highlight any delayed episode of gastroesophageal reflux [13].

The radiographic examination should also include the stomach, focusing on the pyloric region. In a small number of cases, in fact, it is possible to observe reflux and hypertrophic pyloric stenosis or pyloric spasm (Fig. 2).

14.3
Radiologic Features

During the barium swallow, the esophagus has a ribbon-like appearance with irregular caliber due to the presence of narrowing and enlargement.

The general direction of the esophagus is vertical, but it presents two slight curves in its course. First it runs down the middle line, then it deviates to the left side as far as the root of the neck, gradually passes to the middle line again at the level of the fifth thoracic verte-

bra and finally deviates to the left as it passes forward to the esophageal hiatus in the diaphragm. The esophagus also describes anteroposterior flexures corresponding to the curvatures of the cervical and thoracic portions of the vertebral column.

The major radiologic features regarding the use of barium swallow in the diagnostic work-up of gastroesophageal reflux focus on the demonstration of the anatomopathologic substrate, the event of reflux and its complications such as esophagitis, strictures and on the demonstration of a hiatal hernia. Other important elements can be demonstrated by barium swallow, such as presence of atypical anatomic causes of recurrent vomiting as for pyloric stenosis or duodenal web.

The most frequent anatomic condition that predisposes to reflux is the calasia of the cardia, characterized by the reduction or disappearance of the abdominal segment of the esophagogastric junction, enlargement of the angle of His, and patent cardia [7].

According to the height reached by the column of barium during the episode of reflux, six grades of radiologic GER have been described [11]. Grade 1 is reflux

Fig. 2.
The barium esophagogram demonstrates a Grade 1 reflux with a patent cardias and evidence of pyloric stenosis

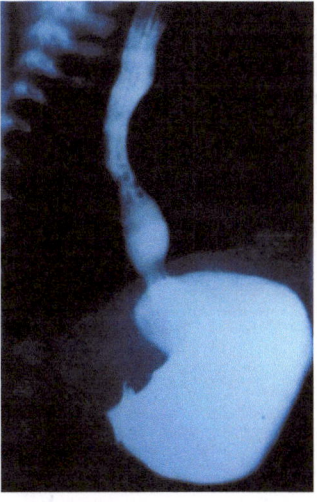

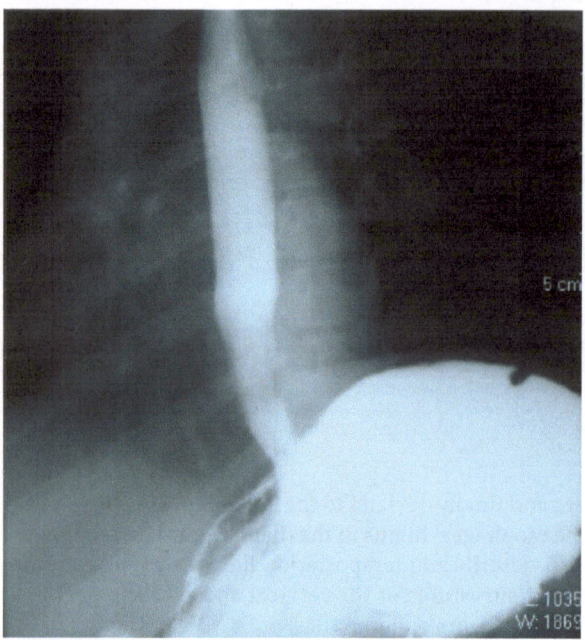

Fig. 3. Grade 2 reflux demonstrated by barium esophagogram. The barium column reaches the thoracic esophagus

that reaches the distal esophagus below the level of the carina; Grade 2 is reflux that reaches the thoracic esophagus but is below the clavicles (Fig. 3); Grade 3 is reflux that reaches the cervical esophagus; Grade 4 is a condition of continuous reflux to the neck with a widely opened gastroesophageal junction; Grade 5 is aspiration of barium into the tracheobronchial tree. The last grade is called Grade D (delayed) because reflux persists at the radiograph taken 30 min after the end of the study.

The hiatal hernia can be demonstrated by barium swallow. Three different types of hernia can be observed. Type 1 or sliding hernia: the cardia and part of the stomach migrate through a widening of the muscular hiatal opening with circumferential laxity of the phreno-esophageal membrane (Fig. 4). This is the most frequent type, and its radiological features are represented by an enlargement of the esophageal diaphragmatic hiatus, by the presence of a hernia that simulates the epiphrenic ampulla but is characterized by gastric mucosa inside, and by the esophago-gastric junction positioned above the diaphragm. Type 2 or paraesophageal hernias are characterized by the maintenance of the angle of His; the hernia is formed by the gastric fundus that migrates through the hiatus laterally to the esophagus. Type 3 is characterized by a shortened and straightened esophagus and the esophagogastric junction clearly above the diaphragm. This type is usually secondary to esophagitis but can be also congenital.

The esophagitis can be recognized only in later stages of GER disease (GERD). The images can display linear defects (*minus*) or small collections of barium (*plus*). The mucosa can appear thickened by edema.

The real value of barium swallow as a diagnostic tool in determining gastroesophageal reflux is still not well established. Different studies have tried to correlate the sensitivity and specificity of the contrast esophagogram to other diagnostic techniques. Usually the barium swallow is compared to 24-h pH monitoring. In adults with GER, the contrast study has demonstrated a high specificity (100%) and a moderate sensitivity (52%) compared to 24-h pH monitoring [1, 12]. The sensitivity increased to 79% in the presence of more severe complications such as mild-type esophagitis or Barrett's esophagus [8]. This suggests that barium swallow could identify patients where complications could be expect-

Fig. 4.
The barium esophagogram demonstrates a sliding hernia with the esophagogastric junction above the diaphragm (*arrows*)

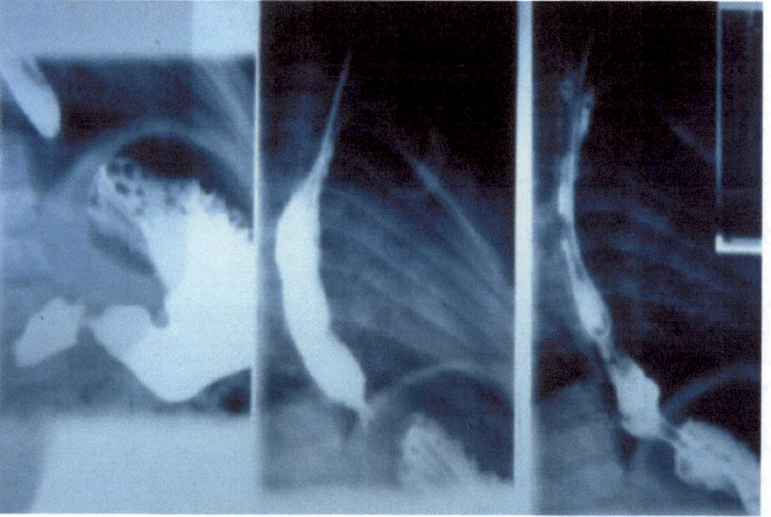

ed; this is not possible with pH monitoring. The same investigators studied GER in infants less than 1 year old, and correlates the radiographic demonstration of GER with 24-h pH monitoring. In this group of patients, the specificity of barium swallow was low (50%) and the sensitivity was even worse (29%) [2]. In children under 2 years of age barium swallow was diagnostic in 79% of cases, whereas pH-metry demonstrated reflux in 98% of the patients studied [6]. Another series showed better sensitivity and specificity for the barium swallow in children; 86% and 69% respectively. In the same study, the results for pH monitoring were 88% and 94%, respectively [9].

Another study attempted to correlate the barium swallow with ultrasonography (US)[4]. US studies the esophagogastric junction and gives a classification of the severity of reflux depending on the number of episodes correlated with the age of patient. In this investigation, US and barium swallow results were in agreement in 93% of the cases. In the other 7%, the US described more severe cases than the barium swallow. The study concluded that since US is less invasive and is a more physiological method of investigation, it should be recommended as the test of choice for screening reflux in children with suspected GER and for the follow-up [4]. According to the same authors, the radiographic study still has a place in the examination of patients with rib or vertebral malformations and in cases of abnormal gastric distention in which a clear ultrasonographic image cannot be achieved [4].

In recent years an important role of hiatal hernia in causing severe GERD has been noted [16]. This was suggested by the observation that children with Barrett's esophagus have hiatal hernia [5], and that hiatal hernia is associated with the more severe degrees of reflux esophagitis [3]. It follows that severe GERD is more likely to be associated with anatomic malformations such as hiatal hernia; patients with less severe GERD probably have more functional abnormalities such as transient lower esophageal sphincter relaxation [16]. The role of barium swallow has then regained importance for the morphological evaluation of the esophagus in particular for the demonstration of a hiatal hernia [10].

Despite the availability of highly sophisticated diagnostic tools, the standard radiologic study of the esophagus with contrast still maintains a definite role in the diagnostic workup of children with suspected GER. Barium swallow allows a clinician to obtain a morphological evaluation of the entire esophagus with the esophagogastric junction, to highlight any anatomical alteration and/or upward migration of the esophagogastric junction itself and to correlate with the severity of the disease in the presence of aspiration of refluxed gastric content or signs of esophagitis or stricture. Barium swallow also has a pivotal role in the evaluation of complicated forms of GERD, where it displays a higher sensitivity, superior even to pH-metry.

References

1. Aksglaede K, Funch-Jensen P, Thommesen P (1999) Radiological demonstration of gastroesophageal reflux. Diagnostic value of barium and bread studies compared with 24-hour pH monitoring. Acta Radiol 40:652–655
2. Aksglaede K, Pederesen JB, Lange A, Funch-Jensen P, Thommesen P (2003) Gastroesophageal reflux demonstrated by radiography in infants less than 1 year of age. Comparison with pH monitoring. Acta Radiol 44:136–138
3. Ben Rejeb M, Bouche O, Zeiton P (1992) Study of 47 consecutive patients with peptic esophageal stricture compared with 3880 cases of reflux esophagitis. Dig Dis Sci 37:733–736
4. Di Mario M, Bergami G, Fariello G, Vecchioli Scaldazza A (1995) Diagnosis of gastroesophageal reflux in childhood. Comparison of ultrasonography and barium swallow. Radiol Med 89:76–81
5. Hassal E (1993) Barrett's esophagus: new definitions and approaches in children. J Pediatr Gastroenterol Nutr 16:345–364
6. Kazerooni NL, VanCamp J, Hirschl RB, Drogowski RA, Coran AG (1994) Fundoplication in 160 children under 2 years of age. J Pediatr Surg 29:677–681
7. Lelli Chiesa PL (1993) Ernia iatale e reflusso gastro-esofageo. In: Domini R, Lima M (eds) Chirurgia delle malformazioni digestive. Piccin, Padova, pp 169–196
8. Madsen E, Aksglaede K, Jacobsen NO, Funch-Jensen P, Thommesen P (2001) Gastro-oesophageal reflux demonstrated by radiography. A supplement to 24-h pH monitoring. Acta Radiol 42:521–525
9. Meyers WF, Roberts CC, Johnson DG, Herbst JJ (1985) Value of tests for evaluation of gastroesophageal reflux in children. J Pediatr Surg 20:515–520
10. Mattioli S, Lugaresi ML, Pierluigi M, Di Simone MP, D'Ovidio F (2003) Review article: indications for antireflux surgery in gastro-oesophageal reflux disease. Aliment Pharmacol Ther 17:60–67
11. McCauley RG, Darling DB, Leonidas JC (1979) Gastroesophageal reflux in infants and children: A useful classification and reliable physiologic technique for its demonstration. Am J Roentgenol 130:47–50
12. Nellemann H, Aksglaede K, Funch-Jensen PF, Thommesen P (2000) Bread and barium. Diagnostic value in patients with suspected primary esophageal motility disorders. Acta Radiol 41:145–150
13. Ramenofsky ML (1986) Gastroesophageal reflux: clinical manifestations and diagnosis. In: Aschcraft KW (ed) Pediatric esophageal surgery. Saunders, Philadelphia, pp 151–179
14. Romeo G, Zuccarello B, Gentile C (1988) Alterazioni funzionali della giunzione esofagocardiale. In: Montanari M, Leggio A, Pipino F, Romeo G (eds) Chirurgia pediatrica e ortopedia–metodologia clinica. USES Edizioni Scientifiche, Firenze, pp 284–304
15. Sty JR, Wells RG, Srashak RJ, Gregg DC (1996) Apparato genitourinario e gastrointestinale. Diagnostica per immagini nel bambino. Momento Medico, Salerno
16. Vandenplas Y, Hassall E (2002) Mechanisms of gastroesophageal reflux and gastroesophageal reflux disease. J Pediatr Gastroenterol Nutr 35:119–136

Chapter 15

Scintigraphic Assessment of GER in Pediatric Patients

15

Andrea Soricelli · Emanuele Nicolai · Marco Salvatore

Contents

15.1
Introduction

Nuclear medicine techniques have been widely employed in the assessment of gastroesophageal dysfunction. Scintigraphic evaluation of the upper gastrointestinal tract includes esophageal transit time, gastroesophageal reflux, and gastric emptying [4, 16].

Gastroesophageal reflux scintigraphy was introduced in 1976 by Fisher and Malmud to detect the presence of the reflux, to quantitate it, and to assess the effectiveness of medical and surgical treatment [1, 2].

The availability of other diagnostic procedures such as endoscopy, esophageal manometry, acid infusion test, and 24-h pH monitoring has reduced the number of procedures performed in adults. However, because of its physiologic and non-invasive character, scintigraphy has gained wide acceptance in the detection and evaluation of gastroesophageal reflux in infants and children [3, 8].

15.2
Nuclear Medicine Procedures

The transit of the bolus in the esophagus depends on several factors such as forces generated by the bolus, esophageal peristalsis, gravity, etc. It should be kept in mind that a pharyngeal contraction transfers the radio-active bolus through a relaxed upper esophageal sphincter into the esophagus. The sphincter then contracts and the radiolabeled bolus proceeds into the stomach due to a primary peristaltic wave through a relaxed lower esophageal sphincter. A secondary peristaltic wave is present along the esophagus due to residual food or refluxed gastric content.

Nonperistaltic contractions may be induced by intramural reflex mechanisms and can also be seen as a variant phenomenon.

The scintigraphic procedure can be performed in two phases: the first for the assessment of esophageal transit time, and the second for the detection of gastroesophageal reflux, eventually continued to determine the gastric emptying. If the patient's clinical condition is critical, only the detection of the gastroesophageal reflux can be performed [5]

15.2.1
Patient Preparation and Bolus Material

The procedure must be performed after an overnight fast and after withdrawal of any medication likely to interfere with esophageal motility. The administered bolus can be solid or liquid. Chicken liver, labeled during cooking with ^{99m}Tc-sulfur colloid, was introduced in 1976 to insure tracer binding to the solid food [12].

Numerous solid foods, including whole eggs, egg whites, liver paté, hamburgers, fibers, and non-digestible particles have been used with or without a liquid component, usually water [9]. Radiolabeled eggs are now routinely used as solid boluses due to the availability, low cost, and stability of the compound.

Solid boluses are theoretically more physiologic in the assessment of esophageal function but are fragmented along the length of the organ and are inadequate for esophageal transit studies. In addition, these solid boluses cannot be administered to pediatric patients. Liquid boluses are homogeneous, not fragmented along the esophagus, and easy to prepare, and they have been shown to provide more reproducible results. Moreover, liquid boluses can be used in very small infants. Gelatin can be used occasionally as an alternative [3, 5].

At present, due to the previous considerations, liquid boluses are preferred for the scintigraphic assessment of esophageal transit time and gastroesophageal reflux in children.

15.2.2
Radiopharmaceuticals

[99m]Technetium (^{99m}Tc) sulfur colloid is usually employed to label solid or liquid boluses. The reasons to use this compound are related to its constant availability, ease of preparation, low cost, and the fact that it is neither absorbed nor secreted by the esophageal mucosa [12]. Furthermore, ^{99m}Tc compounds have optimal physical characteristics for imaging using conventional gamma cameras and relatively low dosimetry compared to other tracers. Some theoretical limitations to the use of ^{99m}Tc tracers are related to the scattered activity from the stomach. [111]Indium-DTPA has been used successfully to radiolabel both liquid and solid boluses, but due to the non-constant availability of this tracer and higher radiation dosimetry compared to ^{99m}Tc compounds, this tracer is not routinely used.

3.7–37 Mega Bequerel (MBq) of ^{99m}Tc sulfur colloid is added to the bolus. The amount of the dose added to the bolus is decreased according to the age and weight of the patient. In infants, the radiopharmaceutical is added to milk feeding, since it has been shown to remain stable. In cases of milk allergy, a substitute may be used.

In older patients, water or other liquid material (i.e. 300 mL of acidified orange juice – 150 mL of orange juice and 150 mL 0.1 N hydrochloric acid) can be used. If [111]Indium is the tracer employed, 3.7–7.4 MBq of tracer is labeled to the bolus. Each center should standardize the volume of the bolus according to age and size of the patient.

If the evaluation of the gastroesophageal scintigraphy continues with the assessment of gastric emptying, it must be kept in mind that the emptying rate differs according to the bolus composition. The assessment of gastric emptying is not always possible, since many ill patients are on modified feeding schedules or are not able to prolong the study due to their clinical condition.

Some centers in the past have performed a double-isotope labeling technique to assess gastric emptying: the solid bolus is labeled with ^{99m}Tc and the liquid one with [111]In.

15.2.3
Positioning

The patient is placed on the table in a supine position. This position is preferred for the early characterization of the esophageal motor disorders because it eliminates the effect of gravity and avoids the counterreflux effect of gravity. The gamma camera is positioned anteriorly or posteriorly, beneath the table. The anterior position is preferred, if the patient is cooperative, because small reflux may be missed using the posterior view due to the attenuation of the spine [3, 6, 7]. If the instrument is a double-head camera, simultaneous anterior and posterior images can be acquired.

Before the administration of the radiolabeled bolus for the evaluation of the esophageal transit time of the tracer, an external radioactive marker (i.e. [57]Cobalt) is placed over the cricoid cartilage and/or the xiphoid process to facilitate the correct positioning and to ensure that all of the esophagus is included in the field of view. After the first dynamic acquisition, the patient may be moved so that the mid-distal portion of the esophagus and the stomach are centered in the field of view of the gamma camera.

15.2.4
Acquisition

Analogic acquisitions are not indicated. The gamma camera must be connected with a computer. If ^{99m}Tc compounds are used, a general-purpose collimator must be used and the photopeak settings should be 140 keV ±20% window. For ^{111}In, 20% energy windows should be established around both the 172 and 246 keV photopeaks, and a medium energy collimator must be used for image acquisition.

If the scintigraphic evaluation of the esophageal transit time is performed, 10 mL of the overall bolus is given. The administered volume is reduced according to age and weight of the infant. Immediately after the bolus administration a dynamic acquisition is started: high-speed framing is required to image esophageal transit. Usually a set of 64×64 pixels images are acquired at the frame rate of 2 or – better – 4 images per second for 2 min.

At the end of this initial acquisition, the remaining bolus can be administered, optimally within 10 min from the beginning of the procedure. After the administration of the whole bolus, a first static image is acquired to assure complete clearance of the radiolabeled material from the esophagus.

The physician or the technologist should record how long it took for the patient to ingest the whole radiolabeled bolus, and if any amount of the meal was not eaten. As stated earlier, each laboratory should standardize the method as to patient positioning and environmental conditions, such as ambient noise, lighting, or other factors affecting patient comfort. The normal values should be based on this standard methodology.

If needed, 30 mL of water is given to clear any residual activity.

Computerized dynamic images are then acquired in the supine position using a 15 s/frame interval (4 frames/min). If the reflux episodes are brief and of relatively small volume, a 5 s/frame interval (12 frames/min) is suggested for better assessment of the frequency of the reflux and the rate at which it clears. The total acquisition time is 60 min, but it can continue up to 120 min if the assessment of gastric emptying is also required and can be performed.

Two additional procedures can be used to enhance the sensitivity of the test to detect the presence of gastroesophageal reflux in cooperative children and adults [15]:

a) An acid load to the stomach to decrease the tone of the lower esophageal sphincter.

b) An inflatable abdominal binder positioned around the lower abdomen to increase the pressure gradient across the lower esophageal sphincter, at baseline and at each 20 mmHg pressure gradient from 0–100 mmHg. Each 20-mmHg increase corresponds to a 5-mmHg increase at the level of the lower esophageal sphincter. In infants, the examiner's hand can be used to create pressure on the abdomen.

A 24-h post-bolus administration static image can be acquired for direct evidence of pulmonary aspiration of refluxed gastric material in the lungs [11].

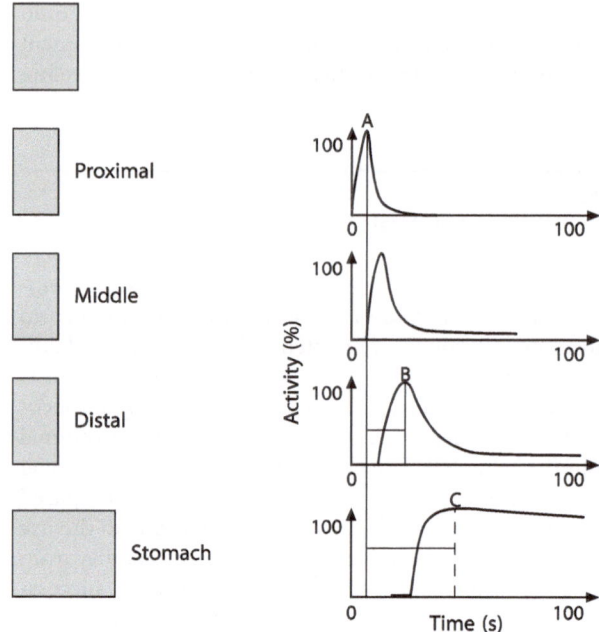

Fig. 1. Schematic positioning of the regions of interest for the creation of time-activity curves on the esophagus and stomach. Regions of interest are drawn over the esophagus and stomach, and esophageal transit time (AB) and esophagogastric transit time (AC) can be calculated

15.2.5
Data Analysis and Imaging Interpretation

Once the study has been completed, the images are reviewed in a one-to-one single-frame analysis and then are played back in a cine display mode. Using the visual analysis, the presence of delayed transit time along the esophagus and the number, rate of clearance, and severity of the reflux episodes can be depicted.

Further, if there has been no movement of the patient, a quantitative assessment of the esophageal transit and presence of gastric reflux can be done. Time-activity curves are generated drawing regions of interest on the esophagus and the upper, mid-, and lower portions of the organ and the stomach (Fig. 1). In normal subjects, the transit of the radioactive bolus from the pharynx into the upper portion of the esophagus takes less than 0.5–1 s. Esophageal transit time for liquid or semisolid boluses varies from 5.5±1.1 to 9.5±1.5 s, depending on the definition and calculation methods used [1, 7, 5].

Due to the compression by the aortic arch or tracheal bifurcation, there can be a slowing of bolus progression at the mid-portion of the esophagus. Abnormal esophageal motility caused by aging (the so-called "presbyesophagus") and delayed esophageal transit in obese patients' reflux have been described [10, 7].

Mainly two parameters can be obtained from the segmental time-activity curves to assess the transit bolus through the esophagus:
- the esophageal transit time calculated as the time interval between the peak activity of the proximal esophageal curve and the peak activity of the distal esophageal curve;
- the esophagogastric transit time, defined as the time interval between peak activity of the proximal esophageal curve and maximal gastric activity [3].

The presence of gastroesophageal reflux can be quantified using the formula:

$$R = E(t) - E(b) \times 100/Go$$

where
- R is the percentage of reflux material into the esophagus.
- E(t), the esophageal counts at time t.
- E(b), the para-esophageal background counts.
- Go, the gastric counts at the beginning of the study.

R and E(t) refer to the entire organ and to the upper, mid-, and lower portions.

According to this formula, the presence of a reflux >4% is considered abnormal. This value corresponds to the minimal radioactivity seen on the gamma-camera screen during the visual analysis, and it should be kept in mind that the volume of the refluxed material is proportional to the radioactivity seen with the scintigraphic method.

For the assessment of esophageal transit time in the visual analysis and in the observation of the time-activity curves, under normal conditions there is a regular progression of the bolus along the esophagus, with early appearance of the stomach. Abnormal patterns in the bolus progression are seen in various clinical conditions such as esophagitis due to gastroesophageal reflux (Fig. 2), achalasia, scleroderma, etc. [3, 8, 10, 13]. In these patients the time-activity curves demonstrate a slow-down in the bolus progression (Fig. 3).

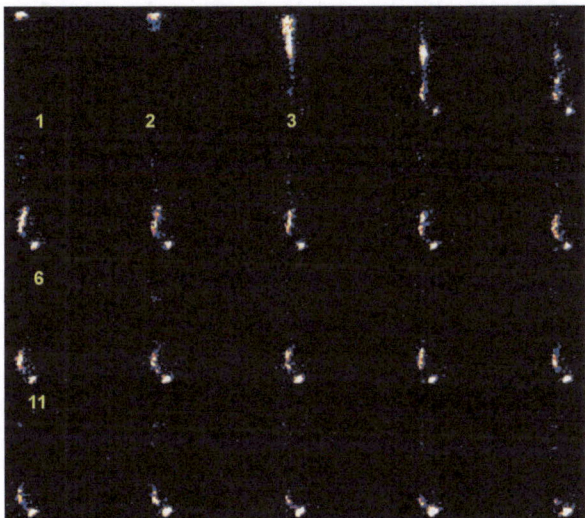

Fig. 2. Dynamic scintigraphic acquisition for the assessment of esophageal transit time (4 images per second). Normal transit of the radioactive bolus through the upper and mid-portions of the esophagus and a delayed transit along the distal portion, due to esophagitis induced by gastroesophageal reflux, are evident

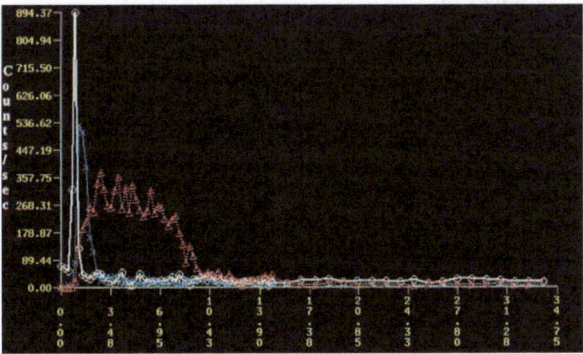

Fig. 3. Time-activity curves of the same patient as in Fig, 2: Regular transit is evident through the upper and mid-portions of the esophagus (*white and blue curves*), whereas transit is delayed in the distal portion (*red curve*)

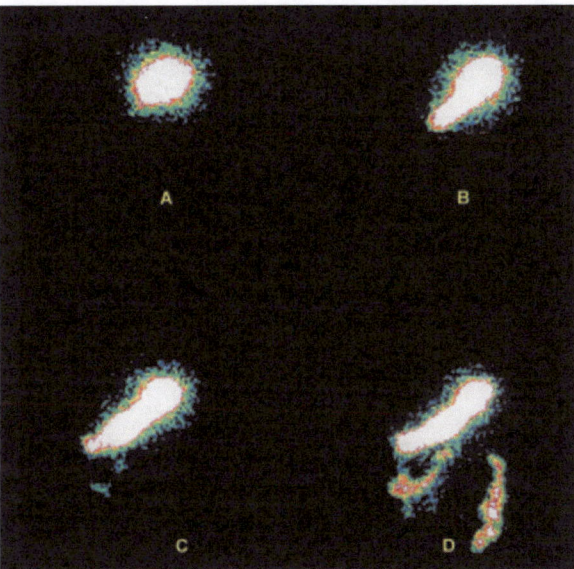

Fig. 4. Normal case. Anterior images at 3 (A), 15 (B), 20 (C), 35 (D) min from the bolus administration. There is no evidence of gastroesophageal reflux

In the second phase of the procedure in normal patients, there is no migration of the radioactive bolus from the stomach to the esophagus (Fig. 4). The presence of the reflux is seen on the scintigraphic images as radioactivity that temporarily migrates from the stomach towards the upper esophageal portion (Figs. 5, 6) or even to the oropharyngeal region. In patients without gastroesophageal reflux this cannot be seen, even by in-

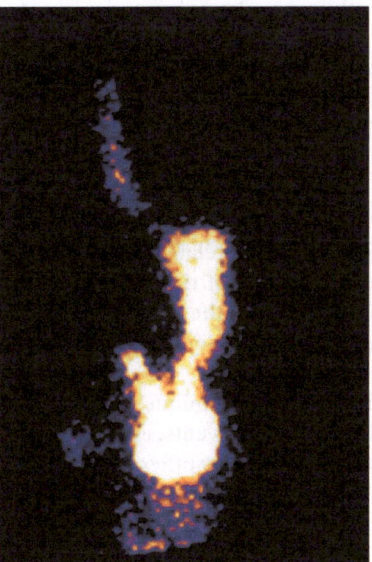

Fig. 5. Anterior image at 25 min from the radiolabeled bolus. The tracer distribution in the stomach and the presence of a reflux that reaches the mid/upper portion of the esophagus are shown

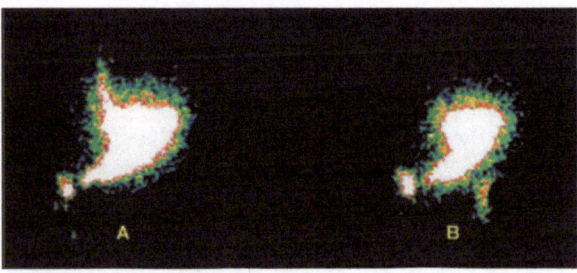

Fig. 6. Anterior image at 15 (**A**) and 25 (**B**) min after the radiolabeled bolus administration. Reflux is evident at 15 min, and is no longer visible in the later image

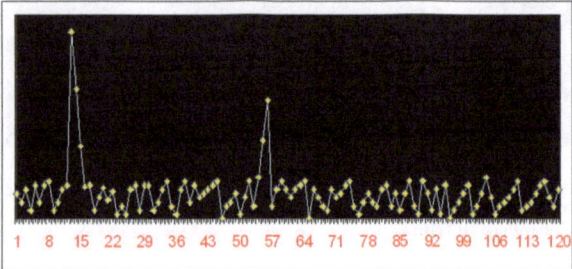

Fig. 7. Time-activity curve of the same patient as in Fig. 6. The presence of two refluxes is evident: one at 15 min and the other at 60 min

creasing pressure up to 100 mmHg [15]. In patients with reflux, an increase in the amount of reflux material is observed as the gradient across the lower esophageal sphincter is increased.

The time-activity curves (Fig. 7) and the calculated reflux indices have been used in an attempt to quantitate each reflux episode as an expression of the gastric content at time zero. These indices can quantify correctly of the number of refluxed episodes over time, the refluxed radioactivity, and the clearance time of each episode. Furthermore, these indices are extremely useful in the follow-up of patients and for the evaluation of treatment.

The sensitivity of the scintigraphic detection of gastroesophageal reflux is related to the radioactive concentration and volume of the refluxed material. Moreover for the detection of the reflux, the residence time of the radioactivity in the esophagus and the tissue attenuation are important.

The scintigraphic technique permits a continuous monitoring of possible events, even those that are very brief and can be missed by other methods. In particular it has been shown that the sensitivity of the nuclear medicine technique is higher compared to other diagnostic imaging techniques such as barium radiography or cineradiography, where the radiation dose to the patients, especially infants and young children, is very high [3]. The overall sensitivity of the technique using both the visual and quantitative techniques is in the range of 88%–91% [16]. Several authors have compared the results obtained with the scintigraphic methods and esophageal pH methods. Tolia et al. [14] showed that nuclear medicine techniques were more sensitive in the detection of reflux during the first 60 min postprandially, whereas pH monitoring was more sensitive in the detection of the reflux beyond the first postprandial hour. These findings can explain the lack of correlation between these two procedures and the good sensitivity of the scintigraphic method in small infants.

Dual-head gamma cameras allow contemporary acquisition in anterior and posterior projections, with an increased sensitivity of the instrument and better clinical results. This technique is also able to detect pulmonary aspiration, which is considered one of the most important complications of the gastroesophageal reflux. This finding can be obtained by performing a 24-h delayed acquisition [11].

Although the relationship between respiratory disease and gastroesophageal reflux has been noted, it is still poorly understood. It has been suggested that the reflux can cause respiratory problems such as recurrent infections, asthma, apnea, etc., and a possible relationship between gastroesophageal reflux and sudden infant death syndrome has also been described. [5, 11]

15.2.6
Dosimetry

The effective dose equivalent for solid and liquid radiolabeled ^{99m}Tc compounds has been estimated to be 0.024 mSv/MBq for adults, 0.029 mSv/MBq for patients aged 15, 0.047 mSv/MBq for patients aged 10, and 0.13 mSv/MBq for patients aged 1 [15, 16]. The effective dose equivalent for ^{111}Indium is 0.31 mSv/MBq for solid bolus and 0.3 mSv/MBq for liquid bolus. All of these effective dose equivalents are extremely low, even for newborns, and cannot be considered a limitation to perform the exam.

15.3
Conclusions

Gastroesophageal scintigraphy for the assessment of esophageal transit and detection of the reflux is a simple, nontraumatic, and easy to perform technique. This procedure is physiological in nature and is sensitive because of the continuous and prolonged monitoring, and can be easily repeated over time. In addition, the visual analysis and the quantitative parameters available have proven to be useful tools to increase the sensitivity in the detection of delayed transit time and presence of gastroesophageal reflux, even of small volume.

References

1. DeVincentis N, Lenti R, Pona C et al (1984) Scintigraphic evaluation of the esophageal transit time for the non-invasive assessment of esophageal motor disorders. J Nucl Med 28: 137–142
2. Fischer RS, Malmud LS Roberts GS et al (1976) Gastro-esophageal (GE) scintiscan to detect and quantitate GE reflux. Gastroenterology 70:301–308
3. Heyman S (1997) Assessment of gastroesophageal dysfunction in children. Q J Nucl Med 41:269–280
4. Heyman S, Reich H (1997) Gastric emptying of milk feeding in infants and children–anterior versus conjugate counting. Clin Nucl Med 22:303–305
5. Heyman S, Eicher PS, Alavi A (1995) Radionuclide studies of the upper gastrointestinal tract in children with feeding disorders. J Nucl Med 36: 351–354
6. Klein HA (1990) The effect of projection in esophageal transit scintigraphy. Clin Nucl Med 15:157–162
7. Klein HA, Wald A (1987) Normal variation in radionuclide esophageal transit studies. Eur J Nucl Med 13:115–120
8. Latini G, Del Vecchio A, De Mitri B et al (1999) Scintigraphic evaluation of gastroesophageal reflux in newborns. Pediatr Med Chir 21:115–117
9. Meyer JH, MacGregor IL, Gueller R et al (1976) 99mTc-tagged chicken liver as marker of solid food markers in vivo. Am J Dig. Dis 21(4):296–304
10. Orenstein SR (1992) Controversies in gastroesophageal reflux. J Pedriat Gastroenterol Nutr 14:338–48
11. Ruth M, Carlsson M, Mansson I et al (1993) Scintigraphic detection of gastro-pulmonary aspiration in patients with respiratory disorders. Clin Physiol 13:19–33
12. Taillefer R, Beauchamp G, Devito M et al (1983) Radionuclide esophagogram (99mTc sulphur colloid) in experimental esophagitis: manometric and histopathologic correlations. J Nucl Med 24:100
13. Thomas EJ, Kumar R, Dasan JB et al (2003) Radionuclide scintigraphy in the evaluation of gastro-oesophageal reflux in postoperative oesophageal atresia and tracheo-oesophageal fistula patients. Nucl Med Commun 24:317–320
14. Tolia V, Kuhns L, Kauffman RE (1993) Comparison of simultaneous esophageal pH monitoring and scintigraphy in infants with gastroesophageal reflux. Am J Gastroenterol 88:661–664
15. Urbain JLC, Charker ND (1995) Recent advances in gastric emptying scintigraphy. Sem Nucl Med 25:318–325
16. Urbain JLC, Vekemans MCM, Malmud LS (1996) Esophageal transit, gastroesophageal reflux and gastric emptying. In: Sandler MP, Coleman RE, Patton JA, Gottschalk A (eds) Diagnostic nuclear medicine. Williams and Wilkins, Philadelphia, pp 733–747

Ultrasonography and Bronchoalveolar Lavage for the Diagnosis of Children with Gastroesophageal Reflux

16

Jacob C. Langer · Stephen Miller

Contents

16.1
Introduction

The diagnosis of gastroesophageal reflux (GER) may be suspected on the basis of clinical history and physical examination, and is confirmed with the aid of a number of other investigations. Most cases are diagnosed based on barium radiography and extended pH studies, with the support of endoscopy with biopsies, nuclear scans, and esophageal manometry. All of these are dealt with in other chapters. This chapter will deal with several other modalities for diagnosing GER which are used more infrequently: ultrasonography and bronchoalveolar lavage (BAL).

16.2
Ultrasonography

The evaluation of children with suspected GER comprises a significant portion of all pediatric radiological examinations. To date, this has been accomplished by the radiographic upper gastrointestinal series (UGI), in which the child is administered a liquid suspension of barium sulfate and is imaged fluoroscopically. This technique establishes the anatomy of the esophagus, stomach, and proximal small bowel, including the position of the ligament of Treitz. Furthermore, the UGI allows evaluation of swallowing, gastric peristalsis, gastric emptying, and gastrointestinal reflux. However, as this is a fluoroscopic technique utilizing ionizing radiation, the total time that the patient may be studied is quite limited. Traditionally, GER is assayed by brief (1–3 s) fluoroscopy performed intermittently every 15–20 s for several minutes at the end of the standard UGI. Therefore, the total period of time in which GER is potentially visualized is only 10–45 s. This is an admittedly brief microcosm; lack of visualization of "known" GER with UGI is quite common. Furthermore, the radiation administered to the child, while as little as is feasible, is not negligible; the standard UGI with 2 min of fluoroscopy time incurs a radiation administered dose (RAD) of 2 rad (2 cGy).

Ultrasonography has gained wide acclaim for its ability to depict anatomy and pathology in the pediatric gastrointestinal tract, including pyloric stenosis, inflammatory bowel disease, and intussusception. Major advantages of ultrasound over fluoroscopy include its lack of ionizing radiation and portability. Ultrasound studies can be performed for fairly protracted periods of time due to the former, while portability renders ultrasound useful in critical situations. Ultrasound is somewhat operator-dependent, however, as is high-quality fluoroscopy.

Despite the lack of a standard technique for evaluating GER by ultrasound, several reports in the literature attest to the ability of ultrasound to depict GER in children [1–8] and in adults [9]. Ultrasound appears to compare quite favorably with gold-standard 24-h pH monitoring, especially with the addition of color Doppler imaging to gray-scale or B-mode sonography [2]. In a large series directly comparing 24-h pH monitoring with gray-scale ultrasound without and with color Doppler, there was 87% agreement between pH monitoring and gray-scale ultrasound, and 94% agreement between pH monitoring and color Doppler sonography. Sensitivity for the detection of GER increased from 84.4% to 98% with the addition of color Doppler imaging to gray-scale ultrasound [2].

Sonography, with or without color Doppler imaging, can provide excellent imaging of rapid, transient, and low-volume reflux episodes. After a milk or formula meal, episodes of GER are seen on standard ultrasound as transient, linear or clustered, retrograde mobile bright echoes within the distal esophagus. After clear liquids, GER may be slightly more difficult to visualize as a bolus of anechoic fluid with few echoic foci propagating within the distal esophagus in a retrograde fashion. The addition of color Doppler imaging affords visualization of very transient, clustered, rapid, or low-volume episodes, due to its high sensitivity for motion. This same sensitivity may prove detrimental, however, in the crying, mobile, or agitated child.

While quite sensitive for GER, ultrasound (with or without color Doppler) cannot accurately depict the volume or proximal extent of GER, as the majority of the thoracic esophagus cannot be seen due to lack of an appropriate sonographic window. Furthermore, sonography is inferior to the UGI in the demonstration of normal and pathologic anatomy of the upper gastrointestinal tract that may predispose to GER. Therefore, while safe, effective, and of low cost, ultrasound (with the addition of color Doppler when available) appears to be most useful as a screening test and as a complementary procedure in patients with symptoms attributable to GER but in whom prior studies, such as pH monitoring and UGI, have been normal.

16.3
Bronchoalveolar Lavage

The principle underlying the use of BAL for the diagnosis of GER is identification of lipid-laden macrophages within the lavage fluid. The assumption is that chronic aspiration of lipid-containing food substances results in uptake of the lipid by alveolar macrophages, which can then be identified and quantitated in the BAL fluid. This technique was first described in the 1970s [10], and has been used by many centers as a test for "silent aspiration" for many years. Animal experiments instilling milk into the lungs confirms that alveolar macrophages take up the lipid, that the lipid can be identified on cytological examination, and that repeated aspiration results in lipid-laden macrophages over a prolonged period of time [11].

The technique involves instilling a saline solution into the bronchial tree at the time of either rigid or flexible bronchoscopy, and recovering the fluid in a suction trap. Usually, some of the fluid is sent for culture, and some is sent to the cytologist for identification of lipid-laden alveolar macrophages. The fluid is centrifuged and the pellet is resuspended and placed on microscope slides. The slides are fixed and then stained with hematoxylin and eosin, and then counter-stained with standard oil-red-O. Using this technique, the macrophages which have taken up lipid contain obvious red material within them (Fig. 1). Some authors have developed methods for quantifying the amount of lipid taken up, using a lipid-laden macrophage index which takes into account both the number of macrophages which contain lipid and the amount of lipid within them [12].

The identification of lipid-laden macrophages in BAL fluid has been correlated with GER in a number of studies. Initial experience suggested a correlation in adults [13], and more recently these findings have been reproduced in the pediatric population [14, 15]. In particular, this technique has been used to investigate the role of GER in the pathogenesis of lung disease in children with other potential causes of lung disease such as tracheomalacia [16], bronchopulmonary dysplasia [17], and recalcitrant undiagnosed respiratory symptoms [18].

A number of authors have expressed concern about the accuracy of BAL in making the diagnosis of GER. In some cases, the lipid-laden macrophage index has not correlated well with the results of extended pH monitoring [18], which is usually considered the "gold-standard" test for reflux. Others have noted that lipid-laden macrophages can also be found in a number of other diseases where there is no evidence of aspiration, such as fat embolism, acute chest syndrome, administration of intravenous lipids, cystic fibrosis, and endogenous lipoid pneumonia [19, 20], as well as iatrogenic conditions such as administration of mineral oil [21] or the antiarrhythmia drug amiodoron [22]. Aspiration may occur in the absence of GER, particularly in children with pharyngeal dyscoordination and impaired swallowing. Finally, some authors have found that the lipid-laden macrophage index does not correlate with indicators of lung inflammation, suggesting that the finding may in part reflect processes other than aspiration [20].

Further studies will be necessary to further refine the technique currently used for quantifying lipid-laden macrophages and for correlating this finding with the presence of GER. Although the presence of lipid-laden macrophages is currently the only way to test for GER

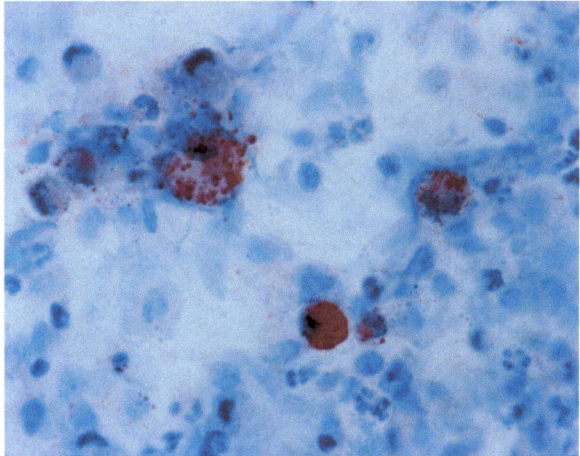

Fig. 1. Fluid from a BAL stained with hematoxylin and eosin, and counter-stained with standard oil-red-O. The lipid is seen within the cytoplasm of the macrophages

using BAL fluid, other techniques may be developed in the future, including the use of surfactant protein analysis [23] or other indicators more specific for the presence of aspiration-induced inflammation.

References

1. Gomes H, Menanteau B (1991) Gastro-esophageal reflux: comparative study between sonography and pH monitoring. Pediatr Radiol 21:168–174
2. Hirsch W, Kedar R, Preis U (1996) Color Doppler in the diagnosis of the gastroesophageal reflux in children: comparison with pH measurements and B-mode ultrasound. Pediatr Radiol 26:232–235
3. Westra SJ, Derkx HHF, Taminiau JAJM (1994) Symptomatic gastroesophageal reflux: diagnosis with ultrasound. J Pediatr Gastroenterol Nutr 19:58–64
4. Yamada M, Kobayashi I, Kawamura N, Okano M, Sakiyama Y, Kobayashi K (1988) Color Doppler ultrasonography for evaluation of gastroesophageal reflux in a sick child. Acta Paediatr 98:229–230
5. Gomes H, Lallemand P (1992) Infant apnea and gastroesophageal reflux. Pediatr Radiol 22:8–11
6. Wynchank S, Mann MD, Fisher R, Dwyer E (1997) Ultrasound as a screening study for gastroesophageal reflux in children. Ann Trop Pediatr 17:343–348
7. Milocco C, Salvatore CM, Torre G, Guastalla P, Ventura A (1997) Sonography versus continuous 24 hours esophageal pH-monitoring in the diagnosis of infants with gastroesophageal reflux. Pediatr Med Chir 19:245–246
8. Westra S, Wolf BH, Staalman CR (1990) Ultrasound diagnosis of gastroesophageal reflux and hiatal hernia in infants and young children. J Clin Ultrasound 18:477–485
9. Madi-Szabo L, Kocsis G (2000) Examination of gastroesophageal reflux by transabdominal ultrasound: can a slow, trickling form of reflux be responsible for reflux esophagitis? Can J Gastroenterol 14:588–592
10. Williams HE, Freeman M (1973) Milk inhalation pneumonia, the significance of fat-filled macrophages in tracheal secretions. Aust Paediatr J 9:286–288
11. Colombo JL, Hallberg TK, Sammut PH (1992) Time course of lipid-laden pulmonary macrophages with acute and recurrent milk aspiration in rabbits. Pediatr Pulmonol 12:95–98
12. Colombo JL, Hallberg TK (1987) Recurrent aspiration in children: lipid-laden alveolar macrophage quantitation. Pediatr Pulmonol 3:86–89
13. Corwin RW, Irwin RS (1985) The lipid-laden alveolar macrophage as a marker of aspiration in parenchymal lung disease. Am Rev Resp Dis 132:576–581
14. Nussbaum E, Maggi JC, Mathis R, Galant SP (1987) Association of lipid-laden alveolar macrophages and gastroesophageal reflux in children. J Pediatr 10:190–194
15. Ahrens P, Noll C, Kitz R, Willigens P, Zielen S, Hofmann D (1999) Lipid-laden alveolar macrophages (LLAM): a useful marker of silent aspiration in children. Pediatr Pulmonol 28:83–88
16. Bibi H, Khvolis E, Shoseyov D et al. (2001) The prevalence of gastroesophageal reflux in children with tracheomalacia and laryngomalacia. Chest 19:409–413
17. Radford PJ, Stillwell PC, Blue B, Hertel G (1995) Aspiration complicating bronchopulmonary dysplasia. Chest 07:185–188
18. Sacco O, Fregonese B, Silvestri M, Sabatini F, Mattioli G, Rossi GA (2000) Bronchoalveolar lavage and esophageal pH monitoring data in children with "difficult to treat" respiratory symptoms. Pediatr Pulmonol 30:313–319
19. Knauer-Fischer S, Ratjen F (1999) Lipid-laden macrophages in bronchoalveolar lavage fluid as a marker for pulmonary aspiration. Pediatr Pulmonol 7:419–422
20. Kazachkov MY, Muhlebach MS, Livasy CA, Noah TL (2001) Lipid-laden macrophage index and inflammation in bronchoalveolar lavage fluids in children. Eur Respir J 8:790–795
21. Bandla HP, Davis SH, Hopkins NE (1999) Lipoid pneumonia: a silent complication of mineral oil aspiration. Pediatrics 103:E19
22. Jacobson W, Stewart S, Gresham GA, Goddard MJ (1997) Effect of amiodarone on the lung shown by polarized light microscopy. Arch Pathol Lab Med 121:1269–1271
23. Griese M, Maderlechner N, Ahrens P, Kitz R (2002) Surfactant proteins A and D in children with pulmonary disease due to gastroesophageal reflux. Am J Respir Crit Care Med 65:1546–1550

The Bronchoalveolar Lavage Technique to Evaluate Silent Aspiration in Children with Reflux-Associated Respiratory Disease

17

Peter Ahrens

Contents

There is a great deal of data suggesting a high incidence of gastroesophageal reflux (GER) in intrinsic asthma, pulmonary fibrosis, recurrent pneumonia, recurrent obstructive bronchitis, chronic nocturnal cough, near missed sudden infant death syndrome, and even recurrent otitis, laryngitis, and vocal cord dysfunction [1–9]. Although this association is well documented, the clinical management of reflux-associated respiratory diseases (RARD) remains difficult. At present, there is no test available which allows the identification of children suffering from silent aspiration due to GER. Moreover, the various pulmonary symptoms associated with GER make the diagnosis of silent aspiration difficult, especially when recurrent vomiting is absent. Chronic lung disease often is the only symptom of GER, because even only one single reflux episode per day reaching the lung may cause pulmonary damage – but not signs or symptoms of gastroesophageal reflux disease (GERD). RARD, therefore, is more often a borderline illness closer to physiological rather than to pathological reflux. It is mild reflux which causes severe respiratory disease and only a minority of patients suffering from severe GERD also suffer from respiratory symptoms. Therefore, it is necessary to discuss the problems concerning diagnosis and management of RARD in another way than it is usually discussed. It is necessary to emphasize the pulmonological aspect in contrast to that of gastroenterology, because obviously a diagnosis of RARD is not easily made using classical gastroenterologic methodology.

Extended pH monitoring, which is considered to be the "gold standard," is a very sensitive method to detect GERD [10, 11]; however, it cannot prove pulmonary aspiration secondary to GER.

Detection of pharyngeal reflux episodes during double-probe pH monitoring, with the second probe being placed behind the larynx, is indicative of laryngopharyngeal reflux and silent aspiration [12]. Double-probe pH monitoring therefore is necessary and recommended in otorhinolaryngological- and pulmonological-diseased patients because the higher probe definitively documents acid reflux into the upper esophagus – near the respiratory system.

Contrast studies are not a sensitive way to diagnose RARD. A barium swallow may demonstrate significant structural abnormalities (hiatal hernia, stricture) but not aspiration. Sensitivities reported in the literature range from 20% to 73%, with an average of 39% for detecting free reflux [13].

The reported sensitivity of technetium-99 scintiscanning is poor and ranges from 14% to 90% with an average of 65% [14]. Additionally, this test suffers from its relatively short monitoring period and the fact that reflux by nature occurs intermittently and frequently after meals.

Usually, endoscopy is the first test used to identify the presence of esophagitis. A number of endoscopic criteria have evolved helping to diagnose reflux esophagitis. Unfortunately, the interpretation of these signs is subject to interobserver and even intraobserver variability [15], when minimal inflammation exists. Microscopic changes indicative of reflux injury may occur even when the mucosa appears normal endoscopically [16]. The most sensitive histological markers of reflux disease are reactive epithelial changes characterized by an increase in the basal cell layer greater than 15% of the epithelial thickness, papilla elongation into the upper third of the epithelium, and cellular infiltration of neutrophils and eosinophils.

None of these methods has been shown to be sensitive or specific for pulmonary aspiration, and a gold standard for the diagnosis of silent aspiration is still lacking.

17.1
Lipid-Laden Alveolar Macrophages

As gastric contents often contain lipid material that will be taken up by macrophages if introduced into the respiratory system, it has been postulated that the lipid content of alveolar macrophages may be a useful indicator for pulmonary aspiration [17–23] and has been suggested as being indicative and even diagnostic of lipid aspiration. The association of lipid-filled vacuoles in the cytoplasm of alveolar macrophages in patients suspected of having pulmonary aspiration led to the development of the quantitative lipid-laden macrophage index. Assessment of the lipid-laden macrophage index rests on its ability to determine whether chronic aspiration is truly present or not. Because there is no gold standard for diagnosing reflux-associated respiratory disease, to date there are no data concerning the accuracy of the test, nor can sensitivity or specificity be precisely calculated; therefore, its value is a matter of discussion.

17.2
Collection Technique and Staining

Bronchoscopy is carried out using a rigid or a flexible pediatric bronchoscope. Bronchoalveolar Lavage (BAL) is performed by wedging the flexible bronchoscope or a suction catheter in the lobe that appears most affected by the underlying disease process, or in a right lower lobe bronchus whenever the disease is not localized. Lavage is performed three or four times with 1 mL 0.9% saline per kg body weight. BAL fluid is collected separately and processed immediately: after filtration through double gauze the material is centrifuged for 10 min at 1,200 rpm. The pellet is resuspended in normal saline to a density of 250,000 cells/ml. Two hundred microliters are centrifuged for 10 min at 1,000 rpm (Cytospin, Shandon GmbH). The slides are stained with Sudan Red (0.2% in 70% alcohol) for 15 min. This is followed by rinsing the slides in 50% alcohol and distilled water. After this, the slide is put in Hämalaun Mayer solution for 5 min and placed under running water for 10 min. Glycerine-gelatin is used as an embedding medium. Each macrophage is graded according to the amount of lipid in the cytoplasm with a number of 0–4 (0= no lipids, 4= filled with lipids; Fig. 1A–D) using the method described by Colombo and Hallberg [17]. The total score is determined by taking the summed total

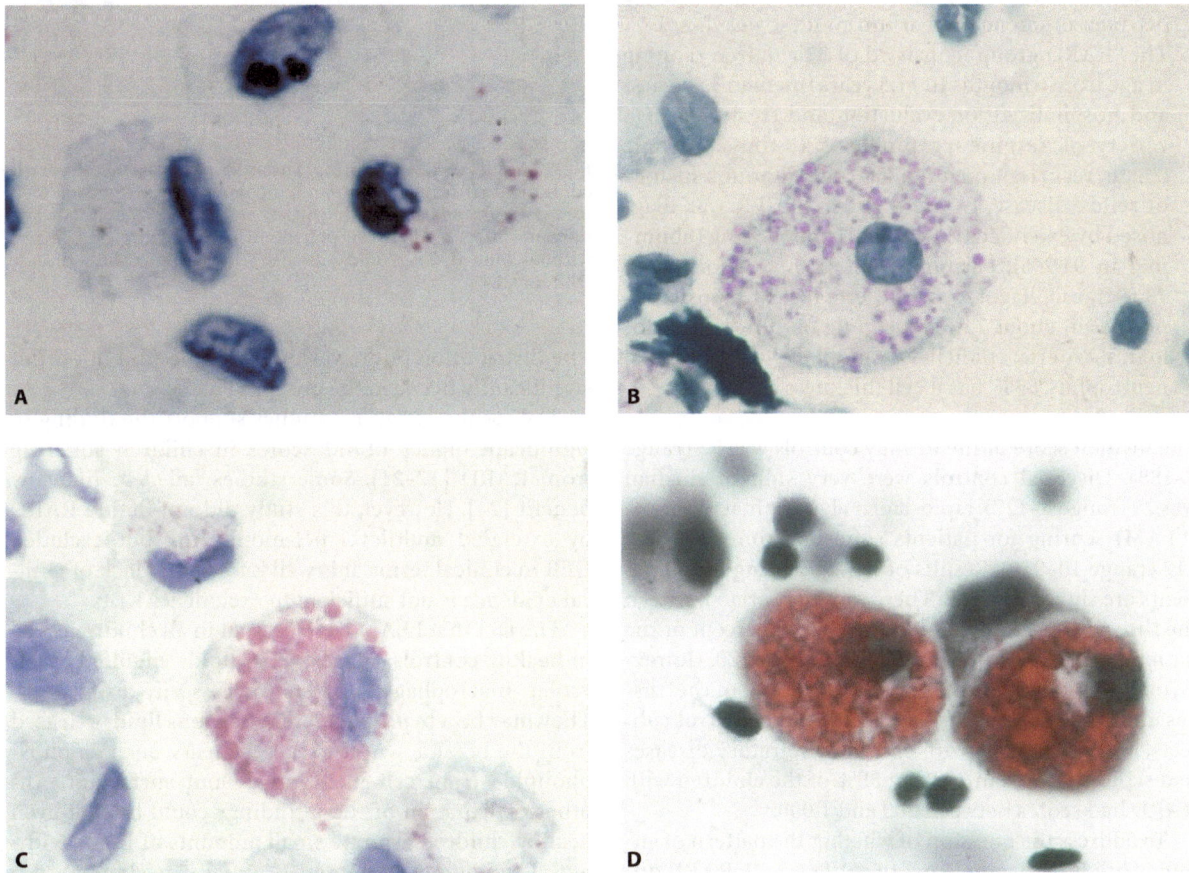

Fig. 1A–D. Lipid laden alveolar macrophages stained with sudan red and filled with different amounts of lipid in the cytoplasm [grade 0 (no lipids) up to grade 4 (filled with lipids)]

grades of 100 cells. Thus, a score with a potential maximum of 400 is obtained for each specimen.

Worldwide there is only one study which compares healthy children, children with different chronic respiratory diseases without GER, and children suggestive for RARD [21]. A total of 900 macrophages per BAL were scored. Therefore, the potential maximum was 3,600 for each specimen.

Patients were divided into three groups:

1. The "Healthy controls" consisted of 20 children aged 1.5–14.7 years (median 5.3 years). These children had no history of allergy or chronic lung disease or any infectious disease of the upper or lower airway for at least 6 weeks prior to the study. They underwent general anesthesia for elective surgery (hernia, varicocele, lipoma, bone fracture, arthroscopy, burns). Children undergoing ear, nose, and throat surgery were not included.

2. "Diseased controls" consisted of 14 children aged 10 months to 9.9 years (median 3.4 years) suffering from recurrent pneumonia due to stenosis of main stem bronchus, foreign body aspiration, immunodeficiency, and bronchiectasis caused by primary ciliary dyskinesia. There was no evidence of pathological reflux activity in any of these patients (dual-probe pH-measurement and barium swallow was done).

3. The "RARD group" consisted of 32 children ranging in age from 6 months to 11.8 years (median 3.4 years) and hospitalized for evaluation and treatment of a variety of respiratory problems (asthma, chronic cough, recurrent pneumonia) and without a history of reflux disease. In these children, GER was diagnosed by extended two-level pH-monitoring (abnormal in 91.2%), barium esophagram (abnormal in 73.5%), esophagoscopy, and esophageal biopsy (abnormal in about 75% depending on different histological criteria: epithelial eosinophils, 46%; epithelial neutrophils, 83%, basal cell thickness, 89%).

The median score of the healthy controls was 37 (range 5–188). Diseased controls were very similar: median was 29 (range 5–127). Lipid-laden alveolar macrophages (LLAM) scoring for patients suffering from GER was 117 (range 10–956). Results of LLAM scoring for all patients are shown in Fig. 2. There was an overlap between the three groups in the lipid scores. Fifty percent of the patients with RARD had a score exceeding 120. However, only 15% out of the controls and 7.1% out of the "diseased controls" exceeded 120. Neither the control subjects, nor the patients with chronic respiratory diseases had scores more than 200, but 38% of the children with RARD had scores between 200 and 1,000.

To address the question of whether the pattern of engulfed lipids in macrophages in patients with RARD differ from healthy or diseased controls, analysis of LLAM scores belonging to the different cell types was done.

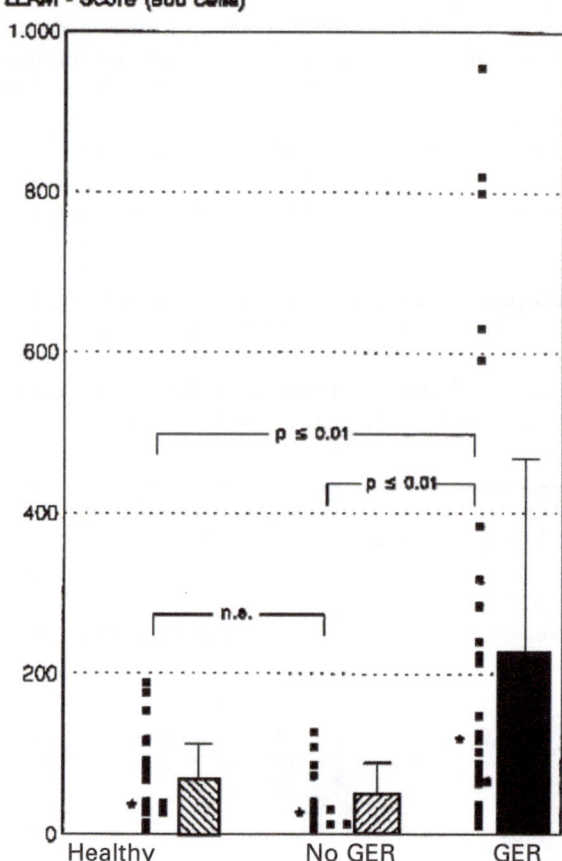

LLAM - Score (900 cells)

Fig. 2. Results of LLAM-scoring. The score refers to 900 cells graded. Individual results (*solid box*), median (*asterisk*), means (*columns*) and standard deviation (*bars*) are shown. There was a significant difference between patients with GER, surgical controls without lung diseases and patients with chronic chest disease without GER

The distribution of the various cell types did not differ significantly between the groups (Fig. 3).

The results of several studies support the finding of significant higher LLAM scores in children suffering from RARD [17–21]. Some studies failed to find any benefit [24]. However, this study did not define RARD by extended multilevel pH-monitoring but excluded GER in clinical terms. It is well known that lack of clinical evidence is not sufficient to exclude RARD!

The fact that LLAM were present in all children, even in healthy controls, suggests that lipids engulfed by alveolar macrophages are not necessarily exogenous. They may be a byproduct of endogenous lipids released from the breakdown of tissue elements, such as phospholipids from cell membranes, and surfactant. Another explanation of these findings could be that even healthy children aspirate small amounts of lipids without showing any symptoms. Animal experiments suggest that one single aspiration can cause an incorporation of lipid into alveolar macrophages for 2–3 days

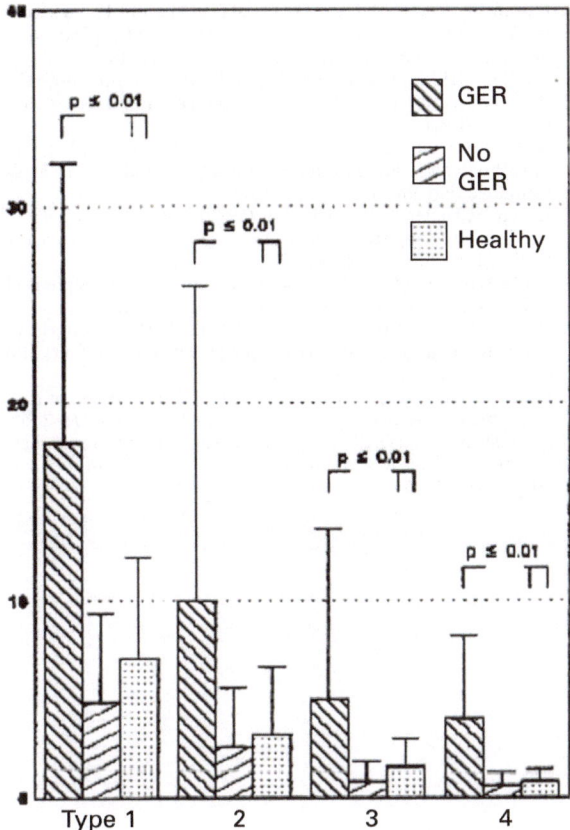

Fig. 3. Distribution of LLAM cell-types. Shown are the number of Sudan red mounted cells of type 1–4 out of 900 cells counted. Means and standard deviations are given

from vagally mediated bronchospasm, in patients with silent aspiration surgery may be the therapy of choice (Hemifundoplication according to Thal). Improvement after surgery and good long-term results justify this therapy [25–29]. In addition, treatment of these patients with acid suppression may not prevent aspiration of nonacidic gastric contents.

In conclusion, BAL and scoring the lipid-laden alveolar macrophages is an important tool to help in diagnosing silent aspiration. There is a significant portion of patients who are identified. It is not a gold standard of diagnosis and there is up to now not any single method to confirm this diagnosis. It is necessary to perform BAL, dual-probe, 24-h pH-monitoring, bronchoscopy, esophago-gastroscopy, esophageal biopsy and sometimes barium esophagram to decide whether or not a reflux associated problem exists. Furthermore it is necessary to exclude diseases such as immunodeficiency, cystic fibrosis, primary ciliary dyskinesia, and allergic diseases. By using all these methods – including LLAM score – it is possible to establish the diagnosis of RARD in children with high precision.

[20]. LLAM, therefore, are a nonspecific finding. Otherwise none of the healthy controls and none of the patients suffering from chronic respiratory disease not caused by reflux had a score more than 200, while 38% of the patients suffering from RARD exceeded a score of 200. These 38% are likely to suffer from chronic aspiration and the score helps to confirm a diagnosis of chronic aspiration. On the other hand, chronic aspiration cannot be excluded by a score less than 200, because the amount of LLAM depends on the time that has passed since aspiration occurred.

The high rate of low LLAM scores in children with documented RARD is not totally unexpected. It is apparent that only a minority of children with RARD develop lung injury due to silent aspiration. Stimulation of esophageal vagal afferents is another mechanism by which reflux is able to cause bronchoconstriction and airway hyperreactivity. Nevertheless, it is clinically very important to distinguish children with silent aspiration from those with pulmonary symptoms triggered solely by acid irritation of the esophagus. While conservative therapy with proton pump inhibitors or H-2-blockers may be useful in treating RARD in children suffering

References

1. Berquist WE, Rachelefsky GE, Kadden M et al (1981) Gastro-esophageal reflux-associated recurrent pneumonia and chronic asthma in children. J Pediatr 68:29–35
2. Malfroot A, Vandenplas Y, Verlinden M et al (1987) Gastro-esophageal reflux and unexplained chronic respiratory disease in infants and children. Pediatr Pulmonol 3:208–213
3. Danus O, Casar C, Larrain A et al (1976) Esophageal reflux: an unrecognized cause of recurrent obstructive bronchitis in children. J Pediatr 89:220–224
4. Mays EE (1976) Intrinsic asthma in adults. Association with gastroesophageal reflux. JAMA 236:2626–2628
5. Buts JP, Barudi D, Moulin D et al (1986) Prevalence and treatment of silent gastroesophageal reflux in children with recurrent respiratory disorders. Eur J Pediatr 145:396–400
6. Ing AJ, Ngu MC, Breslin AB (1991) Chronic persistent cough and gastroesophageal reflux. Thorax 46:476–483
7. Herbst JJ, Monton SD, Books LS (1979) Gastroesophageal reflux causing respiratory distress and apnea in newborn infants. J Pediatr 95:763–768
8. Macfayden UM, Hendry GM, Simpson H (1983) Gastroesophageal reflux in near missed sudden infant death syndrome or suspected recurrent aspiration. Arch Dis Child 58:87–91
9. Ahrens P, Seibt Y, Kitz R (2001) Vocal cord dysfunction bei Kindern und Jugendlichen. Pneumologie 55:378–384
10. Euler AR, Byrne WJ (1981) Twenty-four-hour esophageal intraluminal pH-probe testing: a comparative analysis. Gastroenterology 80:957–961
11. Jolley SG, Herbst JJ, Johnson DG et al (1981) Esophageal pH-monitoring during sleep identifies children with respiratory symptoms from gastroesophageal reflux. Gastroenterology 80:1501–1506
12. Wiener GJ, Koufmann JA, Wu WC et al (1989) Chronic hoarseness secondary to gastroesophageal reflux disease: documentation with 24-h ambulatory pH monitoring. Am J Gastroenterol 84:1503–1508
13. Ott DJ (1994) Gastroesophageal reflux disease. Radiol Clin North Am 32:1147–1166
14. Jenkins AF, Cowan RJ, Richter JE (1985) Gastroesophageal scintigraphy: is it a sensitive screening test for gastroesophageal reflux disease? J Clin Gastroenterol 7:127–131

15. Bytzer P, Havelund T, Moller-Hansen J et al (1993) Interobserver variation of the endoscopic diagnosis of reflux esophagitis. Scand J Gastroenterol 28:119–125

16. Funch-Jensen P, Kock K, Christensen LA et al (1986) Microscopic appearance of the esophageal mucosa in a consecutive series of patients submitted to upper endoscopy. Correlation with gastroesophageal reflux symptoms and macroscopic findings. Scand J Gastroenterol 21:65–69

17. Colombo J, Hallberg TK (1987) Recurrent aspiration in children: Lipid-laden alveolar macrophage quantitation. Pediatr Pulmonol 3:86–89

18. Nussbaum E, Maggi JC, Mathis R et al (1987) Association of lipid-laden alveolar macrophages and gastroesophageal reflux in children. J Pediatr 110:190–194

19. Corwin RW, Irwin RS (1985) The lipid-laden alveolar macrophage as a marker of aspiration in parenchymal lung disease. Am Rev Respir Dis 132:576–581

20. Colombo J, Hallberg TK, Sammut PH et al (1992) Time course of lipid-laden pulmonary macrophages with acute and recurrent milk aspiration in rabbits. Pediatr Pulmonol 12:95–98

21. Ahrens P, Noll C, Kitz R et al (1999) Lipid-laden alveolar macrophages (LLAM(: A useful marker of silent aspiration in children. Pediatr Pulmonol 28:83–88

22. Moran JR, Block SM, Lyerly AD et al (1988) Lipid-laden alveolar macrophage and lactose assay as marker of aspiration in neonates with lung disease. J Pediatr 112:643–645

23. Williams HE, Freeman M (1973) Milk inhalation pneumonia, the significance of fat-filled macrophages in trachea secretions. Aust Paediatr J 9:286–288

24. Knauer-Fischer S, Ratjen F (1999) Lipid-laden macrophages in bronchoalveolar lavage fluid as a marker for pulmonary aspiration. Pediatr Pulmonol 27:419–422

25. Ahrens P, Heller K, Beyer P et al (1999) Antireflux surgery in children suffering from reflux-associated respiratory diseases. Pediatr Pulmonol 28:89–93

26. Fonkelsrud EW (1987) Surgical treatment of gastroesophageal reflux disease in childhood. Z Kinderchir 42:7–11

27. Harnsberger JK, Corey JJ, Johnson DG et al (1983) Long-term followup of surgery for gastroesophageal reflux in infants and children. J Pediatr 102:505–508

28. Johnson D, Herbst J, Oliveros M et al (1977) Evaluation of gastroesophageal reflux surgery in children. Pediatrics 59:62–68

29. Dedinsky G, Vane D, Black T et al (1987) Complications and reoperations after Nissen fundoplication in childhood. Am J Surg 153:177–183

Chapter 18

Gastric Emptying and Pediatric Gastroesophageal Reflux

18

José Estevão-Costa

Contents

18.1
Role of the Stomach in the Antireflux Barrier and Gastroesophageal Reflux Pathogenesis

The gastroesophageal antireflux barrier in humans depends on the interaction of three components: a valvular mechanism, the lower esophageal sphincter (LES); a propulsive "pump", the esophagus; and a reservoir, the stomach [12, 38, 39, 50, 95] (Fig. 1). Although the controversial issues concerning the valvular mechanism, such as the real existence and role of an anatomic sphincter [41, 95], a well-functioning gastric reservoir would certainly be crucial for the efficacy of the antireflux barrier.

In the presence of an incompetent LES, the stomach can contribute to gastroesophageal reflux (GER) by providing aggressive fluid to reflux, but it can also challenge directly the LES. The stomach may induce episodes of reflux if the intraluminal pressure overrides the LES pressure. Gastric distension can produce an incompetent valve by the shortening of the LES length or by inducing transient LES relaxations, as has been demonstrated in both healthy volunteers and patients [30, 33, 50, 70, 79, 108, 113]. Thus, gastric emptying dysfunc-

tion could conceivably play an important role in GER by intensifying these mechanisms [69, 103, 112].

18.2
Physiology of Gastric Emptying

The stomach is not a simple muscular bag that stores large quantities of food. Its motor functions also include fragmentation and mixing of food with gastric secretions to form the chyme and emptying of gastric contents into the duodenum at a controlled rate [9, 60, 104]. The stomach is composed of three distinct muscular components: the fundic reservoir, the antral pump, and the pyloric sieve. These components act in concert with duodenal peristalsis to regulate gastric emptying (GE); there are several programs of emptying, such as a rapid emptying of bland meals and a slow emptying of nutrient-rich meals [104].

GE is regulated by both neural and humoral mechanisms, the vagus nerve being particularly important [9, 104]. The current opinion that contraction of the fundus is responsible for the emptying of liquids, whereas antral contractions control the propulsion of solids is simplistic and not entirely correct [104]. In fact, GE promoted by vigorous antral contractions is opposed by varying degrees of resistance to passage of chyme through the pylorus [60].

To summarize, GE is only moderately controlled by weak gastric factors that promote emptying (local myenteric reflexes and release of gastrin due to stretch and some types of food) and strongly inhibited by duodenal signals, including both the enterogastric nervous system feedback reflexes and hormonal feedback (probably cholecystokinin) [60]. The latter work together to slow the rate of emptying in the presence of fatty acids or monoglycerides, amino acids and peptides, hypertonic solutions and pH less than 3.5 [9]. Therefore, the rate of GE is limited to that amount of chyme that the small intestine can process [9, 60]. Another important issue related to GE is the effect of consistence; viscous solutions empty more slowly from the stomach than nonviscous ones, because their greater inertia resists propulsive contractions [104].

Fig. 1.
Integrated concept of gastro-esophageal antireflux barrier. The valve (LES), the pump (esophageal clearance), and the reservoir (stomach)

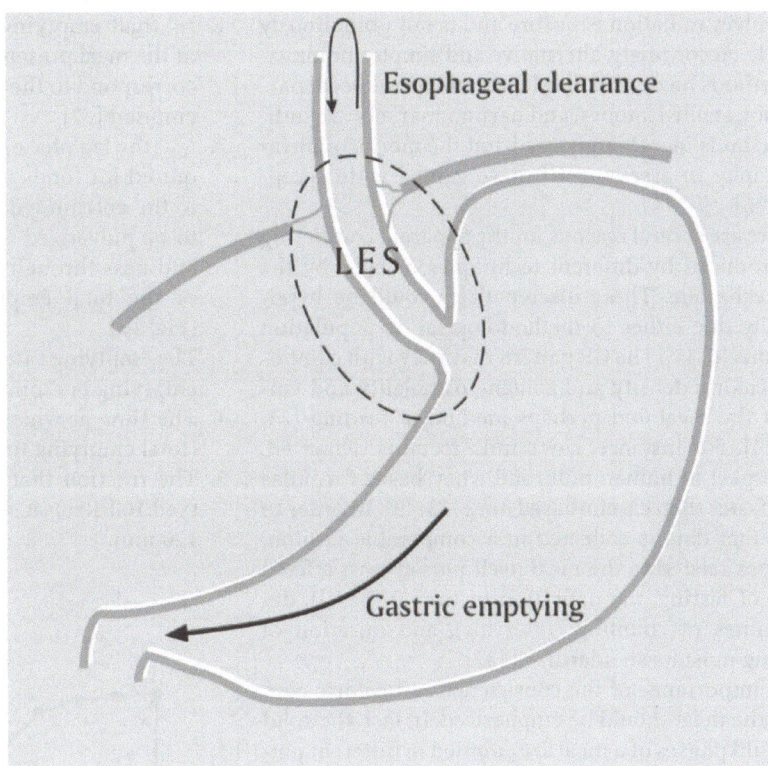

18.3
Delayed Gastric Emptying and Gastroesophageal Reflux

Delayed gastric emptying (DGE) has been documented in a high proportion of patients with GER [6, 33, 42, 91, 108, 120, 126]. In children with GER disease related to esophageal atresia or neurologic impairment, DGE has been recorded in approximately or even more than half of the cases [33, 38, 39, 47, 120, 126]. On the other hand, DGE has assumed clinical relevance because it has been recognized as the main cause of operative treatment failure [33, 91, 120, 126]. In fact, poor gastric emptying is probably partially responsible for postoperative gas-bloat syndrome and for failure of antireflux procedures due to breakdown or slipping of the fundic wrap [13].

Despite its high prevalence, the pathophysiologic role of DGE has not yet been entirely established. Recently, it was suggested that DGE could be an important contributor to GER by increasing esophageal exposure in the postprandial period [31, 42]; it seems to accentuate postprandial reflux probably by increasing the volume of refluxate per episode of reflux through an underlying incompetent lower esophageal sphincter [42]. These findings support that enhancement of GE may be useful in GER disease with DGE and the belief that reduction in meal size is helpful in dealing with GER. However, the primary defect in DGE might be related to

a gastric motility disorder, such as antral hypomotility or impaired coordination of contractions, rather than to an outflow obstruction [32, 67, 75, 101, 120], which explains the well-known efficacy of prokinetics drugs and justifies the controversy about gastric drainage procedures [17, 18, 126]. Nevertheless, therapeutic enhancement of GE has been used with apparent success in GER disease with DGE [18, 22]; actually, adding a pyloroplasty to fundoplication has been associated with lower postoperative complications and recurrence of GER [18, 47, 108].

18.4
Evaluation of Gastric Emptying

Although DGE would not be necessarily a marker of severe GER disease [6, 36, 42, 123], the abovementioned issues dictate the need for evaluation of GE, especially in children in whom antireflux surgery is contemplated. Measurement of GE is therefore important not only to the physiologist investigating gastric motility but also to the clinician who deals with upper gastrointestinal dysfunctions such as GER.

Studies to evaluate GE are being conducted using a variety of techniques, but many of these present limitations that preclude their clinical application. Gastric scintigraphy is currently the gold standard to assess GE but involves radiation exposure and is not ubiquitously available. Accordingly, alternative and simpler noninvasive methods have been developed and introduced; paracetamol, stable isotopes, and barium markers are indirect methods increasingly used, but the merits of ultrasonography in assessing GE have gained wide acceptance [96].

There are several reasons for the apparent conflicting data produced by different techniques or even by the same technique. These discrepancies could be hypothetically due either to methodological or population variations [6, 45]. The GE pattern may vary with composition, caloric density and content, osmolality and volume of the meal and perhaps method of feeding [21, 117, 124]. For instance, cow's milk formula delays GE with respect to human milk, and whey-based formulas empty faster than casein-based ones [23, 49]. In order to ensure that data is collected in a comparable fashion, the issues related to the meal itself plus at least a fixed period of fasting, the definition of time 0 (basal), defined times of counting (intervals), and duration of sampling must be standardized [37].

The importance of the consistence and caloric content of the meal should be emphasized. In fact, the solid and liquid phases of a meal are emptied in different patterns and pathological conditions may affect GE in different ways, the solid phase being usually the first one to be affected [14]. This is therefore an overwhelming issue to be taken into account when a comparison between groups or techniques is performed. The majority of patients with GE disorders have delayed emptying of both solid and liquids, but a substantial subset of patients, such as those with GER disease, presents a normal or even rapid emptying of liquids [5, 22, 28, 29, 44, 76, 126]; thus, methods measuring solid phase are much more sensitive to detect DGE in patients with GER.

Volume is the main determinant of the GE rate of liquids; saline, neutral, isosmolar, and calorically inert solutions empty in a single exponential course [27, 89, 124] (Fig. 2a). GE of solids is biphasic in character. The stomach requires a period of time to process solid food to particles small enough to be handled as liquid; after this initial delay, both solids and liquids have similar emptying rates [118]. The GE curve for solid food is sigmoidal in shape with an initial shoulder with little emptying (lag phase), followed by a prolonged linear phase with a constant rate and, finally, a much slower phase (Fig. 2a) [124].

Another crucial issue is the approach to the analysis and reporting of GE data. From the viewpoint of analysis, all quantitative techniques result in data of the same type, i.e., percent or fraction of the meal remaining in the stomach (or emptied) at defined times after ingestion of the meal [37]. Standard data are usually expressed as:

1. $t_{1/2}$ (half-emptying time), the time at which one-half of the meal present at time 0 has emptied. It may not correspond to the time at which 50% of the meal has emptied [37].
2. t_{lag} (the lag phase) has been assumed as the time required for foods to be transported from the fundus to the antrum within the stomach and for the foods to be pulverized to particles less than 2 mm in size and pass through the pyloric ring, usually 5%–10% of the total emptying time [2, 93, 94, 118, 125] (Fig. 2b).
3. The emptying rate (postlag for solids), i.e., percent of emptying per minute (Fig. 2b) [19, 118, 124].
4. The time at which a specific fraction or the whole (total emptying time) meal has emptied.
5. The fraction that has remained (R%, or has emptyed:100-R%) at a defined time, usually at 60 and 120 min.

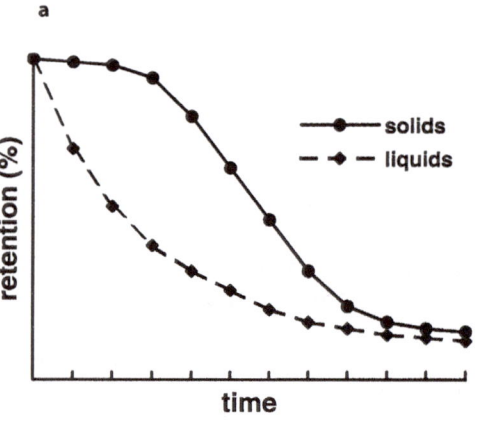

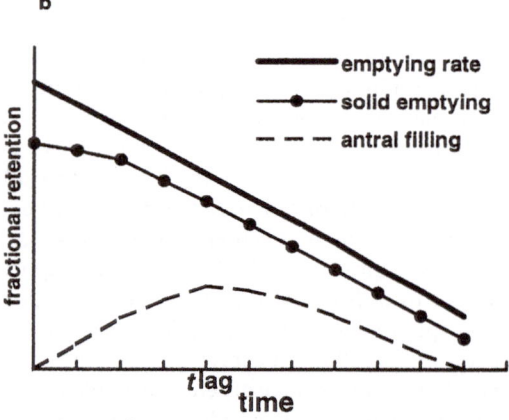

Fig. 2. a Gastric emptying curves for liquids (single exponential) and for solids (sigmoidal). b Power exponential fitting model for an emptying curve of solids. Note that the lag phase (t_{lag}) coincides with the peak antral filling and with the inflection point of the emptying curve

In the context of GER disease the question to be addressed is whether patients have or do not have DGE. For this purpose the method of analysis should take into account the whole emptying curve rather than focusing separately on a specific time point [37]; therefore, individual emptying curves are characterized by one or two parameters that describe the total time course and can be compared statistically. Analysis of GE by fitting a mathematical curve (e.g., the Elashoff or the Siegel power exponential models) using nonlinear least squares has been recommended (Fig. 2b) [1, 37, 118]. A standard method to assess the lag phase is important to study certain motility disorders and therapeutic drugs that mainly affect it [86, 118]. Milk usually empties in a monoexponential or biexponential manner, thus $t_{1/2}$ may be meaningful [67].

The values for normal GE have been difficult to establish, especially in infants and children because of the lack of normal controls [67]. The importance of standardization is amplified in children because age influences the remaining factors. It seems that normal GE rate is age-related, thus one must consider the age range when determining the normal range for GE [109].

Apart from the intersubject variability in a skewed distribution, motility measurements of the stomach are rendered more difficult by substantial day-to-day variability [88]. Although reproducibility is better using solid rather than liquid tests [84], the intrasubject variability has coefficients of variation of almost 15% or even higher [15, 35].

The administration of drugs and concurrent conditions that may modify gastric motility should also be considered in the evaluation of GE [8, 20, 89, 104, 122]; the former should be stopped at least 48 h prior to the GE study (Table 1).

Lastly, there are several factors that may alter GE assessment, which are frequently overlooked. The meal should be appetizing and easy to ingest because gastric motility could be influenced by the cephalic phase [34]; meal temperature, posture, and exercise may also affect GE [16, 59, 121].

Table 1. Medications and diseases that may affect gastric emptying

Medications	Diseases
Delay	
Anticholinergics	Celiac disease
Tricyclic antidepressants	Diabetes mellitus
Narcotic analgesics	Neuromuscular disorders
Calcium channel blockers	Helicobacter pylori infection
Adrenergic agents	Chronic gastritis
Accelerate	
Metoclopramide, Cisapride, Domperidone	Dumping (early liquid phase), Pyloroplasty
Erytromycin	Hyperthyroidism

18.5
Indirect Assessment of Gastric Emptying

18.5.1
Stable Isotopic Techniques

Although gamma scintigraphy is still regarded as the reference method, stable nonradioactive isotopic labeling of the test meal has been increasingly reported as a feasible alternative technique to assess GE.

Breath tests are based upon the absorption in the duodenum of a test meal labeled with [^{13}C or ^{14}C]-octanoic acid or acetate and the hepatic oxidation of this fatty acid to [^{13}C or ^{14}C]-dioxide, which is loaded in expired air. [^{13}C]-glycine has been used as a marker of the liquid phase because it is easily solubilized in water [87]. Isotopic enrichment is analyzed in collected breath samples, which after mathematical evaluation allows the calculation of the standard parameters in much the same way as radioscintigraphy [20].

There are, however, some pitfalls. These methods assume that GE is the rate-limiting step in the ultimate delivery of [*C]-dioxide to the breath; moreover, the tests may not be accurate in the presence of pancreatic, liver, or pulmonary diseases as well as in patients with visceral hemodynamic disorders [20].

Stable isotope breath tests have been validated against scintigraphy and ultrasonography for solid and/or liquid phases with a significant correlation and similar reproducibility [14, 53, 73, 87]. However, a good agreement has not been always observed, because [*C] breath tests have a tendency to underestimate the measurements probably because of the time needed for absorption and metabolism of the fatty acid [2]. Although it cannot assess the GE of solids as accurately as scintigraphy, [*C]-fatty acid breath tests are a noninvasive and reliable modality increasingly used to study GE rate because of the low substrate price and radiation burden is 50–100 times less than scintigraphy (^{14}C) or totally absent (^{13}C). It can be therefore performed repeatedly in short periods of time with less discomfort for the patients and is applicable to field testing as breath samples can be stored and sent to reference laboratories [14, 20, 53, 116]. Increasing availability of equipment to measure breath [^{13}C]-dioxide for detection of Helicobacter infection will certainly result in an increased application for measurement of GE [20].

Breath tests based on ethanol and with ^{13}C-bicarbonate have been also used [10, 46].

18.5.2
Paracetamol Absorption Test

Paracetamol (acetaminophen) absorption kinetics after oral ingestion of the drug has been proposed to estimate GE. It is based on the assumption that the rate of paracetamol absorption, which occurs mainly and rapidly in the small intestine, assessed by plasma sampling exclusively represents GE rate [48, 63]. The safety, simplicity, reproducibility, and good acceptance by patients justify the popularity of this method [110]. However, the validity of the test is not consensual, as the most suitable index for the rate of paracetamol absorption remains inconclusive [110]. Although paracetamol absorption test could be reproducible when the drug is given together with a semi-solid meal in healthy volunteers [100], it has not gained wide clinical application because reliability has been assumed mainly for the liquid phase [110]. In conclusion, paracetamol tracer technique is a noninvasive (except for an indwelling intravenous catheter), relatively inexpensive, and easy to perform test that may yield a good approximation but not detailed information of GE [98].

18.5.3
Other Indirect Methods

Radiopaque barium markers has recently been suggested as a simple, cost-effective, low-invasive test for evaluation of GE, since it only requires standard x-ray equipment and a capsule of barium markers [24, 65, 80]. However, it is controversial whether emptying of indigestible material truly reflects physiologic GE [24]. Because of the poor correlation with scintigraphy, the radiopaque marker method may only be useful as a screening test to assess whether GE is rapid or delayed [114].

Cutaneous electrogastrography (EGG) techniques are becoming increasingly standardized [25, 112]. Gastric electrical abnormalities such as postprandial dysrhythmias and lack of a postprandial increase in the power of the EGG signal have been advocated as a reliable method to detect DGE [25, 26, 32]. In patients with GER, it may be able to predict postfundoplication complications [20, 107]. However, the clinical role of EGG is not yet established [20].

Derived parameters from extended esophageal pH-monitoring were recently proposed as an accurate method to predict the type of GE in patients with GER [40]. The postprandial to fasting *ratio* for reflux index seems to have high sensitivity and negative predictive value, whereas the distribution of the occurrence of the longest episode of reflux presents high specificity and positive predictive value [40]. The combination of a postprandial to fasting *ratio* for reflux index higher than 1 (i.e., a reflux index greater in the postprandial period) plus occurrence of the longest episode of reflux in the postprandial period was associated with a significantly high probability of DGE in the scintigraphic study [40].

18.6
Direct Measurement of Gastric Emptying

18.6.1
Scintigraphy

GE scintigraphy was introduced almost four decades ago by Griffith et al. [58]. After several refinements and optimization, it has become the gold standard for the evaluation of GE in many gastrointestinal diseases and for assessing the efficacy of medical and surgical treatment [64, 92, 124]. Its noninvasiveness and physiological character, along with high accuracy for liquid, solid, and combined phases, have favored functional scintigraphy as the best method for measuring GE [14, 108, 124].

Conventional scintigraphy is a relatively simple procedure that requires static imaging at defined time intervals and minimal processing and analysis, usually measuring $t_{1/2}$ [124] (Fig. 3).

Technical Details. A large field-of-view gamma camera with a dedicated computer for analysis is preferable for quantification of radioactivity in the region of interest [27]. The measurements should start immediately after meal ingestion. Usually, frequent images are taken to allow measurement of the lag time and the postlag fractional emptying rate. Counts should be corrected for isotope decay and tissue attenuation [20, 27]. In children, however, anterior image alone may be satisfactory [67]. The radiation burden should be considered in the choice of the isotope; since the $t_{1/2}$ of ^{99m}Tc is approximately 6 h (64 h for ^{111}In), it is preferred for labeling meals in single phase studies [62]. Because some variation in GE has been demonstrated between upright and supine positions, the imaging geometry must be standardized [119].

Scintigraphic studies presents some pitfalls [20, 100]. Some sources of potential error have been recognized, such as a small overlap of gastric and duodenal activity and posteroanterior movement of the contents [20, 43, 67]. The isotope may separate from the solid phase and empty with the liquid phase, resulting in erroneous assessment of solid emptying [20]. When the emptying does not reach 50%, the extrapolated value for $t_{1/2}$ may be unreliable [20].

Normal values have not been established for children. As a guide, reported normal control values for young adults using the anterior projection may be appropriate [66, 89].

Gastric scintigraphy has also gained acceptance in the detection and evaluation of GER in infants and children [124]. GER can be quantified and the positions and circumstances at which it occurs can be determined using the same radionuclide [36, 68]. In addition, pulmonary scanning to document aspiration of refluxed material is useful in children [52].

Fig. 3a, b.
$t_{1/2}$ calculated by linear fitting.
a Normal and b Delayed emp-
tying studies, taking into account the patient's age and
the issues related to test meal,
technique and methodology
of analysis

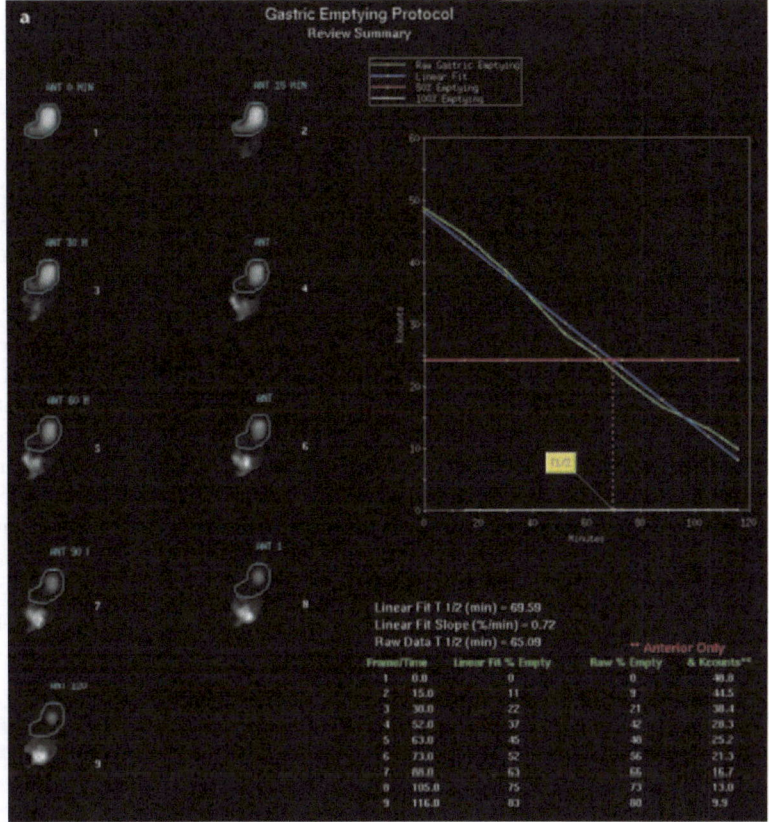

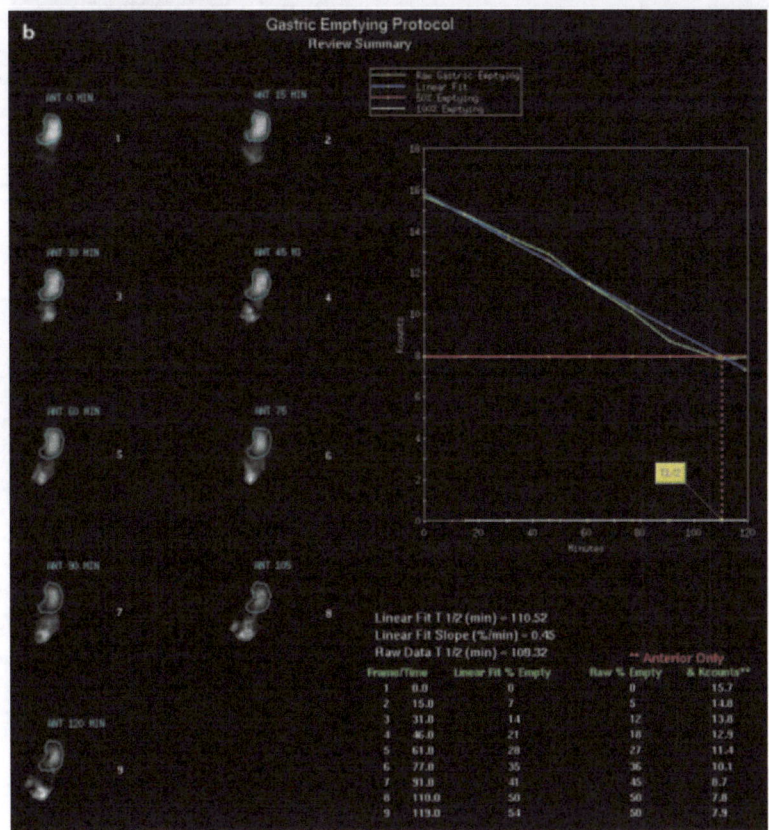

Scintigraphy presents however a relatively high cost-benefit ratio and involves radiation hazards for patients and personnel [37, 53]. It is a time-consuming study not often readily available and not suitable for repeated examinations [14]; avoidance of movements is a limitation especially relevant in children [14, 57].

Besides its common use in the assessment of GE, scintigraphy has experienced recent developments such as compartmental analysis of the stomach and digital antral dynamics that provide much more information on gastric physiology and pathophysiological mechanisms [78, 124].

18.6.2
Ultrasonography

Real-time ultrasonography (US) is useful for assessing GE and has major advantages over scintigraphy in that it is simple, noninvasive, does not entail radiation, and is widely available [11]. The rationale for using US is based upon the assumption that the calculation of the antral cross-sectional area (ACSA) in a serial manner after a feed provides an estimation of GE [21, 34]. In fact, there is passive distention of the antrum with gastric filling and linear relation between antral cross-sectional area and intragastric volume [4, 11, 34, 99, 106].

Technical Details. An ultrasound probe is positioned vertically (sagittal plane) to permit simultaneous visualization of the antrum, the left lobe of the liver, the superior mesenteric artery, and the abdominal aorta (Fig. 4); although the superior mesenteric vein [11] has been used as an anatomic landmark to standardize the position of the scan, the artery is easier to demonstrate [2]. The measurements are single (unique) or repeated several times and averaged to allow for variations in peristalsis [21]. The areas are traced using the (built-in) internal caliper and calculation program [2, 21, 34, 73] or calculated using the formula $\pi AB/4$ (A-longitudinal, B-anteroposterior diameters) assuming an elliptical shape [11, 34]. A prefeeding (basal) and serial measurements at defined postprandial intervals are usually per-

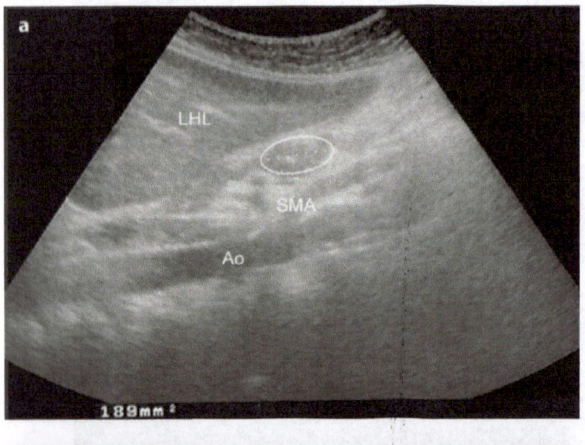
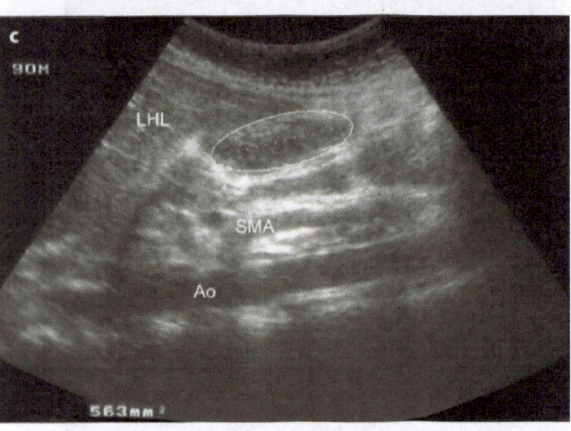
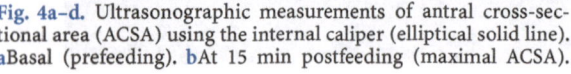

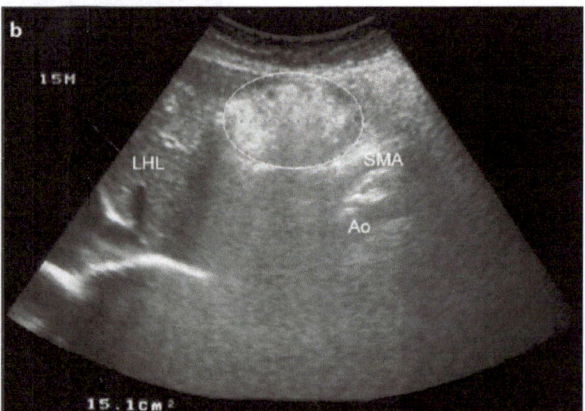
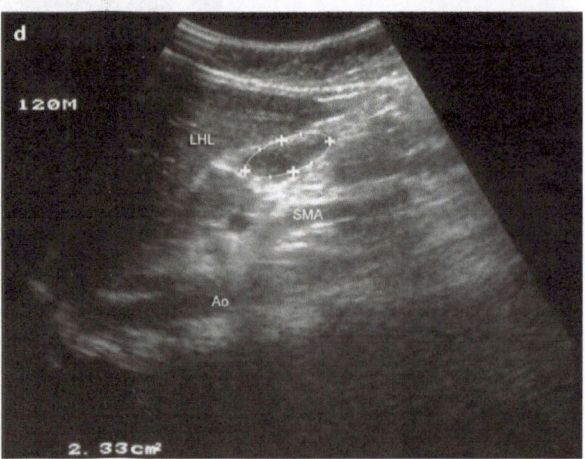

Fig. 4a–d. Ultrasonographic measurements of antral cross-sectional area (ACSA) using the internal caliper (elliptical solid line). **a** Basal (prefeeding). **b** At 15 min postfeeding (maximal ACSA). **c** At 90 min. **d** At 120 min. LHL, left hepatic lobe; Ao, Aorta; SMA, superior mesenteric artery

formed sequentially until the ACSA returns to the basal value (Fig. 4). After plotting them against time, it is possible to calculate the standard GE parameters [7, 21, 82, 118]. A measurement (e.g. at 90 min) smaller than the basal one may be found as a result of the secretion of gastric juice prior to meal ingestion due to the cephalic phase [34]. The test meal should be echogenic to achieve clear images of the gastric contents and a good depiction of the stomach wall [34].

US presents some limitations. Methodological difficulty of the procedure causes observer variance, thus a skilled and experienced operator is required to obtain reliable results [52, 82]. In addition, it may not be feasible because of air in the stomach, obesity, or partial gastrectomy [61, 72, 82] and is generally impractical for prolonged observations [20].

However, US has been suggested as a valid alternative to scintigraphy. In fact, measurements of ACSA have been validated against scintigraphy [73, 90] with a good inter- and intraobserver agreement [74, 106] and a variability lower than 9.5% [34, 45, 54, 90]. These measurements are also reproducible and viable with small feeding volumes making US a suitable method to investigate GE even in premature infants [21, 45, 83, 85]. US is therefore a noninvasive and inexpensive method that allows an evaluation of the whole "realistic" meal [6]. Additionally, transabdominal US has proved to be useful for evaluating GER in children [127] and dynamic imaging permits the study of gastric contractions and antroduodenal motility [31, 61, 71, 81].

Three-dimensional US has been recently introduced for assessing GE, but it is not as easy to introduce in general practice as real-time US [55, 56].

18.6.3
Other Direct Techniques

Magnetic resonance imaging after administration of an oral marker is a promising method to evaluate GE [115]. It has been advocated as a noninvasive, radiation-free technique providing both functional and anatomical information, i.e., measurement of GE and gastric morphology [115]. As additional advantages, there is no need to inhibit gastric acid secretion or to perform mathematical corrections; the technique is feasible even in the presence of aerogastria, obesity, or partial gastrectomy [115]. However, MRI has been used mainly in research studies because it involves expensive equipment not widely available and specialized personnel. *Potential tomography* has not gained substantial clinical application [3].

Intubation techniques such as the double-sampling polyethylene glycol dilution provide quantitative and accurate data of the liquid GE; as they may alter gastric physiology and require a specific liquid meal and the placement of a nasogastric catheter, their use has been mostly limited to research purposes [51, 77, 97, 98, 105].

18.7
Conclusion

Delayed gastric emptying (DGE) is frequent in children with gastroesophageal reflux (GER) disease. Since it seems logical that poor gastric emptying (GE) would contribute to pathological GER [69, 103, 112, 43], therapeutic enhancement of GE has been used with apparent success in this subset of patients [18, 22, 47, 108]. These features dictate the necessity of additional investigation to assess GE mainly in children who are candidates for surgical treatment [108].

The lack of standards for GE studies regarding registration technique and meal composition has been a problem, especially in pediatric patients; accordingly, no reference data are available for healthy children of all ages. Apart from the standardization of the numerous factors aforementioned, the evaluation of GE in children should emphasize the importance of age and type of meal used for the study [36].

The method of choice for evaluating GE is dependent on several factors such as the study population, the cost, the degree of invasiveness, whether detailed information on the different phases of GE is required, and whether the goal is to study liquid and/or solid GE [98]. Children with GER may empty liquids in a normal or even rapid fashion [126]. Since scintigraphy is the most precise method in the determination of the solid emptying phase in a physiological and noninvasive manner, it remains the gold standard for assessing GE in GER disease; however, scintigraphy has disadvantages, such as the inherent risk of radiation exposure, that limit its application [37, 111]. Novel alternatives to measure GE are being increasingly used, especially US and stable isotopic techniques. Real-time US has proved to be a reliable, reproducible, inexpensive, and widely available method but it cannot discriminate between solid and liquid components of the meal [73]. Breath [^{13}C]-dioxide is an extremely promising radiation-free method particularly suitable to standard hospital practice [20, 87]. Studies comparing different techniques performed under equivalent conditions of implementation and methodology of analysis are really needed.

GE data display significant intersubject variability that should be taken into consideration in clinical practice [55]. GE measurements also present substantive coefficients of intrasubject variability [15, 35]; this fact influences the interpretation of a single test and therefore only unequivocal results are clinically important [20].

■ **Acknowledgements.** To José Luis Carvalho, MD, for his cooperation; to Ana Maria Brazão, MD, and Maria José Pinheiro, PhD, for their advice on radioisotopic techniques and mathematical interpretation respectively; to António José Madureira, MD, for his help on ultrasonography.

References

1. Andres JM, Mathias JR, Clench MH, Davis RH (1988) Gastric emptying in infants with gastroesophageal reflux. Measurement with a technetium-99m-labeled semisolid meal. Dig Dis Sci 33:393–399
2. Aoki S, Haruma K, Kusunoki H, et al (2002) Evaluation of gastric emptying measured with the ^{13}C-octanoic acid breath test in patients with functional dyspepsia. Scan J Gastroenterol 37:662–666
3. Avill R, Mangnall YF, Bird NC et al (1987) Applied potential tomography: a new noninvasive technique for measuring gastric emptying. Gastroenterology 92:1019–1026
4. Bateman DN, Whittingham TA (1982) Measurement of gastric emptying by real-time ultrasound. Gut 23:524–527
5. Behar J, Rambsy G (1978) Gastric emptying and antral motility in reflux esophagitis. Gastroenterology 74:253–256
6. Benini L, Sembenini C, Castellani G et al (1996) Gastric emptying and dyspeptic symptoms in patients with gastroesophageal reflux. Am J Gastroenterol 91:1351–1354
7. Benini L, Sembenini C, Heading RC et al (1999) Simultaneous measurement of gastric emptying of a solid meal by ultrasound and by scintigraphy. Am J Gastroenterol 94:2861–2865
8. Benini L, Sembenini C, Salamandini L et al (2001) Gastric emptying of realistic meals with and without gluten in patients with celiac disease. Effect of jejunal mucosal recovery. Scand J Gastroenterol 36:1044–1048
9. Berne RM, Levy MN (1988) Gastrointestinal motility. In: Physiology. C.V. Mosby, St. Louis, pp 649–681
10. Bjorkman DJ, Moore JG, Klein PD, Graham DY (1991) ^{13}C bicarbonate breath test as a measure of gastric emptying. Am J Gastroenterol 86:821–823
11. Bolondi L, Bortolotti M, Santi V et al (1985) Measurement of gastric emptying time by real-time ultrasonography. Gastroenterology 89:752–759
12. Bonaniva L, DeMeester TR, Evander A (1988) Role of the overall length of the distal esophageal sphincter in the antireflux mechanism. In: Siewert JR, Hölscher AH (eds) Diseases of the esophagus. Springer-Verlag, Berlin, pp 1031–1036
13. Borgstein ES, Heij HA, Beugelaar JD et al (1994) Risks and benefits of antireflux operations in neurologically impaired children. Eur J Pediatr 53:248–251
14. Braden B, Adams S, Duan L-P et al (1995) The [^{13}C]acetate breath test accurately reflects gastric emptying of liquids in both liquid and semisolid test meal. Gastroenterology 108:1048–1055
15. Brophy CM, Moore JG, Christian PE et al (1986) Variability of gastric emptying measurements in man employing standardized radiolabeled meals. Dig Dis Sci 31:799–806
16. Brown BP (1995) The effects of exercise on gastric emptying. Motility 31:4
17. Brown RA, Wynchank S, Rode H et al (1997) Is a gastric drainage procedure necessary at the time of antireflux surgery? J Pediatr Gastroenterol Nutr 25:377–380
18. Bustorff-Silva J, Fonkalsrud EW, Perez CA et al (1999) Gastric emptying procedures decrease the risk of postoperative recurrent reflux in children with delayed gastric emptying. J Pediatr Surg 34:79–83
19. Camillieri M, Malagelada J-R, Brown ML et al (1985) Relation between antral motility and gastric emptying of solids and liquids in humans. Am J Physiol 249:G580–G585
20. Camillieri M, Hasler WL, Parkman HP et al (1998) Measurement of gastrointestinal motility in the GI laboratory. Gastroenterology 115:747–762
21. Carlos MA, Babyn PS, Marcon MA, Moore AM (1997) Changes in gastric emptying in early postnatal life. J Pediatr 130:931–937
22. Carroccio A, Iacono G, LiVoti GL et al (1992) Gastric emptying in infants with gastroesophageal reflux. Ultrasound evaluation before and after cisapride administration. Scand J Gastroenterol 27:799–804
23. Cavell B (1979) Gastric emptying in preterm infants. Acta Pediatr Scand 68:725–730
24. Chang CS, Chen GH, Kao CH et al (1997) Correlation between patterns of antral contractility and gastric emptying of radiopaque markers. Am J Gastroenterol 92:830–834
25. Chen JDZ, Lin Z, Pan J, MaCallum RW (1996) Abnormal gastric myoelectrical activity and delayed gastric emptying in patients with symptoms suggestive of gastroparesis. Dig Dis Sci 41:1538–1545
26. Chen JZ, McCallum RW (1993) Clinical applications of electrogastrography. Am J Gastroenterol 88:1324–1336
27. Collins PJ, Horowitz M, Cook DJ et al (1983) Gastric emptying in normal subjects–a reproducible technique using a single scintillation camera and computer system. Gut 24:1117–1125
28. Corinaldesi R, Stanghellini V, Paparo GF et al (1989) Gastric acid secretion and gastric emptying of liquids in 99 male duodenal ulcer patients. Dig Dis Sci 34:251–256
29. Csandes A, Henriquez A (1978) Gastric emptying in patients with reflux esophagitis or benign strictures of the esophagus secondary to reflux compared to controls. Scand J Gastroenterol 13:205–207
30. Cucchiara S, Bortolotti M, Minella R et al (1993) Fasting and postprandial mechanisms of gastroesophageal reflux in children with gastroesophageal reflux disease. Dig Dis Sci 38:86–92
31. Cucchiara S, Minella R, Iorio R et al (1995) Real-time ultrasound reveals gastric motor abnormalities in children investigated for dyspeptic symptoms. J Pediatr Gastroenterol Nutr 21:446–453
32. Cucchiara S, Salvia G, Borrelli O et al (1997) Gastric electrical dysrhythmias and delayed gastric emptying in gastroesophageal reflux disease. Am J Gastroenterol 92:1103–1108
33. Cunningham KM, Horowitz M, Riddell PS et al (1991) Relations among autonomic nerve dysfunction, oesophageal motility, and gastric emptying in gastro-oesophageal reflux disease. Gut 32:1436–1440
34. Darwiche G, Almér L-O, Björgell O et al (1999) Measurement of gastric emptying by standardized real-time ultrasonography in healthy subjects and diabetic patients. J Ultrasound Med 18:673–682
35. Degen LP, Philips SF (1996) Variability of gastrointestinal transit in healthy women and men. Gut 39:299–305
36. Di Lorenzo C, Piepsz A, Ham H, Cadranel S (1987) Gastric emptying with gastro-oesophageal reflux. Arch Dis Child 62:449–453
37. Elashoff JD, Reedy TJ, Meyer JH (1982) Analysis of gastric emptying data. Gastroenterology 83:1306–1312
38. Estevão-Costa J (1997) Refluxo gastro-esofágico. Contribuição para a sua caracterização fisiopatológica. Medisa, Porto
39. Estevão-Costa J (2000) Gastroesophageal reflux. Surgical treatment in children. Arq Port Cirurgia 9:93–99
40. Estevão-Costa J, Trindade E, Carvalho JL et al (2000) Can esophageal pH-monitoring predict delayed gastric emptying? J Pediatr Gastroenterol Nutr 31:S37–S38
41. Estevão-Costa J, Morales L, Parri FJ, Albert A (2001) Antireflux role of free muscle transplantation. Experimental study in a reflux esophagitis rat model. Eur J Pediatr Surg 11:295–299
42. Estevão-Costa J, Campos M, Dias JA et al (2001). Delayed gastric emptying and gastroesophageal reflux. A pathophysiologic relationship. J Pediatr Gastroenterol Nutr 32:471–474

43. Euler AR, Ament ME (1977) Value of esophageal manometry studies in the gastroesophageal reflux of infancy 59:58–61
44. Euler AR, Byrne WJ (1983) Gastric emptying times of water in infants and children: comparison of those with and without gastroesophageal reflux. J Pediatr Gastroenterol Nutr 2:595–598
45. Ewer AK, Durbin GM, Morgan MEI, Booth IW (1994) Gastric emptying in preterm infants. Arch Dis Child 71:F24–F27
46. Finch JE, Kendall MJ, Mitchard M (1974) An assessment of gastric emptying by breathalyzer. Br J Clin Pharmacol 1:233–236
47. Fonkalsrud EW, Foglia RP, Ament ME et al (1989) Operative treatment for gastroesophageal reflux syndrome in children. J Pediatr Surg 24:525–529
48. Forrest JAH, Clements JA, Prescott LF (1982) Clinical pharmacokinetics of paracetamol. Clin Pharmacokinet 7:93–107
49. Fried MD, Khoshoo V, Secker DJ et al (1992) Decrease in gastric emptying time and episodes of regurgitation in children with spastic quadriplegia fed a whey based formula. J Pediatr 120:569–572
50. Galmiche JP, Janssens J (1995) The pathophysiology of gastro-oesophageal reflux disease: an overview. Scand J Gastroenterol Suppl 211:7–18
51. George JD (1968) New clinical method for measuring the rate of gastric emptying: the double sampling test method. Gut 9:237–242
52. Ghaed N, Stein MR (1979) Assessment of a technique for scintigraphic monitoring of pulmonary aspiration of gastric contents in asthmatics with gastroesophageal reflux. Ann Allergy 42:306–308
53. Ghoos Y, Maes BD, Geypens BJ et al (1993) Measurement of gastric emptying rate of solids by means of a carbon-labeled octanoic acid breath test. Gastroenterology 104:1640–1647
54. Gilja OH, Hausken T, Odegaard S, Berstad A (1995) Monitoring postprandial size of the proximal stomach by ultrasonography. J Ultrasound Med 14:81–89
55. Gilja OH, Detmer PR, Jong JM et al (1997) Intragastric distribution and gastric emptying assessed by three-dimensional ultrasonography. Gastroenterology 113:38–49
56. Gilja OH, Hausken T, Odegaard S, Berstad A (1999) Gastric emptying measured by ultrasonography. World J Gastroenterol 5:93–94
57. Glowniak JV, Whal RL (1985) Patient motion artifacts on scintigraphic gastric emptying studies. Radiology 154:537–538
58. Griffith GH, Owen GM, Kirkman S et al (1966): Measurement of rate of gastric emptying using Chromium-51. Lancet 1:1244–1245
59. Gulsrud PO, Taylor IL, Watts ND et al (1980) How gastric emptying of carbohydrate affects glucose tolerance and symptoms after truncal vagotomy and pyloroplasty. Gastroenterology 78:1463–1471
60. Guyton AC, Hall JE (1996) Transport and mixing of food in the alimentary tract. In: Textbook of medical physiology. W.B. Saunders, Philadelphia, pp 803–813
61. Hausken T, Odegaard S, Berstad A (1991) Antroduodenal motility studied by real-time ultrasonography. Effect of enprostil. Gastroenterology 100:59–63
62. Heading RC, Bolondi L, Camilleri M et al (1992) Working team report: gastric emptying. Gastroenterol Int 5:203–215
63. Heading RC, Nimmo J, Prescott LF et al (1973) The dependence of paracetamol absorption on the rate of gastric emptying. Br J Pharmacol 47:415–421
64. Heading RC, Tothill P, McLoughlin GP et al (1976) Gastric emptying rate measurement in man. Gastroenterology 71:45–50
65. Hebbard GS, Fone DR, Zwar R et al (1995) Emptying of radiopaque markers as a measure of gastric emptying. Gastroenterology 108:A612
66. Heyman S (1988) Gastric emptying, gastroesophageal reflux and esophageal motility. In: Gelfand MJ, Thoman SR (eds) Effective use of computers in nuclear medicine. McGraw-Hill, New York, pp 412–437
67. Heyman S (1995) Gastroesophageal reflux, esophageal transit, gastric emptying, and pulmonary aspiration. In: Treve ST (ed) Pediatric nuclear medicine. Springer-Verlag, New York, pp 430–452
68. Hillemeier AC, Lange R, McCallum RW (1981) Delayed gastric emptying in infants with gastroesophageal reflux. J Pediatr 98:190–193
69. Holloway RH, Dent J (1990) Pathophysiology of gastroesophageal reflux. Lower esophageal sphincter dysfunction in gastroesophageal reflux disease. Gastroenterol Clin North Am 19:517–535
70. Holloway RH, Hongo M, Berger K et al (1985) Gastric distention: A mechanism for postprandial gastroesophageal reflux. Gastroenterology 89:779–784
71. Holt S, McDicken WN, Anderson T, et al (1980) Dynamic imaging of the stomach by real-time ultrasound: a method for the study of gastric motility. Gut 21:597–601
72. Holt S, Cervantes J, Wilkinson AA, Wallace JH (1986) Measurement of gastric emptying rate in humans by real-time ultrasound. Gastroenterology 90:918–923
73. Hveem K, Jones KL; Chatterton BR, Horowitz M (1996) Scintigraphic measurement of gastric emptying and ultrasonographic assessment of antral area: relation to appetite. Gut 38:816–821
74. Irvine J, Tougas G, Lappalainem R, Bathurst NC (1993) Relationship and intraobserver variability of ultrasonographic measurement of gastric emptying rate. Dig Dis Sci 38:803–810
75. Johnson DG, Reid BS, Meyers RL et al (1998) Are scintiscans accurate in the selection of reflux patients for pyloroplasty? J Pediatr Surg 33:573–579
76. Jolley SG, Leonard JC, Tunnell WP (1987) Gastric emptying in children with gastroesophageal reflux. I. An estimate of effective gastric emptying. J Pediatr Surg 22:923–926
77. Jolley SG, Tunnell WP Leonard JC et al (1987) Gastric emptying in children with gastroesophageal reflux. II. The relationship to retching symptoms following antireflux surgery. J Pediatr Surg 22:927–930
78. Jones K, Edelbroek M, Horowitz M et al (1995) Evaluation of antral motility in humans using manometry and scintigraphy. Gut 37:643–648
79. Kawahara H, Dent J, Davidson G (1997) Mechanisms responsible for gastroesophageal reflux in children. Gastroenterology 113:399–408
80. Kikuchi K, Kusano M, Kawamura O et al (2000) Measurement and evaluation of gastric emptying using radiopaque barium markers. Dig Dis Sci 45:242–247
81. King PM, Adam RD, Pryde A et al (1984) Relationships of human antroduodenal motility and transpyloric fluid movement: noninvasive observations with real-time ultrasound. Gut 25:1384–1391
82. Kusunoki H, Haruma K, Hata J et al (2000) Real-time ultrasonographic assessment of antroduodenal motility after ingestion of solid and liquid meals by patients with functional dyspepsia. J Gastroenterol Hepatol 15:1022–1027
83. Lambrecht L, Robberecht E, Deschynkel K, Afschrift M (1988) Ultrasonic evaluation of gastric clearing in young infants. Pediatr Radiol 18:314–318
84. Lartigue S, Bizais Y, des Varannes SB et al (1994) Inter- and intrasubject variability of solid and liquid gastric emptying parameters: a scintigraphic study in healthy subjects and diabetic patients. Dig Dis Sci 39:109–115
85. LiVoti G, Tulone V, Bruno R et al (1992) Ultrasonography and gastric emptying: evaluation in infants with gastroesophageal reflux. J Pediatr Gastroenterol Nutr 14:397–399
86. Lood FD, Palmer DW, Soergel KH et al (1984) Gastric emptying in patients with diabetes mellitus. Gastroenterology 86:485–494
87. Maes BD, Ghoos YF, Geypens BJ et al (1994) Combined carbon-13-glycine/carbon-14-octanoic acid breath test to monitor gastric emptying rates of liquids and solids. J Nucl Med 35:824–831
88. Maes BD, Ghoos YF, Hiele MI, Rutgeerts PJ (1997) Gastric emptying rate of solids in patients with nonulcer dyspepsia. Dig Dis Sci 42:1158–1162
89. Malmud LS, Fisher RS, Knight LC, Rock E (1982) Scintigraphic evaluation of gastric emptying. Semin Nucl Med 12:116–125

90. Marzio L, Giacobbe A, Conoscitore P et al (1989) Evaluation of the use of ultrasonography in the study of liquid gastric emptying. Am J Gastroenterol 84:496–500

91. McCallum RW, Berkowitz DB, Lerner E (1981) Gastric emptying in patients with gastroesophageal reflux. Gastroenterology 80:285–291

92. Meyer JH, MacGregor IL, Gueller R et al (1976) 99m Tc-tagged chicken liver as a marker of solid food in the human stomach. Am J Dig Dis 21:296–304

93. Meyers JH, Thomson JB, Cohen MB et al (1979) Sieving of solid food by the canine stomach and sieving after gastric surgery. Gastroenterology 76:804–813

94. Meyers JH, Ohashi H, Jehan D et al (1981) Size of liver particles emptied from the human stomach. Gastroenterology 80:1489–1496

95. Mittal RK (1990) Current concepts of the antireflux barrier. Gastroenterol Clin N Am 19:501–516

96. Miwa H, Sato N (2000) A long way toward understanding the pathogenesis of functional dyspepsia, but we should go forward with the accumulation of clinical evidence. J Gastroenterol Hepatol 15:967–968

97. Muller-Lissner SA, Schattenmann G et al (1983) Effect of a transpyloric tube on gastric emptying and duodenogastric reflux in the dog. Digestion 28:176–180

98. Näslund E, Bogefors J, Grybäck P et al (2000) Gastric emptying: comparison of scintigraphic, polyethylene glycol dilution, and paracetamol tracer assessment techniques. Scand J Gastroenterol 35:375–379

99. Newel SJ, Chapman S, Booth IW (1993) Ultrasonic assessment of gastric emptying in the preterm infant. Arch Dis Child 69:32–36

100. Paintaud G, Thibault P, Queneau P-E et al (1998) Intraindividual variability of paracetamol absorption kinetics after a semi-solid meal in healthy volunteers. Eur J Clin Pharmacol 53:355–359

101. Parkman HP, Fisher RS (1997) Contributing role of motility abnormalities in the pathogenesis of gastroesophageal reflux disease. Dig Dis 15(Suppl)1:40–52

102. Parkman HP, Harris AD, Krevsky B et al (1995) Gastroduodenal motility and dysmotility: an update on techniques available for evaluation. Am J Gastroenterol 90:869–892

103. Penagini R, Hebbard G, Horowitz M et al (1998) Motor function of the proximal stomach and visceral perception in gastro-oesophageal reflux disease. Gut 42:251–257

104. Read NW, Houghton LA (1989) Physiology of gastric emptying and pathophysiology of gastroparesis. Gastroenterol Clin North Am 18:359–373

105. Read NW, Janabi MN, Bates TE et al (1983) Effect of gastrointestinal intubation on the passage of a solid meal through the stomach and small intestine in humans. Gastroenterology 84:1568–1572

106. Ricci R, Bontempo I, Corazziari E et al (1993) Real time ultrasonography of the gastric antrum. Gut 34:173–176

107. Richards CA, Andrews PLR, Spitz L, Milla PJ (1998) Nissen fundoplication may induce gastric myolectrical disturbance in children. J Pediatr Surg 33:1801–1805

108. Richter JE (1997) Delayed gastric emptying in reflux patients: to be or not to be? Am J Gastroenterol 92:1077–1078

109. Rosen PR, Treves S (1984) The relationship of gastroesophageal reflux and gastric emptying in infants and children: concise communication. J Nucl Med 25:571–574

110. Sanaka M, Kuyama Y, Yamanaka M (1998) Guide for judicious use of the paracetamol absorption technique in a study of gastric emptying rate of liquids. J Gastroenterol 33:785–791

111. Scarpignato C (1990) Gastric emptying measurement in man. Front Gastrointest Res 17:198–246

112. Schoeman MN, Tippett MD, Akkermans LM et al (1995) Mechanisms of gastroesophageal reflux in ambulant healthy human subjects. Gastroenterology 108:83–91

113. Schwizer W, Hinder RA, DeMeester TR (1989) Does delayed gastric emptying contribute to gastroesophageal reflux disease? Am J Surg 157:74–80

114. Schwizer W, Maecke H, Fried M (1992) Measurement of gastric emptying by magnetic resonance imaging in humans. Gastroenterology 103:369–376

115. Schwizer W, Fraser R, Borovicka J et al (1996) Measurement of proximal and distal gastric motility with magnetic resonance imaging. Am J Physiol 271:G217–G222

116. Siegel J, Wu R, Knight L et al (1983) Radiation dose estimates for oral agents used in upper gastrointestinal disease. J Nucl Med 24:835–837

117. Siegel M, Krantz B, Lebenthal E (1985) Effect of fat and carbohydrate composition on the gastric emptying of isocaloric feedings in premature infants. Gastroenterology 89:785–790

118. Siegel JA, Urbain J-L, Adler LP et al (1988) Biphasic nature of gastric emptying. Gut 29:85–89

119. Signer E, Fredrich R (1975) Gastric emptying in newborns and young infants. Acta Pediatr Scand 64:525–530

120. Soykan I, Lin Z, Jones S et al (1997) Gastric myoelectrical activity, gastric emptying and correlations with dyspepsia symptoms in patients with gastroesophageal reflux. J Investig Med 45:483–487

121. Sun WM, Houghton LA, Read NW et al (1988) Effect of meal temperature on gastric emptying of liquids in man. Gut 29:302–305

122. Talley NJ (1994) A critique of therapeutic trials in Helicobacter pylori-positive functional dyspepsia. Gastroenterology 106:1174–1183

123. Urbain D, Muls V, Caucheteur B et al (1997) Gastric emptying in patients with gastroesophageal reflux disease. Am J Gastroenterol 92:724

124. Urbain J-L, Charkes ND (1995) Recent advances in gastric emptying scintigraphy. Semin Nucl Med 25:318–325

125. Urbain J-LC, Siegel JA, Charkes ND et al (1989) The two-component stomach: Effects of meal particle size on fundal and antral emptying. Eur J Nucl Med 15:254–259

126. Velasco N, Hill LD, Gannan RM et al (1982) Gastric emptying and gastroesophageal reflux. Effects of surgery and correlation with esophageal motor function. Am J Surg 44:58–61

127. Westra SJ, Wolf BH, Staalman SR (1990) Ultrasound diagnosis of gastroesophageal reflux and hiatal hernia in infants and young children. J Clin Ultrasound 18:477–485

Chapter 19

Current Concepts in the Medical Treatment of GER in Children

19

Yvan Vandenplas · Silvia Salvatore · Bruno Hauser

Contents

19.1
Introduction

Gastroesophageal reflux (GER) is a common phenomenon occurring at any age with a benign prognosis in the majority of cases, but requiring prompt evaluation and treatment when presenting with alarm symptoms or when persisting [1]. The involuntary passage of gastric contents into the esophagus is the definition of GER. Since every individual has a number of episodes of GER, it is a physiological phenomenon. Most reflux episodes are limited to the distal esophagus, are brief and asymptomatic. The difference between physiologic reflux and reflux disease is to a lesser extent defined by the frequency, duration, content, and severity of the reflux episodes. The occurrence of symptoms, manifestations severe enough to impair quality of life, or complications suggest GER disease (GERD) [2, 3]. When this occurs, and the forces overcome the defense, the esophageal mucosa may become damaged, with significant consequences for the affected individual [3].

The passive passage of refluxed gastric contents into the oral pharynx and the mouth accompanied by gastric content drooling out of the mouth is referred to as regurgitation or spitting-up. In case of vomiting, the refluxed gastric content is expulsed with force from the mouth [4, 5]. Only few reflux episodes are accompanied by regurgitation or vomiting. Rumination is characterized by the voluntary, habitual regurgitation of recently ingested food that is subsequently spitted up or re-swallowed.

GER is a normal esophageal function serving a protective role, and thus functional. During meals, or in the immediate postprandial period, if the stomach is overdistended, GER serves to decompress the stomach. Thus, regurgitation is physiological in healthy, thriving, happy infants. Functional or symptomatic GER is successfully treated by conservative measures and does not require diagnostic investigations. Primary GER results from a primary disorder of function of the upper gastrointestinal tract. In secondary GER, reflux results from dysmotility occurring in systemic disorders such as neurologic impairment or systemic sclerosis. It may also result from mechanical factors at play in chronic lung disease or upper airway obstruction such as in chronic tonsillitis. Other causes include systemic or local infections (urinary tract infection, gastroenteritis), food allergy, metabolic disorders, intracranial hypertension, and medications such as chemotherapy. In some cases, secondary reflux results from stimulation of the vomiting center by afferent impulses from circulating bacterial toxins, or stimulation from sites such as the eye, olfactory epithelium, labyrinths, pharynx, gastrointestinal and urinary tracts, and testes [4, 5]. These stimuli usually cause vomiting. The symptoms and signs of primary and secondary reflux are similar, but a distinction is conceptually helpful in determining a therapeutic approach. Secondary GER is not further discussed.

Because symptoms suggesting GERD are frequent and nonspecific, especially during infancy, and because there is no "golden-standard" diagnostic technique, many infants are exposed to antireflux treatment.

Therefore, attention in the paragraphs below on therapeutic possibilities is focused on safety aspects. Therapeutic intervention should always be a balance between intended improvement of symptoms and risk of side effects. The choice of therapy for GERD depends upon the severity of signs and the degree of esophagitis.

19.2
Complications of Nonintervention

Complications of GER may be severe [1]. Untreated GERD results in complications such as esophagitis, failure to thrive in children, esophageal stricture, and Barrett's esophagus. The natural history of GER in infants and children is difficult to know, since treatment is common. The natural history of untreated patients from the initial studies, when medical treatment was unavailable, is not well described. The absence of pathognomonic symptoms for GERD) and its complications makes it impossible to predict, on an individual basis, which child will continue to have GERD into and during adult life.

Recent observations suggest a decreased quality of life in regurgitating infants and their parents, even if the regurgitation has disappeared. A 10-year follow-up of esophagitis showed that over 70% of the patients had persisting symptoms, and 2% strictures [6]. Untreated or uncontrolled GERD is associated with severe complications such as esophagitis, Barrett's mucosa, stricture formation, and even esophageal adenocarcinoma. The frequency, severity, and duration of reflux symptoms are related to the risk of esophageal cancer. It is not known whether mild esophagitis or GERD symptoms persisting from childhood into adulthood carry an increased risk of severe complications in adult life. Spontaneous improvement and healing of nonulcerated esophagitis may actually exist. Nevertheless, complications and side effects of medication must be considered in relation to the natural evolution of untreated GERD.

19.3
Nonpharmacological and Nonsurgical Therapies for GER

The different steps in therapeutic approach are listed in Table 1. Efficacy was not demonstrated for nonpharmacological (and nonsurgical) therapies for GER, although some may decrease the incidence of regurgitation. Lifestyle changes (in adults) are rarely beneficial [7]. Despite gravity, the upright seated position leads to significantly more and larger reflux episodes than the simple prone and 30° elevated prone positions, both when the infant is awake or asleep [8, 9]. This is likely due to increased abdominal or intragastric pressure.

Table 1. Different steps in the treatment of GER and GERD

Nonpharmacological and nonsurgical therapies
　Parental reassurance
　In nonbreastfed infants: milk-thickening agents or antiregurgitation formula
　(Allergic origin/eosinophilic esophagitis and gastroenteritis:
　　In non breast-fed babies: extensive hydrolysate or amino-acid formula
　　In breast-fed babies: hypoallergenic diet mother)
Pharmacological therapies
　Prokinetics
　　Cisapride, domperidone, metoclopramide, erythromycin, …
　　Tegaserod, baclofen, (prucalopride, alosetron, ondansetron)
　Alginates and antacids
　H2-recepter antagonists (ranitidine, nizatidine, etc.)
　Proton pump inhibitors (lansoprazole, omeprazole, esomeprazole, pantoprazole, etc.)
　Other molecules: sucralfate
　(Eosinophilic esophagitis: steroids, cromolyn sodium, montelukast, fluticasone,…)
Endoscopic procedures
　Endoscopic gastroplasty (Endocinch system)
　Radiofrequency delivery at the cardia (Stretta system)
　Injection therapy (Enteryx procedure)
Surgical procedures
　Open versus laparoscopic surgery
　Nissen, Thal, and other procedures

The supine (lying on back) and lateral positions (lying on left or right side) usually result in intermediate pH-metric GER values and do not appear to influence GER [8, 10]. However, there is now ample evidence that the prone sleeping position is a risk factor in sudden infant death, independent of overheating, smoking, or way of feeding. The impact of pacifier use on reflux frequency was equivocal and dependent on infant position.

The protein content of formula was not found to affect reflux. Another study suggested that the lower the osmolality, the less acid reflux. Larger food volume and higher osmolality increase the rate of transient lower esophageal sphincter (LES) relaxations and drifts in LES pressure; a reduction of the food volume results in a decrease in the number of regurgitations but no change in acid reflux [11]. The data of 10 randomized controlled trials of nonpharmacological and nonsurgical GERD in healthy infants were recently reviewed [12]. Although no study demonstrated a significant reflux-reducing benefit of thickened formula compared to placebo, one study detected a significant benefit of formula thickened with carob bean gum compared to rice flour. Milk-thickening agents include bean gum preparations prepared from St. John's bread, a galactomannan, carboxymethylcellulose, a combination of pectin and cellulose, cereals and starch from rice, potato, corn, etc. There are as many different compositions of antiregurgitation formulas as there are formula companies: some are casein-predominant, others contain protein hydrolysates. Milk thickeners have been reported to reduce regurgitation in infants [8]. However, their effects on the esophageal acid exposure are inconsistent. Increased coughing has also been demonstrated in infants receiving milk thickeners [8]. According to in vitro models testing the effect on one meal, bean gum may cause malabsorption of minerals and micronutrients [13]. Studies of various thickening agents, including guar gum, carob bean gum, and soybean polysaccharides indicate the potential for deceased intestinal absorption of carbohydrates, fats, calcium, iron, zinc, and copper [14]. Abdominal pain, colic, and diarrhea may ensue from fermentation of bean gum derivatives in the colon. Carob bean gum induces frequent, loose, gelatinous stools. In some, but not all, animal studies, adding carob bean gum to the diet decreased growth [14]. However, growth and nutritional parameters in infants receiving a casein-predominant formula thickened with bean gum were normal [15]. Serious complications such as acute intestinal obstruction in newborns have been reported, although rarely [8]. Milk thickeners are often wrongly considered 'inexpensive'. Allergic reactions to carob bean gum have been reported in adults exposed to it at their workplaces and in infants after exposure to formula thickened with carob bean gum [14]. Milk thickeners remain a valuable first-line measure in relieving regurgitation in many infants, in view of their safety and efficacy in decreasing regurgitation. In contrast, their efficacy in GERD is questionable.

GER and cow's milk allergy (CMA) occur frequently in infants less than 1 year of age [16]. In recent years, the relation between these two entities has been investigated and relevant conclusions have been reached: in almost half of the cases of GER in infants less than 1 year of age, there is an association with CMA. In a high proportion of cases, GER is not only CMA-associated but also CMA-induced. The frequency of this association should induce pediatricians to screen for possible concomitant CMA in all infants with GER less than 1 year old. With the exception of some patients with mild typical CMA manifestations (diarrhea, dermatitis, or rhinitis), the symptoms of GER associated with CMA are the same as those observed in primary GER. Immunological tests and esophageal pH monitoring (with a typical pH pattern characterized by a progressive, slow decrease in esophageal pH between feedings) may be helpful if an association between GER and CMA is suspected, although the clinical response to an elimination diet and challenge is the only clue to the diagnosis. Abundant infiltration of the esophageal mucosa with eosinophils as occurs in eosinophilic gastroenteritis

and eosinophilic esophagitis is increasing and necessitates proper treatment (hypoallergenic feeding, corticoids, etc.). Patients with allergic esophagitis seem to have a younger age and common atopic features (allergic symptoms or positive allergic tests), but no specific symptoms. In children, eosinophilic esophagitis account for almost 1.0% of esophagitis in some selected series [17]. Atopic features are reported in more than 90% and peripheral eosinophilia in 50% of patients. At endoscopy, a pale, granular, furrowed, and occasional ringed esophageal mucosa may appear [18]. In reflux esophagitis, the distal and lower eosinophilic infiltrate is limited to less than 5 eosinophils per high-power field (HPF) with 85% positive response to GER treatment, compared to primary eosinophilic esophagitis with >20 eosinophils per HPF [17–19]. In adults, allergic esophagitis and eosinophilic esophagitis are rarely found, suggesting an age-related regression or a possible underinvestigation. Different approaches have been proposed in the treatment of eosinophilic esophagitis. Dietary treatment with extensive hydrolysates or amino acid-based formulas is recommended and successful [16]. Although amino acid-based formulas are clearly more effective than extensive hydrolysates, there is not yet consensus regarding which therapeutic option is the first choice. If dietary treatment fails, there is a place for medication.

19.4
Prokinetics

Metoclopramide, domperidone, erythromycin, and cisapride are considered to be prokinetic drugs. Metoclopramide and domperidone also have anti-emetic properties due to their dopamine-receptor blocking action, whereas cisapride is a prokinetic mainly acting via indirect release of acetyl choline from the myenteric plexus.

19.4.1
Cisapride

Critical evaluations of published reports on the efficacy of different prokinetics (cisapride, domperidone, and metoclopramide) concluded that cisapride is the preferred agent [20, 21]. According to these assessments, the vast majority of clinical trials on the efficacy of cisapride demonstrated that at least one of the end-points changes favorably as a result of the intervention [20]. Cisapride is more effective than metoclopramide [21]. A Cochrane review on cisapride in children analyzed data from seven trials including 236 patients comparing cisapride to placebo on the effect on symptom presence and improvement [22]. It was concluded that there was a significant difference for the parameter symptoms "present/absent" but there was no significant difference for "symptom change" between placebo and cisapride. The Cochrane review also concluded that cisapride compared to placebo significantly reduced the number and duration of acid reflux episodes, since there was a significant decrease in reflux index, which is the percent time that the esophageal pH is below 4.0 [22]. Cisapride increases saliva secretion, and increases the buffering capacity of saliva [23, 24]. Cisapride is superior to placebo in patients with functional dyspepsia [25]. In general, cisapride is well tolerated. The most common adverse events at therapeutic doses are transient diarrhea and colic (in about 2%). The effect of cisapride on relevant cardiac events such as QT prolongation and arrhythmia is dose- and risk factor-related. Isolated reports on more serious adverse events such as extrapyramidal reactions, seizures in epileptic patients, and cholestasis in very premature infants have been reported.

The relation between cisapride, P-450 cytochrome, and cardiac effect was considered in 1996 [26]. The cytochrome P450 system and especially CYP3A4 metabolizes cisapride in the liver [27]. There is little doubt that cisapride has a QT-prolonging effect [20], as do many other drugs and clinical situations [28]. Cisapride possesses class III antiarrhythmic properties and prolongs the action potential duration delaying cardiac repolarization [29], although many studies do not report an increase in duration of QTc, in neonates as well as in older children. Torsades de pointes have been reported with cisapride use, especially in those receiving high doses or macrolides [30]. Co-treatment of cisapride and macrolides such as clarithromycin and erythromycin clearly prolongs the QT duration [31]. Underlying cardiac disease, drug interactions, and electrolyte imbalance are clearly interfering factors [32]. . Cisapride causes prolongation of ventricular repolarization without causing increased heterogenicity of repolarization (QT dispersion), but all patients in the study remained asymptomatic without dysrhythmia [33]. The QT-prolonging effect of cisapride may be related to age [34]. The cytochrome P4503A4, which is involved in the metabolism of cisapride, is immature at birth and reaches adult-level activity by the age of 3 months. Cisapride accumulation occurs in newborns due to enzymatic immaturity. A significant QTc prolongation occurs especially in infants younger than 3 months, but not in the older infants [35, 36]. This effect was related to higher plasma levels. A more frequent administration of lower doses (resulting in a recommended daily dose of 0.8 mg/kg per day) in premature infants results in lower peak levels [37]. Consumption of grapefruit juice also alters cisapride metabolism [38]. According to recent data, gene mutation may be the fundamental culprit [39]. Molecular screening may allow identification among family members of gene carriers potentially at risk if treated with I(Kr) blockers [40].

19.4.2
Domperidone

The studies supporting efficacy of domperidone in improving GER in infants are limited [41]. The ability of oral domperidone to increase the pressure of the LES or to promote healing of reflux esophagitis is poorly documented in placebo-controlled trials. Most studies have been performed in older children, or investigate the effects of domperidone co-administered with other anti-reflux agents [41–43]. The combination of Gaviscon and domperidone was effective in infants with GERD not responding to parental reassurance, positional treatment, and milk-thickening [43]. Domperidone alone was not better than placebo [42]. In a comparison of domperidone and metoclopramide, elicited adverse effects on the central nervous system were more severe and more common with metoclopramide [43]. Because very little domperidone crosses the blood-brain barrier, reports of central nervous system adverse effects, such as dystonic reactions, are rare [44]. Domperidone is better tolerated than metoclopramide, since dystonic reactions (tremors) and anxiety are infrequent. Prolactin plasma levels may increase, due to pituitary gland stimulation [45]. Somnolence was acknowledged by 49% of patients after 4 weeks of metoclopramide treatment compared with 29% of patients after 4 weeks of domperidone [45]. A reduction in mental acuity was acknowledged by 33% of patients compared to 20% in the domperidone group. Akathisia, asthenia, anxiety, and depression were also acknowledged less often, and at a lower severity after 4 weeks of domperidone, although these differences were not significant. Domperidone possesses cardiac electrophysiological effects similar to those of cisapride and class III antiarrhythmic drugs [41]. Intravenous administered domperidone clearly causes QT-prolongation and ventricular fibrillation [46, 47]. Only few efficacy data for oral domperidone in the treatment of GERD alone are available, but efficacy seems very poor according to the few data. However, in children with insulin-dependent diabetes mellitus complicated by dyspeptic symptoms and gastroparesis, domperidone was superior to cisapride in reversing gastric emptying delay and gastric electrical abnormalities, as well as in improving dyspeptic symptoms and diabetic metabolic control [48].

19.4.3
Erythromycin

Only two randomized placebo-controlled trials have been conducted with this molecule in children [49, 50]. Both trials were in preterm infants with feeding intolerance [50]. Both randomized trials use erythromycin at a dose higher than 12 mg/kg/day [50]. Both trials did not show a significant difference in the incidence of necrotizing enterocolitis, in number of days needed to reach full enteral feeding, length of hospital stay, or adverse events [50]. Erythromycin has a prokinetic activity if it is administered intravenously, although clinical efficacy was also suggested after oral administration [49]. However, according to a recently published randomized trial using 10 mg/kg per day of erythromycin, the number of days needed to reach full enteral feeding was reduced by 25%, from 7.9 days to 6.0 days, and the number of large residual gastric volumes after a feeding was also reduced [51].

Erythromycin is reported to cause QT-prolongation and ventricular fibrillation [8, 52]. Pretreatment with erythromycin prevents octeotride-induced inhibition of antral contractions [53]. No serious adverse effects have as yet been reported in studies in which erythromycin was used for its prokinetic effects, although fatal reactions have followed the intravenous administration of erythromycin to neonates in antibiotic doses [49]. Systemic administration of erythromycin in young infants increases the risk for the infants to develop hypertrophic pyloric stenosis [54]. Similarly, a possible association exists with maternal macrolide therapy in late pregnancy [54]. The use of erythromycin at doses far below the concentrations necessary for an inhibitory effect on susceptible bacteria provides close to ideal conditions for the induction of bacterial mutation and selection [55]. Emergence of bacteria increasingly resistant to macrolide antibiotics has been reported [56]. New erythromycin-like molecules without the antibiotic properties are in development.

19.4.4
Metoclopramide

Data supporting the efficacy of metoclopramide are contradictory, and positive results are limited to observations with intravenous administration [41]. Oral metoclopramide did not decrease the frequency or duration of GER in children with GERD [57]. Application in infants is limited because of severe adverse events that occur quite frequently (in more than 20% of patients) including central nervous system effects and interactions with the endocrine system [41]. Pharmacokinetics of metoclopramide in infants and adults differ: plasma clearance is prolonged in infants, and the steady-state volume of distribution in a neonate is twice that of an adult [58].

The adverse effects regarding the central nervous system are mainly related to its dopamine-receptor blocking properties in the substantia nigra, and include extrapyramidal effects (dystonic reactions, irritability) and drowsiness, but also asthenia and sleepiness. Isolated cases of metoclopramide-induced methemoglobinemia and sulfhemoglobinemia have been reported [41,

59]. Neuroendocrine side effects such as galactorrhea do occur [60]. Metoclopramide has also been reported to induce Torsade de pointes [61].

19.4.5
Other Prokinetics

From the pathophysiologic point of view, prokinetics seems a logic therapeutic approach. However, efficacy data for the whole group of prokinetic drugs are disappointing. Cisapride was shown to have some efficacy on esophageal acid-exposure duration [62], but is now banned because of cardiac side effects. Prucalopride, a 5HT4 agonist, has been suggested as a possible option, but although the drug seems effective in adult constipation [63], its use was prohibited for children because of the extrapyramidal side effects. Ondansetron is a 5HT3 receptor antagonist that accelerates gastric emptying, inhibits chemotherapy-induced emesis or following neurosurgery in the area of the posterior fossa, but prolongs colonic transit time [64, 65]. Ondansetron was also shown to significantly reduce emesis during acute gastroenteritis [66]. However, there are no data of ondansetron in primary GERD in children. The most frequently reported adverse events of ondansetron were mild to moderate headache, constipation, and diarrhea in patients receiving chemotherapy. Tegaserod is a partial 5-HT4 agonist that has been studied mostly in constipation-predominant irritable bowel syndrome in adults [67, 68]. Tegaserod was shown to accelerate small intestinal transit time, and to increase proximal colonic emptying. Tegaserod also improves gastric emptying and decreases GER [69], and may be a promising drug. However, as of today, there are no efficacy data in the treatment in pediatric GER published. Baclofen, 4-amino-3-(-chlorophenyl)-butanoic acid is a gamma-aminobutyric acid (GABA)-B receptor agonist that is used in children with extreme spasticity. Given orally, it has been shown to decrease GER in healthy adults [70]. Administration in eight pediatric patients was reported to be safe [71]. Alosetron is a 5-HT3 antagonist that increases colonic compliance to distension, delays (ascending) colonic transit time, and increases basal fluid absorption [72]. Alosetron induces severe constipation and causes ischemic colitis [72].

19.5
(Alginate-)Antacids

Although antacids, and especially alginates, are used extensively in children, only a very few prospective randomized blinded trials have been performed and published. The efficacy of alginate-antacids in buffering the gastric acidity in infants is strongly influenced by the time of administration and requires multiple administrations. Alginate-antacids form a viscous fluid with surface-active properties, floating as a raft on the surface of the gastric contents, and hence form an artificial protective barrier against reflux [73]. Their efficacy for reflux as monotherapy or in combination with prokinetics is not convincing [57]. However, we reported a good efficacy on symptom decrease and pH-metric parameters with domperidone in combination with alginates [43]. Magnesium hydroxide and aluminum hydroxide in combination with domperidone was more effective than magnesium hydroxide and aluminum hydroxide alone, or domperidone plus alginate, or placebo [42]. In fact, symptoms improved in 16/20 patients in the group with domperidone and magnesium hydroxide and aluminum hydroxide, whereas only 8/20, 9/20, and 7/20 improved with the other therapeutic approaches, magnesium hydroxide and aluminum hydroxide alone, or domperidone plus alginate or placebo, respectively [42]. Important drug interactions with antacids include the prevention of the absorption of antibacterials such as tetracycline, azithromycin, and quinolones [74]. Antacid ingestion decreased the bioavailability of famotidine, ranitidine, and cimetidine by 20–25%, and the bioavailability of nizatidine by 12% [75]. Gaviscon contains a considerable amount of sodium carbonate, so that its administration may increase the sodium content of the feeds to an undesirable degree (1 g of Gaviscon contains 46 mg of sodium, and the suspension contains twice this amount). Algicon, having a better taste than Gaviscon, has a lower sodium load, but a higher aluminum content [73]. Occasional formation of large bezoar-like masses of agglutinated intragastric material has been reported in association with Gaviscon. Side effects include diarrhea with magnesium-rich preparations, and excessive absorption of aluminum in infants [73]. Dimethicone or simethicone is used in some regions for regurgitation, although there are no reliable studies demonstrating its efficacy in the treatment of GER in infants. Although often classified as an antacid, it acts more as a feed thickener, as it contains more than 50% of bean gum and has hardly any acid-neutralizing properties. Simethicone is better than placebo, and better than cisapride after 2 weeks of treatment but not after 4 and 8 weeks in patients with functional dyspepsia [25].

19.6
H2-receptor Antagonists (H2RAs)

Acid suppressant therapy is recommended in severe esophagitis, but this does not rectify primary disordered motility, a major pathophysiologic mechanism underlying GERD in children. Historically, cimetidine was the first H2-receptor antagonist (H^{2}RA) that became available. Ranitidine and nizatidine are the most popular and the best (although quite poorly) studied H^{2}RA in children [76, 77]. Nizatidine has been shown to increase the volume of saliva secreted and the concentration of salivary epidermal growth factor and bicarbonate in healthy volunteers, similar to the effect of cisapride [24]. Famotidine does not increase saliva volume or improve its composition [24]. Experience with other H^{2}RAs such as roxatidine and ebrotidine in children is very limited or nonexistent. In general, H^{2}RAs are considered to be quite safe. Adverse events reported in clinical trials with ranitidine include headache, tiredness, and mild gastrointestinal disturbances, but the incidence is not higher than for placebo [77]. High doses of cimetidine can cause reversible impotence and gynecomastia [77]. The endocrinological side effects associated with long-term administration of cimetidine in adults essentially preclude its long-term use in children [78]. Fatigue, dizziness, headache, dyspepsia, nausea, abdominal pain, flatulence, constipation, and diarrhea occur in 1–6% of patients [79]. H^{2}RAs have been reported to provoke central nervous system dysfunction, but this is poorly documented in children. Ranitidine enhances ischemic neuronal damage [79]. Ranitidine has occasionally been associated with acute interstitial nephritis in native and transplant kidneys [80]. Whereas ranitidine exhibits no clinically significant drug-drug interactions, cimetidine interacts with many drugs metabolized by cytochrome P450. Theophylline plasma levels are 25–32% higher when cimetidine is administered compared to ranitidine. Neither ranitidine nor nizatidine increases theophylline levels [75, 81]. However, minimal decreases in forced expiratory volume after 1 sec and forced vital capacity may be caused by H^{2}RAs, and this may clinically worsen chronic obstructive pulmonary disease in patients with severe obstruction [82]. This hypothesis is of interest, since most patients with severe chronic obstructive pulmonary disease do have GER. H2RAs, PPIs, and prokinetic agents undergo metabolism by the cytochrome P450 system present in the liver and gastrointestinal tract [74]. Cimetidine is an inhibitor of CYP3A, and it may cause significant interactions with drugs of narrow therapeutic range and low bioavailability that are metabolized by those enzymes [74].

Whether ranitidine may exceptionally cause QT prolongation or not is still debated [83]. If ranitidine is administered intravenously after autonomic blockage, the sinus cycle length is prolonged, and the systolic and diastolic blood pressures are decreased [84]. Thus, ranitidine must be administered by a slow intravenous infusion in patients with sinus node dysfunction [84]. The altered cardiac sympathovagal balance after oral administration of the H2RA ranitidine indicates a shift toward sympathetic predominance in heart rate control [85]. Ranitidine modulates the high-frequency power of the heart rate, and this may be the underlying mechanism of cardiovascular side effects [86]. Since H2 receptors are present in the stomach and the heart, they tend to decrease the heart rate and cardiac contractility.

Nizatidine and ranitidine are susceptible to metabolism by colonic bacteria, but famotidine and cimetidine are not (see also the section below on proton pump inhibitors) [87]. Ranitidine alters the gastrointestinal flora [88] and causes significantly more pneumonias in patients in intensive care units [89]. In the majority of patients on H2RAs, there is a relatively important nocturnal breakthrough of acid secretion sometimes limiting therapeutic efficacy, but on the other hand minimizing the side effect related to long-term blockage of acid secretion, as with proton pump inhibitors. There is a rapid development of tachyphylaxis or tolerance to H2RAs, limiting their long-term clinical use [90].

The combination of ranitidine and pirenzepine, a muscarinic receptor antagonist, does not aid the healing of reflux esophagitis, but does improve symptom relief after 4 weeks [91]. However, side effects were reported in 9/75 patients in the ranitidine group and 19/76 patients in the ranitidine and pirenzepine group [91].

19.7
Proton Pump Inhibitors

The superior efficacy and safety of proton pump inhibitors have changed the diagnostic and therapeutic recommendations in adults [1]. Proton pump inhibitors (PPI) belong to a group of chemically related compounds whose primary function is the inhibition of acid production in the final common metabolic pathway of gastric parietal cells [92]. The suppression of gastric acid secretion achieved with H2RAs has proved to be suboptimal [90]. PPIs have been shown to be more effective than H2RAs [7]. Esomeprazole seems to be the most effective PPI commercialized today [93]. Step-down treatment is recommended in adults [94]. Failure to control symptoms with high-dose PPI treatment raises the likelihood of non-acid-related causes of the symptoms. The pharmacokinetics and tolerance of pantoprazole were similar in patients with moderate and severe hepatic impairment [95]. These were also evaluated for famotidine in 150 children [96]. Recent studies with lansoprazole showed its efficacy in reducing symptoms and healing esophagitis in children [97]. The dosage used in children for lansoprazole is 0.73–1.66 mg/kg/day, with a maximum of 30 mg/day [92]. The availability of a syrup facilitates the use of this drug in children [97]. Lansoprazole is probably the best studied PPI in children [98]. After 5 days of lansoprazole, reflux symptoms improve in most children [98]. Adolescents exhibit reductions from baseline in the percentage of days and nights with heartburn or any other predominant symptom of GERD, the severity of heartburn, the percentage of days antacids were used, and the number of antacid tablets used per day [98]. Oral pantoprazole is effective in the treatment of reflux esophagitis in children [99]. Zimmerman and colleagues reviewed the literature on the use and administration of omeprazole in children [100]. In uncontrolled trials and case reports, omeprazole was used in dosage between 0.2–3.5 mg/kg per day for periods ranging from 14 days to 36 months, and was found effective and well tolerated for the acute and chronic treatment of esophageal and peptic ulcer disease in children aged 2 months to 18 years [92, 100]. In the pediatric population, there are very few comparable studies [92].

PPIs are highly selective and effective in their action and have few short- or long-term adverse effects [92]. The following side effects have been reported: allergic reactions, pharyngitis, headache (±3%), neurological and psychiatric side effects. especially fatigue, dizziness, and confusion in patients with hepatic diseases and/or advanced age; cutaneous reactions, generally rash and urticaria; hemolytic anemia, leucopenia, and agranulocytosis; gynecomastia; subacute myopathy; gastrointestinal side effects such as flatulence, constipation, diarrhea (±4%), dyspepsia and nausea (±2%), vomiting, and abdominal pain; hepatic disorders, especially moderate elevation of aminotransferases; excessive urinary sodium loss [8, 73, 98, 101, 102]. Last but not least, the high cost is a quite important albeit not medical "side effect". Omeprazole, esomeprazole, lansoprazole, rabeprazole, and pantaprazole rarely exhibit clinically important interactions with other hepatically metabolized medications or pH-dependent drugs [103]. In a pediatric trial, pantoprazole as found to be safe [99]. The absorption of drugs that are pH-sensitive as is the case with digoxin and ketoconazole will be influenced by PPIs [104]. More pediatric safety data on PPIs are needed [105].

The gastroparietal PPIs lansoprazole, omeprazole. and pantoprazole are all primarily metabolized by a genetically polymorphic enzyme, CYP2C19, that is absent in approximately 3% of Caucasians and 20% of Asians [74]. These drugs may also interact with CYP3A, but to a lesser extent. Esomeprazole has the potential to interact with CYP2C19. The slightly altered metabolism of cisapride was also suggested to be the result of inhibition of a minor metabolic pathway for cisapride mediated by CYP2C19. Esomeprazole did not interact with the CYP3A4 substrates clarithromycin or quinidine [104]. Only 4% of omeprazole is metabolized via the cytochrome P450 3A4 (the CYP causing all the cisapride problems); however, as much as 27% of esomeprazole is metabolized through the P450 3A4. Overall, the potential for drug-drug interactions with esomeprazole is low, and similar to that reported for omeprazole [104]. Salivary secretion is decreased with omeprazole. Prolonged use of a PPI can result in vitamin B12 deficiency as a consequence of impaired release of vitamin B12 from food in a nonacid environment. However, cystic fibrosis patients treated for at least 2 years with a PPI and cystic fibrosis without PPI had higher vitamin B12 levels than healthy controls [106].

The safety of long-term administration of acid-blocking medication needs to be considered in relation to potential consequences of prolonged acid suppression, including the risk of proliferation of gastric flora and the risk of developing enterochromaffin-like cell hyperplasia, which could in turn, theoretically, lead to gastric malignancy. Hypergastrinemia occurs in nearly all patients treated with omeprazole, causing hyperplasia and pseudohypertrophy of the parietal cells, as recently shown in 93% of adult patients on long-term omeprazole. Patients on omeprazole therapy for 5 to 8 years remained without evidence of significant enterochromaffin cell hyperplasia, gastric atrophy, intestinal metaplasia, dysplasia, or neoplastic changes [107]. Because of their excellent efficacy profiles, these drugs tend to be overused [108]. Since PPIs could delay the diagnosis of gastric cancer, the long-term uncontrolled and unnecessary use of these drugs should be avoided. Bacterial proliferation in the gastric content may not only change colonic flora, but may also be a risk factor for the patient to develop nosocomial pneumonia.

19.8
Other Drugs

Sucralfate causes bezoars, especially when given to patients in intensive care units, and diarrhea. Patients with renal failure treated with sucralfate are exposed to aluminum toxicity [109–111]. Other anti-emetic drugs such as batanopride also have a QTc-prolonging effect [112]. Octeotride is a long-acting somatostatin that induces phase 3-like migrating motor complexes response, which is not inhibited by meals (differs from normal), and has an inhibitory effect on gastric antrum (and is therefore indicated in dumping syndrome) [53]. Motilin agonists have been studied with inconsistent results in adults, and are not yet available for pediatric use [113].

Patients with primary eosinophilic esophagitis may respond to dietary elimination, cromolyn sodium, or steroids [18]. Montelukast and fluticasone were also recently reported to be of benefit [114, 115].

19.9
Therapeutic Endoscopic Procedures

In recent years, new endoscopic techniques intended to improve the function of the antireflux barrier were developed. The first results of endoscopic gastroplasty (the Endocinch system), radiofrequency delivery at the cardia (the Stretta system), and injection therapy (the Enteryx procedure) in adults have been reported [116–119]. The first series in adolescents have been performed. Although experience is too limited to recommend broad use, the theoretical concept of these procedures is interesting. Further improvements to the techniques are still being introduced.

19.10
Surgery

While antireflux surgery in certain groups of children may be of considerable benefit, it also has mortality and failure rates [120–123]. Ninety percent of patients remain free of significant reflux symptoms after laparoscopic Nissen, although side effects occur in up to 22% [124]. After a median follow-up of 16 years, the Nissen-Rosetti procedure in 24 consecutive children without congenital or acquired anomalies of the esophagus except for GERD obtained results considered excellent in only 75%, good in 21%, and poor in 4% [125]. Failure rates of 5–20% have been found after objective postoperative follow-up [125]. A protective antireflux surgical procedure in neurologically impaired children needing a gastrostomy increases the morbidity and mortality rates of the gastrostomy procedure itself [126].

19.11
Conclusion

GER and GERD are frequent conditions in infants, children, and adolescents. Symptomatology differs with age, although the main pathophysiologic mechanism, transient relaxations of the lower esophageal sphincter associated with reflux, is identical at all ages. Although infant regurgitation is likely to disappear with age, little is known about reflux. The majority of symptomatic reflux episodes are acid, but nonacid and gas reflux can as well cause symptoms. Complications of reflux disease may be severe and even life-threatening, such as esophageal stenosis and Barrett's esophagus. There is no golden standard diagnostic technique. A simple questionnaire may be among the best diagnostic helps in infants; nonacid reflux is best investigated with impedancometry. Primary GERD is mainly a motility disorder. Guidelines for treatment struggle with the fact that there is no prokinetic drug with a convincing efficacy profile. As a consequence, treatment of GERD focuses on anti-acid drugs. There is little or no information on how to organize follow-up.

References

1. Salvatore S, Vandenplas Y (2003) Gastro-oesophageal reflux disease and motility disorders. Best Pract Res Clin Gastroenterol 17:163–179
2. de Caestecker J (2001) Oesophagus: heartburn. BMJ 323: 736–739
3. Dent J, Brun J, Fendrick AM (1999) An evidence-based appraisal of the reflux disease management – The Genval Workshop Report. Gut 44:S1–S16
4. Rudolph CD, Mazur LJ, Liptak GS, baker RD, Boyle JT, Coletti RB, Gerson WT, Werlin SL (2001) Guidelines for evaluation and treatment of gastroesophageal reflux in infants and children. Recommendations of the North American Society for Pediatric Gastroenterology and Nutrition. J Pediatr Gastroenterol Nutr 32(Suppl 2):S1–S31
5. Vandenplas Y (1992) Oesophageal pH monitoring for gastro-oesophageal reflux in infants and children. Wiley, Chichester, England, pp 27–36
6. McDougall NJ, Johnston BT, Kee F (1996) Natural history of reflux oesophagitis: a 10 year follow up of its effect on patient symptomatology and quality of life. Gut 38:481–486
7. Kaynard A, Flora K (2001) Gastroesophageal reflux disease. Control of symptoms, prevention of complications. Postgrad Med 110:42–44
8. Vandenplas Y, Belli D, Benhamou P, Cadranel S, Cezard JP, Cucchiara S, Dupont C, Faure C, Gottrand F, Hassall E, Heymans H, Kneepkens CMF, Sandhu B (1997) A critical appraisal of current management practices for infant regurgitation–recommendations of a working party. Eur J Pediatr 156: 343–357
9. Orenstein SR, Whitington PF, Orenstein DM (1983) The infant seat as treatment for gastroesophageal reflux. N Engl J Med 309:760–763
10. Ewer AK, James ME, Tobin JM (1999) Prone and left lateral positioning reduce gastro-oesophageal reflux in preterm infants. Arch Dis Child Fetal Neonatal Ed 81:F201–F205
11. Khoshoo V, Ross G, Brown S, Edell D (2000) Smaller volume, thickened formulas in the management of gastroesophageal reflux in thriving infants. J Pediatr Gastroenterol Nutr 31: 554–556
12. Carroll AE, Garrison MM, Christakis DA (2002) A systematic review of nonpharmacological and nonsurgical therapies for gastroesophageal reflux in infants. Arch Pediatr Adolesc Med 156:109–113
13. Bosscher D, van Caillie-Bertrand M, van Dyck K (2000) Thickening of infant formula with digestible and indigestible carbohydrate availability of calcium, iron and zinc in vitro. J Pediatr Gastroenterol Nutr 30:373–378
14. Aggett PJ, Agostoni C, Goulet O, Kolezko B, Lafeber HL, Michaelsen KF, Milla P, Rigo J, Weaver LT (2002) Antireflux or antiregurgitation milk products for infants and young children: a commentary by the ESPGHAN Committee on Nutrition. J Pediatr Gastroenterol Nutr 34:496–498
15. Levtchenko E, Hauser B, Vandenplas Y (1998) Nutritional value of an "anti-regurgitation" formula. Acta Gastroenterol Belg 61:285–287
16. Salvatore S, Vandenplas Y (2002) Gastroesophageal reflux and cow's milk allergy: is there a link? Pediatrics 110:972–984
17. Liacouras CA, Wenner WJ, Brown K, Ruchelli E (1998) Primary eosinophilic esophagitis in children: successful treatment with oral corticosteroids. J Pediatr Gastroenterol Nutr 26:380–385
18. Orenstein SR, Shalaby TM, Di Lorenzo C (2000) The spectrum of pediatric eosinophilic esophagitis beyond infancy: a clinical series of 30 children. Am J Gastroenterol 95: 1422–1430
19. Ruchelli E, Wenner W, Voytek T, et al (1999) Severity of esophageal eosinophilia predicts response to conventional gastroesophageal reflux therapy. Pediatr Develop Path 2: 15–18
20. Vandenplas Y, the ESPGHAN Cisapride Panel (2000) Current pediatric indications for cisapride. J Pediatr Gastroenterol 31:480–489

21. Rode H, Millar AJW, Melis J, Cywes S (1987) Esophageal assessment of gastroesophageal reflux in 18 patients and the effect of two prokinetic agents: cisapride and metoclopramide. J Pediatr Surg 22:931–934
22. Augood C, MacLennan S, Gilbert R, Logan S (2000) Cisapride treatment for gastro-oesophageal reflux in children. Cochrane Database Syst Rev 3:CD002300
23. Goldin GF, Marcienkiewicz M, Zborch T, Bityutskiy LP, McCallum RW, Sarosiek J (1997) Esophagoprotective potential for cisapride. An additional benefit for gastroesophageal reflux disease. Dig Dis Sci 42:1362–1369
24. Adache K, Ono M, Kawamura A, Yuki M, Fujishiro H, Kinoshita Y (2002) Nizatidine and cisapride enhance salivary secretion in humans. Aliment Pharmacol Ther 16:297–302
25. Holtmann G, Gschossmann J, Mayr P, Talley NJ (2002) A randomised placebo-controlled trial of simethicone and cisapride for the treatment of patients with functional dyspepsia. Aliment Pharmacol Ther 16:1641–1647
26. Shulman RJ (1996) Report from the NASPGN therapeutics subcommittee. Cisapride and the attack of the P-450s. J Pediatr Gatsroenterol Nutr 23:395–397
27. Desta Z, Zoukhova N, Mahal SK, Flockhart DA (2000) Interaction of cisapride with the human cytochrome P450 system: metabolism and inhibition studies. Drug Metab Dispos 28: 789–800
28. Viskin S (1999) Long QT syndromes and torsades de pointes. Lancet 354:1625–1633
29. Tonini M, De Ponti F, Di Nucci A, Crema F (1999) Review article: cardiac adverse effects of gastrointestinal prokinetics. Aliment Pharmacol Ther 13:1585–1591
30. Hill SL, Evangelista JK, Pizzi AM, Mobassaleh M, Furton DR, Berul CI (1998) Proarrhythmia associated with cisapride in children. Pediatrics 101:1053–1056
31. Ward RM, Lemons JA, Molteni RA (1999) Cisapride: a survey of the frequency of use and adverse events in premature newborns. Pediatrics 103:469–472
32. Levy J, Hayes C, Kern J, Harris J, Flores A, Hyams J, Murray R, Tolia V (2001) Does cisapride influence cardiac rhythm? Results of a US multicenter, double-blind, placebo controlled pediatric study. J Pediatr Gastroenterol Nutr 32:458–463
33. Tutar HE, Kansu A, Kalayci AG, Girgin N, Ataly S, Imamoglu A (2000) Effects of cisapride on ventricular repolarization in children. Acta Paediatr 89:820–823
34. Semama DS, Bernardini S, Louf S, Laurent-Atthalin B, Guyon JB (2001) Effects of cisapride on QTc interval interm neonates. Arch Dis Child Fetal Neonat Ed 84:F44–F46
35. Benatar A, Feenstra A, De Craene T, Vandenplas Y (2001) QTc interval in infants and serum concentrations. J Pediatr Gastroenterol Nutr 33:41–46
36. Benatar A, Feenstra A, Decraene T, Vandenplas Y (2000) Effects of cisapride on corrected QT interval, heart rate, and rhythm in infants undergoing polysomnography. Pediatrics 106:E85
37. Cools F, Benatar A, Bruneel E, Theyskens C, Bougatef A, Casteels A, Vandenplas Y (2003) A comparison of the pharmacokinetics of two dosing regimens of cisapride and their effects on corrected QT interval in premature infants. Eur J Clin Pharmacol. 59:17–22
38. Kivisto KT, Lilja JJ, Backman JT, Neuvonen PJ (1999) Repeated consumption of grapefruit juice considerably increases plasma concentrations of cisapride. Clin Pharmacol Ther 66: 448–453
39. Napolitano C, Schwartz PJ, Brown AM, Ronchetti E, Bianchi L, Pinnavaia A, Acquaro G, Priori SG (2000) Evidence for a cardiac ion channel mutation underlying drug-induced QT prolongation and life-threatening arrhythmias. J Cardiovasc Electrophysiol 11:691–696
40. Walker AM, Szneke P, Weatherby LB, Dicker LW, Lanza LL, Loughlin JE, Yee CL, Dreyer NA (1999) The risk of serious cardiac arrhythmias among cisapride users in the United Kingdom and Canada. Am J Med 107:356–362
41. Vandenplas Y (1998) Clinical use of cisapride and its risk-benefit in paediatric patients. Eur J Gastroenterol Hepatol 10:871–881

42. Carroccio A, Iacono G, Montalto G, Cavataio F, Soresi M, Notarbartolo A (1994) Domperidone plus magnesium hydroxide and aluminum hydroxide: a valid therapy in children with gastroesophageal reflux. A double-blind randomized study versus placebo. Scand J Gastroenterol 29:300–304

43. Vandenplas Y, Sacré L (1987)Gastro-oesophageal reflux in infants. Evaluation of treatment by pH-monitoring. Eur J Pediatr 146:504–507

44. Patterson D, Abell T, Rothstein R, Koch K, Barnett J (1999) A double-blind multicenter comparison of domperidone and metoclopramide in the treatment of diabetic patients with symptoms of gastroparesis. Am J Gastroenterol 94: 1230–1234

45. Barone JA (1999) Domperidone: a peripherally acting dopamine 2-receptor antagonist. Ann Pharmacother 33:429–440

46. Drolet B, Rousseau G, Daleau P, Cardinal R, Turgeon J (2000) Domperidone should not be considered a no-risk alternative to cisapride in the treatment of gastrointestinal motility disorders. Circulation 102:1883–1885

47. Cameron HA, Reyntjes AJ, Lake-Bakaar G (1985) Cardiac arrest after treatment with intravenous domperidone. BMJ 290: 160

48. Franzese A, Borrelli O, Corrado G, Rea P, Di Nardo G, Grandinetti AL, Dito L, Cucchiara S (2002) Domperidone is more effective than cisapride in children with diabetic gastroparesis. Aliment Pharmacol Ther 16:951–957

49. Curry JI, Lander TD, Stringer MD (2001) Review article: erythromycin as a prokinetic agent in infants and children. Aliment Pharmacol Ther 15:595–603

50. Ng E, Shah V (2001) Erythromycin for feeding intolerance in preterm infants. Cochrane Database Syst Rev CD001815

51. Oei J (2001) A placebo-controlled trial low-dose erythromycin to promote oral tolerance in preterm infants. Acta Paediatr 90:904–908

52. Mishra A, Friedman HS, Sinha AK (1999) The effects of erythromycin on the electrocardiogram. Chest 115:983–986

53. Di Lorenzo C, Lucanto C, Flores AF, Idries S, Hyman PE (1999) Effect of sequential erythromycin and octeotride on antroduodenal manometry. J Pediatr Gastroenterol Nutr 29: 293–296

54. Mahon BE, Rosenman MB, Kleiman MB (2001) Maternal and infant use of erythromycin and other macrolides antibiotics as risk factors for infantile hypertrophic pylori stenosis. J Pediatr 139:380–384

55. Guerin JM, Leibinger F (2002) Why not use erythromycin in GI motility. Chest 121:301

56. Gay K, Baughan W, Miller J (2000) The emergence of Streptococcus pneumoniae resistant to macrolide antimicrobial agents: a 6-year population-based assessment. J Infect Dis 182:1417–1424

57. Forbes D, Hodgson M, Hill R (1986) The effects of Gaviscon and metoclopramide in gastroesophageal reflux in children. J Pediatr Gastroenterol Nutr 5:556–559

58. Kearns GL (1998) Pharmacokinetics of metoclopramide in neonates. J Clin Pharmacol 38:122–118

59. Aravindhan N, Chisholm DG (2000) Sulfhemoglobinemia presenting as pulse oximetry desaturations. Anesthesiology 93:883–884

60. Cinquetti M, Bonetti P, Bertamini P (2000) Current role of antidopaminergic drugs in pediatrics. Pediatr Med Chir 22: 1–7

61. Chou CC, Wu D (2001) Torsade de pointes induced by metoclopramide in an elderly woman with preexisting complete left bundle branch block. Chang Gung Med J 4:805–809

62. Augood C, Gilbert R, Logan S, MacLennan S (2002) Cisapride treatment for gastro-oesophageal reflux in children. Cochrane Database Syst Rev (3):CD002300

63. Coremans G, Kerstens R, De Pauw M, Stevens M (2003) Prucalopride is effective in patients with severe chronic constipation in whom laxatives fail to provide adequate relief. Results of a double-blind, placebo-controlled clinical trial. Digestion 67:82–89

64. Culy CR, Bhana N, Plosker GL (2001) Ondansetron: a review of its use as an antiemetic in children. Paediatr Drugs 3: 441–479

65. Neufeld S (2002) Pharmacology review: the role of ondansetron in the management of children's nausea and vomiting following posterior fossa neurosurgical procedures. Axone 23:24–29

66. Ramsook C, Sahagun-Carreon I, Kozinetz CA, Moro-Sutherland D (2002) A randomized clinical trial comparing oral ondansetron with placebo in children with vomiting from acute gastroenteritis. Ann Emerg Med 39:397–403

67. Wagstaff A, Frampton J, Croom K (2003) Tegaserod: a review of its use in the management of irritable bowel syndrome with constipation in women. Drugs 63:1101–1120

68. Jones BW, Moore DJ, Robinson SM, Song F (2002) A systematic review of tegaserod for the treatment of irritable bowel syndrome. J Clin Pharm Ther 27:343–352

69. Kahrilas PJ, Quigley EM, Castell DO, Spechler SJ (2000) The effects of tegaserod (HTF 919) on oesophageal acid exposure in gastro-oesophageal reflux disease. Aliment Pharmacol Ther 14:1503–1509

70. Ciccaglione AF, Marzio L (2003) Effect of acute and chronic administration of the GABA(B) agonist baclofen on 24 hour pH metry and symptoms in control subjects and in patients with gastro-oesophageal reflux disease. Gut 52:464–470

71. Wiersma HE (2003) Pharmacokinetics of a single oral dose of baclofen in pediatric patients with GERD. Ther Drug Monitor 25:93–98

72. Talley NJ (2001) Serotoninergic neuroenteric modulators. Lancet 358:2061–2068

73. Vandenplas Y, Belli DC, Benatar A, Cadranel S, Cucchiara S, Dupont C, Gottrand F, Hassall E, Heymans HS, Kearns G, Kneepkens CM, Koletzko S, Milla P, Polanco I, Staiano AM (1999) The role of cisapride in the treatment of pediatric gastroesophageal reflux. The European Society of Pediatric Gastroenterology, Hepatology and Nutrition. J Pediatr Gastroenterol Nutr 28:518–528

74. Flockhart DA, Desta Z, Mahal SK (2000) Selection of drugs to treat gastro-oesophageal reflux disease: the role of drug interactions. Clin Pharmacokinet 39:295–309

75. Bachmann KA, Sullivan TJ, Jauregui L, Reese J, Miller K, Levine L (1994) Drug interactions of H2-receptor antagonists. Scan J Gastroenterol Suppl 206:14–19

76. Paul K, Redman CM, Chen M (2001) Effectiveness and safety of nizatidine, 75 mg, for the relief of episodic heartburn. Aliment Pharmacol Ther 15:1571–1577

77. Sabesin SM (1993) Safety issues relating to long-term treatment with histamine H2-receptor antagonists. Aliment Pharmacol 7(Suppl2):S35–S40

78. Kelly DA (1994) Do H2 receptor antagonists have a therapeutic role in childhood? J Pediatr Gastroenterol 19:270–276

79. Adachi N, Seyfried FJ, Arai T (2001) Blockade of central histaminergic H2-receptors aggravates ischemic neuronal damage in gerbil hippocampus. Crit Care Med 29:1189–1194

80. Emovon OE, King JA, Holt CO, Browne BJ (2001) Ranitidine induced acute interstitial nephritis in a cadaveric renal allograft. Am J Kidney Dis 38:169–172

81. Boehning W (1990) Effect of cimetidine and ranitidine on plasma theophylline in patients with chronic obstructive airways disease treated with theophylline and corticosteroids. Eur J Clin Pharmacol 38:43–45

82. Hasnoglu HC, Yildirim Z, Hasanoglu A, Ozcan C, Gokirmak M, Koksal N, Kalkan S (2003) Effects of ranitidine on pulmonary function tests of patients with chronic obstructive pulmonary disease. Pharmacol Res 47:535–539

83. Alliet P, Devos E (1993) Ranitidine-induced bradycardia in a neonate–secondary to a congenital long QT interval syndrome. Eur J Pediatr 152:933–934

84. Hu WH, Wang KY, Hwang DS, Ting CT, Wu TC (1997) Histamine 2 receptor blocker-ranitidine and sinus mode dysfunction. Zhonghua Yi Xue Za Zhi 60:1–5

85. Nault MA, Milne B, Parlow JL (2002) Effects of the selective H1 and H2 histamine receptor antagonists loretadine and ranitidine on autonomic control of the heart. Anesthesiology 96:336–341

86. Ooie T, Saaikawa T, Hara M, Ono H, Seike M, Sakata T (1999) H2-blocker modulates heart rate variability. Heart Vessels 14: 137–142

87. Basit AW, Newaton JM, Lacey LF (2002) Susceptibility of the H2-receptor antagonists cimetidine, famotidine and nizatidine, to metabolism by the gastrointestinal microflora. Int J Pharm 237:23–33

88. Cothran DS, Borowitz SM, Sutphen JL, Dudley SM, Donowitz LG (1997) Alteration of normal gastric flora in neonates receiving ranitidine. J Perinatol 17:383–388

89. Messori A, Trippoli S, Vaiani M, Gorini M, Corrado A (2000) Bleeding and pneumonia in intensive care patients given ranitidine and sucralfate for prevention of stress ulcer: meta-analysis of randomised controlled trials. BMJ 321:1103–1106

90. Huang JQ, Hunt RH (2001) Pharmacological and pharmacodynamic essentials of H(2)-receptor antagonists and proton pump inhibitors for the practising physician. Best Pract Res Clin Gastroenterol 15:355–370

91. Londong W, Phillips J, Johnson NJ, Wood JR (1992) The effect of combined therapy with ranitidine and pirenzipine in the treatment of reflux esophagitis. Aliment Pharmacol Ther 6:609–618

92. Gibbons TE, Gold BD (2003) The use of proton pump inhibitors in children: a comprehensive review. Paediatr Drugs 5:25–40

93. Vakil NB, Shaker R, Johnson DA, Kovacs T, Baerg RD, Hwang C, D'Amico D, Hamelin B (2001) The new proton pump inhibitor esomeprazole is effective as a maintenance therapy in GERD patients with healed erosive esophagitis: a 6-month, randomized, double-blind, placebo-controlled study of efficacy and safety. Aliment Pharmacol Ther 15:927–935

94. Jones R, Bytzer P (2001) Acid suppression in the management of gastro-oesophageal reflux disease–an appraisal of treatment options in primary care. Aliment Pharmacol Ther 16:765–771

95. Ferron GM, Preston RA, Noveck RJ, Pockros P, Mayer P, Getsy J, Turner M, Abell M, Paul J (2001) Pharmacokinetics of pantoprazole in patients with moderate and severe hepatic dysfunction. Clin Ther 23:1180–1192

96. James LP, Kearns GL (1996) Pharmacokinetics and pharmacodynamics of famotidine in paediatric patients. Clin Pharmacokinet 31:103–110

97. Scott LJ (2003) Lansoprazole: in the management of gastroesophageal reflux disease in children. Paediatr Drugs 5:57–61

98. Gunasekaran T, Gupta S, Gremse D, Karol M, Pan WJ, Chiu YL, Keith R, Fitzgerald J (2002) Lansoprazole in adolescents with gastroesophageal reflux disease: pharmacokinetics, pharmacodynamics, symptom relief, efficacy and tolerability. J Pediatr Gastroenterol Nutr 35(Suppl 4):S327–S335

99. Madrazo-De la Garza A, Dibildox M, Vargas A, Delgado J, Gonzales J, Yanez P (2003) Efficacy and safety of oral pantoprazole 20 mg given once daily for reflux esophagitis in children. J Pediatr Gastroenterol Nutr 36:261–265

100. Zimmermann AE, Walters JK, Katona BG, Souney PE, Levine D (2001) A review of omeprazole use in the treatment of acid-related disorders in children. Clin Ther 23:660–679

101. Leufkans H, Claessens A, Heerdink E, van Eijk J, Lamers CB (1997) A prospective follow-up study of 5669 users of lansoprazole in daily practice. Aliment Pharmacol Ther 11:887–897

102. Castot A, Bidault I, Dahan R, Efthymiou ML (1993) Evaluation of unexpected and toxic effects of omeprazole A90-reported to the regional centers of pharmacovigilance during the first 22 postmarketing months. Therapie 48:469–474

103. Berardi RR (2000) A critical evaluation of proton pump inhibitors in the treatment of gastroesophageal reflux disease. Am J Manag Care 6(Suppl):S491–505

104. Andersson T, Hanssan-alin M, Hasselgren G, Rohss K (2001) Drug interaction studies with esomeprazole, the (S)-isomer of omeprazole. Clin Pharmacokinet 40:523–537

105. Scaillon M, Cadranel S (2002) Safety data required for proton-pump inhibitor use in children. J Pediatr Gastroenetrol Nutr 35:113–118

106. ter Heide H, Hendriks HJ, Heijmans H, Menheere PP, Spaapen LJ, Bakker JA, Forget PP (2001) Are children with cystic fibrosis who are treated with a proton-pump inhibitor at risk for Vitamin B12 deficiency? J Pediatr Gastroenterol Nutr 33:342–345

107. Singh P, Indaram A, Greenberg R, Visvalingam V (2000) Bank S. Long term omeprazole therapy for reflux esophagitis: follow-up in serum gastrin levels, EC cell hyperplasia and neoplasia. World J Gastroenterol 6:789–792

108. Nuanton M, Peterson GM, Bleasel MD (2000) Overuse of proton pump inhibitors. J Clin Pharm Ther 25:333–338

109. Amaro R, Montelongo PC, Barkin JS (1999) Sucralfate-induced diarrhea in an enterally fed patient. Am J Gastroenterol 94:2328–2329

110. Guy C, Ollagnier M (1999) Sucralfate and bezoars: data from the system of pharmacologic vigilance and review of the literature. Therapie 54:55–58

111. Hemstreet BA (2001) Use of sucralfate in renal failure. Ann Pharmacother 35:360–364

112. Fleming GF, Vokes EE, McEvilly JM, Janisch L, Francher D, Smaldone L (1991) Double-blind, randomized crossover study of metoclopramide and batanopride for prevention of cisplatin-induced emesis. Cancer Chemother Pharmacol 28:226–227

113. Talley NJ, Verlinden M, Snape W, Beker JA, Ducrotte P, Dettmer A, Brinkhoff H, Eaker E; Ohning G, Miner PB, Mathias JR, Fumugalli I, Staessen D, Mack RJ (2000) Failure of a motilin receptor agonist (ABT-229) to relieve the symptoms of functional dyspepsia in patients with and without delayed gastric emptying: a randomized double-blind placebo-controlled trial. Aliment Pharmacol Ther 14:1653–1661

114. Attwood SE, Lewis CJ, Bronder CS, Morris CD, Armstrong GR, Whittam J (2003) Eosinophilic oesophagitis: a novel treatment using Montelukast. Gut 52:181–185

115. Teitelbaum JE, Fox VL, Twarog FJ, Nurko S, Antonioli D, Gleich G, Badizadegan K, Furuta GT (2002) Eosinophilic esophagitis in children: immunopathological analysis and response to fluticasone propionate. Gastroenterology 122:1216–1225

116. Mahmood Z, McMahon BP, Arfin Q, Byrne PJ, Reynolds JV, Murphy EM, Weir DG (2003) Endocinch therapy for gastro-oesophageal reflux disease: a one year prospective follow up. Gut 52:34–39

117. Wolfsen HC, Richards WO (2002) The Stretta procedure for the treatment of GERD: a registry of 558 patients. J Laparoendosc Adv Surg Tech A 12:395–402

118. Johnson DA, Ganz R, Aisenberg J, Cohen LB, Deviere J, Foley TR, Haber GB, Peters JH, Lehman GA (2003) Endoscopic, deep mural implantation of enteryx for the treatment of GERD: 6-month follow-up of a multicenter trial. Am J Gastroenterol 98:250–258

119. Galmiche JP, Bruley des Varannes S (2003) Endoluminal therapies for gastro-oesophageal reflux disease. Lancet 361:1119–1121

120. Fonkalsrud EX, Bustorff-Silva J, Perez CA, Quintero R, Martin L, Atkinson JB (1999) Antireflux surgery in children under three months of age. J Pediatr Surg 34:527–531

121. Pearl RH, Robie DK, Ein SH, Shandling B, Wesson DE, Superina R, Mctaggart K, Garcia VF, O'Connor JA, Filler RM (1990) Complications of gastroesophageal reflux surgery in neurologically impaired versus neurologically normal children. J Pediatr Surg 25:1169–1173

122. Alexander F, Wyllie R, Jirousek K, Secic M, Porvasnik S (1997) Delayed gastric emptying affects outcome of Nissen fundoplication in neurologically impaired children. Surgery 122:690–697

123. Spitz L, Roth K, Kiely EM, Brereton RJ, Drake DP, Milla PJ (1993) Operation for gastro-oesophageal reflux associated with severe mental retardation. Arch Dis Child 68:347–351

124. Booth MI, Jones L, Stratford J, Dehn TC (2002) Results of laparoscopic Nissen fundoplication 8 years after surgery. Br J Surg 89:476–481

125. Bergmeijer JH, Harbers JS, Molenaar JC (1997) Function of pediatric Nissen-Rosetti fundoplication followed up into adolescence and adulthood. J Am Coll Surg 184:259–261

126. Burd RS, Price MR, Whalen TV (2002) The role of protective antireflux procedures in neurologically impaired children: a decision analysis. J Pediatr Surg 37:500–506

Chapter 20

Long-Term Results of Medical Treatment and Indications for Surgery

20

Gabriella Boccia · Renata Auricchio
Annamaria Staiano · Ray E. Clouse

Contents

20.1
Introduction

Gastroesophageal reflux disease (GERD) is being recognized at increasing rates in infants, children, and adolescents. For example, Callahan noted a 20-fold increase in the diagnosis of GERD for infants discharged from a U.S. Army hospital in 1995 compared with those released in 1971 [1]. In a recent review of the Pediatric Health Information System Database, the discharge diagnosis of GERD was found to represent almost 4% of all hospital admissions for children in the United States, with hospitalization rates increasing significantly over the 5-year period from 1995 to 2000 [2]. Whether these increased rates reflect a true increment in disease or are biased by more diligent evaluation of the patients' symptoms through improved technology has not been established.

A very limited amount of long-term outcome information is available in the pediatric literature, and, thus, a full understanding of the prevalence of the problem, the rates of chronic versus limited-duration manifestations, and the likelihood of relevant morbidity related to GERD over time in pediatric subsets has not yet been obtained. Yet this information is important in evaluating the results of long-term medical or surgical interventions. Current estimates of the prevalence based on available literature indicate that recurrent vomiting is reported in two-thirds of 4-month-old infants but is present in only 5%–10% of infants by 1 year of age [3]. Beyond infancy, nearly 15% of adolescents (10–17 years of age) and one-fourth of children (3 to 9 years of age) report adult-like symptoms such as heartburn or dyspepsia [4]. Among children with developmental disabilities or neurological injury, the risk of GERD and other feeding-related difficulties appears much higher. In a recent study of 79 children (mean age 5.8±3.7) with moderate to severe motor and cognitive dysfunction, 56% were found to have GERD by 24-h esophageal pH monitoring [5].

20.2
Rationale for Long-Term Therapy

As in adults, GERD in pediatric patients beyond 1 year of age is a chronic relapsing condition [5, 6]. The motor abnormalities underlying this disease are largely irreversible and not completely corrected by therapy. Consequently, palliative therapeutic goals in children are to relieve symptoms, promote normal weight gain and growth, improve quality of life, heal epithelial injury caused by refluxed gastric content, and avoid complications [7].

Therapy throughout infancy is aimed at preventing pulmonary and growth-related complications. In this age group, GERD typically manifests as recurrent vomiting; a small minority of infants develops anorexia and other symptoms, failure to thrive, hematemesis, or anemia. Gastroesophageal reflux is one cause of apparent life-threatening events (ALTEs) in infants and has been associated with chronic respiratory alterations including recurrent stridor, reactive airway disease, chronic cough, asthma, and recurrent pneumonia. The last of these is uncommon in all but neurologically impaired children [8].

Older children are more likely to have the adult pattern of GERD, and long-term treatment is aimed at the prevention of esophageal epithelial injury, management of atypical manifestations (oral, pharyngeal, pulmonary complications), and control of symptoms (heartburn, chest pain, regurgitation). Erosive esophagitis is a serious complication of chronic reflux. In children it may present as dysphagia or food impaction. Sometimes the associated esophageal pain results in stereotypical, repetitive, stretching and arching movements that are mistaken for atypical seizures or dystonia (Sandifer syndrome) [9]. Significant epithelial damage also may result in anemia, hypoproteinemia, hematemesis, or melena [10]. Esophagitis can be further complicated by stricture or hemorrhage in up to 20% of adult patients and a substantial proportion of children [11, 12]. The epithelial damage of esophagitis also is considered an important intermediary in the development of the potentially malignant epithelium known as a Barrett's metaplasia [13]. Neither long-term medical therapy nor surgical therapy may impact the progression of this metaplasia to malignancy [14], but sustained treatment may prevent extension of the Barrett's segment – an outcome of significance considering the increase in malignancy risk relative to length of affected esophagus.

20.3
Medications Available for Long-Term Therapy

Acid-reducing agents and prokinetic medications represent the two major categories of pharmacological treatment for GERD in children. Of the acid-reducing agents, antacids act by briefly neutralizing gastric acid. Antacids commonly are used in children and adolescents affected by GERD for short-term relief of acid-triggered esophageal and extra-esophageal symptoms, but published data are unavailable concerning their efficacy and safety for long-term use [7].

Acid suppressants [histamine-2 receptor antagonists (H2RAs), proton pump inhibitors (PPIs)] represent the gold standard of short-term GERD treatment and the most studied agents for short- and long-term use. The H2RAs effectively decrease histamine-stimulated acid secretion, but their effect is limited to acid secretion induced by meals or other stimuli [15]. This mode of action in part explains the decreased efficacy in GERD of H2RAs compared with PPIs, the latter affecting both basal and meal-induced acid secretion. Tolerance to the acid-inhibitory effects of H2RAs has been reported in several studies following treatment periods as short as 30 days [16, 17].

PPIs selectively and irreversibly block the final common pathway of acid secretion at the luminal surface of parietal cells by binding H^+,K^+-ATPase, the so-called "proton pump" [7]. Despite the relatively short half-life in plasma of omeprazole (<1 h in most cases), clinically adequate suppression of acid secretion lasts 12–15 h with a single morning dose. This results from the covalent binding of omeprazole with the proton pump exposed at the parietal cell lumen [18]. The more pronounced effects of PPIs on acid secretion has helped establish their superiority to H2RAs in adult patients for initial treatment of esophagitis, maintenance of remission following esophagitis healing, and prevention of GERD complications [6, 19–21]. These factors have helped make PPIs more cost-effective than H2RAs for GERD management in adults.

In children, PPIs have been shown to be safe and effective for short-term treatment of erosive esophagitis and GERD symptoms that are refractory to other measures. Studies using omeprazole and lansoprazole in children have reported endoscopic healing rates ranging from 40% to 100% and symptoms relief rates from 70% to 100% [21–26]. On a body weight basis, the dosages of omeprazole and lanzoprazole used in the treatment of children with GERD are higher then those used in adults. This is because in the first years of life, children exhibit metabolic rates that are several-fold higher than those observed in adults [18]. An initial dosage of 0.7 mg/kg/day has been suggested based on data presented in several studies involving omeprazole and lanzoprazole [26–29]. The dosage may be adjusted based on 24-h intraesophageal/intragastric pH monitoring, persistent symptoms, or endoscopic findings [24]. Widespread awareness of the greater efficacy of PPIs compared with H2RAs in GERD has resulted in a dramatic increase in their use–the number of PPI prescriptions more than tripling in the last 3 years for American children aged 12–17 years [27, 28].

The aims of prokinetic agents are to reduce acid exposure time and amount of refluxate potentially by improving contractility of the esophageal body, increasing lower esophageal sphincter pressure, decreasing the frequency of transient lower esophageal sphincter relaxations, and reducing gastric emptying time. However, a number of studies have failed to demonstrate that prokinetic agents actually decrease the frequency of reflux episodes. Thus, the principal mechanisms of action of prokinetics in GERD may be enhancement of esophageal peristalsis and acceleration of gastric emptying, thereby reducing refluxate quantity. Among prokinetic agents, cisapride has been shown to improve symptoms, esophageal histopathology, and pulmonary function in infants and children with GERD [29–31]. However, the potential for cardiac toxicity has markedly restricted use of this agent [32]. Efficacy and safety of other prokinetic drugs (e.g., metoclopramide, domperidone, bethanechol) in the treatment of GERD in infants and children are not established [7].

20.4
Long-Term Outcome of Treated or Untreated GERD

The largely irreversible pathophysiology of GERD in all but the infant group suggests that it should be considered a chronic, relapsing disease, but little is known about its natural history and the long-term outcome from treatment in most pediatric subgroups. Much of the current information comes from follow-up of studies of patients treated for short periods following an initial GERD diagnosis.

Several studies demonstrate that complete, spontaneous resolution of symptoms following treatment withdrawal is unlikely over modest periods of observation in children (but not infants) with GERD. Treem and colleagues [33] found that fewer than half of 32 otherwise healthy children (age 3.5–16 years at the time of GERD diagnosis) experienced spontaneous resolution or marked improvement in symptoms over a 1- to 8-year follow-up period. Half of this subject group initially had esophagitis. Four (12%) of the patients were unimproved symptomatically despite medical therapy, and two others (6%) required fundoplication for ongoing symptoms and esophagitis. In a separate study, Ashorn and colleagues [34] found that only 24% of children with endoscopically diagnosed GERD became symptom-free following short periods (up to 3 months) of medical therapy. Thus, GERD in children, particularly when accompanied by esophagitis, typically will persist without ongoing intervention.

In contrast, sustained treatment with effective antireflux interventions can maintain symptomatic and endoscopic remission. The first study to examine the utility of long-term omeprazole use (beyond 2–3 months) in children with esophagitis was that of Gunasekaran and Hassal [35]. After initial omeprazole treatment, 10 of the 15 patients studied had a normal-appearing esophageal mucosa (grade 0 or 1). Following up to 6 months of treatment, esophagitis had healed in all patients, and symptoms and signs of GERD had resolved or markedly improved. These patients were then effectively maintained on omeprazole therapy for periods up to 26 months at dosages ranging from 0.7 to 3.3 mg/kg per day. Likewise, in a recently published study by Hassal and colleagues [24], PPIs were able to maintain healing in 95% (54/57) of children with chronic, severe, and endoscopically proven erosive reflux esophagitis for up to 6 months of therapy. The children in this study were aged 1–16 years, and the dose of omeprazole used ranged from 0.7 to 3.5 mg/kg per day.

PPIs also appear to provide effective salvage therapy in patients who do not have adequate or sustained response to other treatments. Karjoo and Kane [36] studied 129 children (6–18 years of age) with esophagitis; 31% had grade 1 esophagitis, whereas the remaining 69% had overt erosions. Patients who remained symptomatic following 4 weeks of H2RAs were treated with omeprazole at a dose of 20 mg daily. Although initial response rates to the H2RA ranged from 37% to 90% depending on esophagitis grade, fully 87% of the nonresponders had symptomatic improvement following as little as 2 weeks of omeprazole therapy. Others have reported the value of long-term PPI treatment in children with GERD manifestations following fundoplication [37]. Charts from one institution were reviewed from all children over a 10-year period who were given omeprazole for evidence of failed fundoplication. Fifteen subjects in this study were followed for a mean 4.4 years on omeprazole, and marked improvement in severity of both symptoms and esophagitis was noted in these patients while on treatment. No patient required further antireflux surgery.

Consequently, the available literature supports the value of sustained treatment (at least 6 months) with PPIs in managing symptoms or esophagitis in children that is unresponsive to or recurs following other interventions and in preventing relapse of symptoms and esophagitis in patients with well-documented GERD. Whether such treatment will have very long, sustained effects is not established. Likewise, it is not known how useful this approach will be in preventing GERD complications. Of particular importance is preventing progression of Barrett's metaplasia to dysplastic epithelium and adenocarcinoma. Encouraging data in adults at least demonstrate that PPI therapy, adjusted with the use of ambulatory pH monitoring, can persistently control acid reflux in these patients [38, 39]. Omeprazole has been shown to heal esophageal erosions associated with Barrett's metaplasia in pediatric patients, but dosages as high as 80 mg/day are required in some subjects for as long as 8 months to completely heal deeper ulceration [40]. Although associated esophagitis and ulceration can be healed with intervention, a well-documented case of complete regression of Barrett's metaplasia with either medical or surgical therapy has not been reported to date [41, 42]. Limited regression has been observed, but a defined reduction in cancer risk has not been observed [14, 43].

20.5
Safety of Long-Term Medical Therapy

Potent and sustained gastric acid suppression, as seen with PPIs in treatment of GERD, may cause elevated levels of serum gastrin, gastric histological changes, advancement of *Helicobacter pylori* infection into more proximal stomach regions, changes in the microbial flora of the gastrointestinal tract, and altered absorption of iron and vitamin B12. Despite the potential diversity of adverse effects, only hypergastrinemia and resultant gastric histological changes have received much attention, particularly in children.

Hypoclorhydia induces hypergastrinemia. Hypergastrinemia is a trophic stimulus for some gastric cells, particularly the enterochromaffin-like (ECL) cells and parietal cells [44]. Thus, concern has been raised that this physiological response to pharmacological agents that significantly reduce acid secretion may ultimately lead to gastric malignancies [24, 40, 44]. This concern was heightened by the observation that rats develop ECL-cell carcinoids if given omeprazole throughout life [45]. This finding was explained by hypergastrinemia, not direct drug toxicity, as similar observations were made in rats following high-dose treatment with H2RAs or when hypergastrinemia was induced following gastric surgical procedures [46]. Fortunately, because of species-specific responses and other fundamental differences between animal models and human subjects (e.g., very large differences in gastric ECL-cell density), it is unlikely that these early rat model findings can be extrapolated to human subjects. Moreover, in the adult literature covering more than a decade of PPI use, no case of an actual carcinoid tumor has been reported [6]. Current views are that the variations that occur in the endocrine cells of the stomach are minimal, benign, reversible, and mainly self-limiting with no progression toward neoplasia [24].

Nevertheless, hypergastrinemia is observed when children are treated with PPIs. Highly variable gastrin response, ranging from normal to 10-times normal, has been observed in several studies involving PPIs in children [6, 18, 24, 25, 47]. Gastrin levels in some children have been noted to rise and then return to the normal range despite continued PPI therapy [48]. Hassal and colleagues [24] found an increase in serum gastrin levels above normal levels (>100 pmol/L) in 18 of 56 children treated with omeprazole; however, the authors were unable to establish any correlation between gastrin level and dose or duration of omeprazole treatment. Franco et al. [25] observed serum gastrin levels that ranged from 200 to 400 ng/l (normal <120 ng/l) in 8 of 35 children with GERD treated with lansoprazole. Endocrine-cell hyperplasia has been rarely observed [24], but no carcinoid tumors have been reported.

Gastrin also has trophic effects on the gastric parietal cells [44]. Studies reporting the use of acid suppressants in children have described parietal-cell hyperplasia and benign gastric polyps [24, 45, 49, 50]. While it may be tempting to ascribe these morphologic alterations to pharmacologically induced hypergastrinemia, normal fasting serum gastrin levels have been noted in some patients exhibiting these changes [49–51]. Other investigations involving both adults and children have found no correlation between dose and duration of PPI therapy, degree or duration of hypergastrinemia, or presence of polyps and parietal-cell changes, if present [47–52]. Consequently, the gastric morphological changes that can be observed with long-term acid suppression therapy, particularly PPIs, do not necessarily relate to the gastrin response. At present, these changes are not considered premalignant or to have other important consequences–although the findings remain under observation.

The bulk of evidence today indicates that maintenance medical therapy for GERD, including maintenance with potent acid suppressant agents, is safe. The physiological and histological changes that can occur with such therapy continue to be monitored for their potential as being important heralds of later complications. Nevertheless, the safety profile currently appears to fare very well against the morbidity and mortality of the alternative, antireflux surgery. A direct objective comparison of very long-term PPI use versus surgery with safety and efficacy considerations in mind has not been performed, however, in children.

20.6
Indications for Antireflux Surgery

Antireflux surgery often is considered of value in patients with severe or complicated reflux, especially in those with symptoms or findings that cannot be managed medically. The most commonly performed operation is the Nissen fundoplication. This procedure as originally described involved posterior passage of the gastric fundus around the esophagus to encircle up to 6 cm of its distal length. Many variations and modifications have since been described. Variables include approach (transthoracic or abdominal), portion of stomach wall used (anterior and posterior or anterior only), combination with other procedures such as vagotomy or gastroplasty, and looseness, completeness, and length of the wrap [53, 54]. Most surgeons choose to perform a loose (floppy) Nissen procedure that is approximately 1 to 2 cm in length and includes a posterior crural repair. A common modification is a 360° fundic wrap without ligation of the short gastric vessels (Rossetti-Nissen). A partial 270° wrap (Toupet) is used for patients with severe associated motor abnormalities who may be at greater risk for postoperative dysphagia. The latest advance has been the introduction of laparoscopic Nissen fundoplication. Several investigators have shown that laparoscopic fundoplication can be safely and efficiently performed in infants and children, with clinical results similar to those achieved by open surgery, little morbidity, and very short hospital stay [54–57].

Benefits of surgery extend beyond the mechanical effect of creating an external valve around the esophagus. The procedure also reduces a hiatal hernia when present, re-establishes anatomical apposition of the distal esophagus to the crura, closes the crura, and restores an intra-abdominal component to the sphincteric region. Likely related to some of these effects, a well-performed fundoplication also may decrease the frequency of reflux-associated transient lower esophageal sphincter relaxations [58].

Indications for surgery vary somewhat with the age of the patient. In most otherwise healthy children under 1 year of age, gastroesophageal reflux is a temporary condition with spontaneous resolution of symptoms occurring in up to 90% of patients [3, 7]. Because the prognosis for resolution of GERD is better in infants than in older children, the risks of antireflux surgery must be carefully considered against this better prognosis in infants without associated anatomic abnormalities and life-threatening events [59]. In contrast, when GERD occurs in association with congenital malformations and/or life-threatening conditions, early operative correction may be necessary. The latter include apnea or aborted episodes of sudden infant death syndrome. Major congenital anomalies seen in the infant group that might influence the development of GERD and require surgical intervention include corrected esophageal atresia, congenital diaphragmatic hernias, malrotations, congenital abdominal wall defects, and congenital cardiac malformations [60–64]. A recent report described the safe performance of antireflux surgery in infants less than 3 months of age with resolution of presenting problems in 79% of the subjects [64].

In infants, as in older children with GERD, pulmonary aspiration of gastric contents causing pneumonia and reactive airway disease, failure to thrive, and complication of esophagitis remain sources of significant morbidity, especially in neurologically impaired children. These complications of GERD are considered appropriate indications for surgery, especially when medical management is ineffective. Neurological impairment currently constitutes one of the principal comorbidities that encourage proceeding with antireflux surgery in pediatric patients. Unfortunately, children with neurological injury tend to have lower success rates and higher rates of complications in the postoperative period, probably because of their tendency to have poorer health, greater anesthesia risk, and less ability to reflect the usual symptoms and signs of GERD complications [65–67].

In older children, antireflux surgery is often considered for those whose GERD symptoms are chronic and persist following medical management and lifestyle changes, or for those who cannot be weaned from medical therapy [7]. This traditional approach is being challenged by the demonstration that effective treatment can be accomplished with chronic medical therapy using PPIs in many patients, a treatment that appears to have a safe track record to date. Complicated GERD or refractory esophagitis remain as reasonable indications in this older patient group, especially if adequate dosages and treatment courses of antisecretory agents have been offered.

Surgical success rates (defined as complete relief of symptoms) have ranged from 57% to 92% [54, 55, 58, 68]. However, the efficacy of surgery in pediatric groups has been derived primarily from results of case series that used different inclusion criteria, focused predominantly on neurologically impaired children, had short follow-up periods, and reported variable endpoints [7].

Documented postoperative complications have included breakdown or migration of the wrap, small bowel obstruction, gas-bloat syndrome, infection, atelectasis or pneumonia, perforation, esophageal stricture, and esophageal obstruction–complications rates ranging from 2% to 45% of patients [54, 58, 66, 68–70]. Operative mortality may be as high as 5%, and death due to comorbid conditions has been reported with rates up to 21% [7, 55, 58]. Re-operation has been required in 3%–19% of patients [7, 71]. In adults, proximal migration of the wrap with reformation of hiatal hernias and physiological failure occurs in a modest minority of patients within the first 5 years, thereby challenging the long-term efficacy of the procedure.

The above-mentioned limitations of surgery, paucity or absence of controlled efficacy trials or systematic reports regarding long-term outcome, and growing respect for the success of contemporary medical approaches have become critical issues for redefining the role of surgery for GERD management in children. Studies in adults have suggested that antireflux operations produce better quality of life and better symptom control than medical regimens, at least in short-term follow-up [72, 73]. These reports may not have used optimal medical treatment regimens in their comparisons. A recent 3-year follow-up report from a randomized clinical trial comparing antireflux surgery with omeprazole showed that surgery and long-term PPI therapy have comparable benefits, provided there is opportunity to increase omeprazole dosage if response to the standard dosage is suboptimal [74]. Another recent randomized controlled trial found that during 10–13 years of postoperative observation, 62% of surgical patients took antireflux medications on a regular basis, and there were no significant differences between the medical and surgical treatment groups in subsequent rates of neoplastic and peptic complications of GERD. Fundoplication unexpectedly was associated with a significant decrease in long-term survival. The authors concluded that antireflux surgery should not be advised with the expectation that patients will no longer take antisecretory medications or that it is clearly a cancer-preventing procedure [75].

Costs also are relevant to this discussion. Patients in the United States may spend as much as 5 billion dollars annually on antireflux medicines [76]. PPIs presently are expensive, but so is surgery, in particular when it fails or has complications that lead to more doctors visits, tests, and repeated operations. In a recent randomized trial comparing omeprazole and open antireflux surgery, the direct medical costs over five years (cost of medication, surgery, visits, and examinations) together with the indirect medical costs (loss of productivity from GERD-related sick leave) were found to be significantly lower with omeprazole treatment than with surgery, although differences between countries were estimated [77]. Laparoscopic fundoplication has been estimated to cost the same as 10 years of omeprazole therapy [78], and, thus, its cost benefits would be limited in those resuming medical treatment or requiring subsequent diagnosis or intervention in shorter time frames.

Fundoplication has led and continues to lead to improved quality and quantity of life in many selected children, and surgery may be preferable to a lifetime of medication when risk factors for relapse are absent (e.g., in the neurologically normal child with no previous esophageal surgery) and necessary in the face of life-threatening events [79, 80]. However, the advent of PPIs has revolutionized the approach to acid-related disorders in both children and adults. It remains the charge of the pediatric gastroenterologist to (1) complete a thorough pre-operative evaluation aimed at avoiding erroneous diagnoses that commonly mimic GERD and are associated with a high likelihood of poor operative outcome (e.g., cyclic vomiting, rumination, eosinophilic esophagitis), (2) present to patients and their families a realistic explanation of possible problems that may arise after intervention, and (3) verify accurately whether pharmacological therapy has been used correctly in duration and dosage, while keeping in mind that the best therapeutic choice should be a safe one for children with GERD.

References

1. Callahan CW (1998) The diagnosis of gastroesophageal reflux in hospitalized infants: 1971–1995. J Am Osteopath Ass 98: 32–34
2. Gibbons TE, et al (2001) The status of gastroesophageal reflux disease in hospitalized US children 1995–2000 (Abstract). J Pediatr Gastroenterol Nutr 33:197
3. Nelson SP, et al.(1997) Prevalence of symptoms of gastroesophageal reflux during infancy: a pediatric practice-based survey. Pediatric Practice Research Group. Arch Pediatr Adolesc Med 151:569–572
4. Nelson SP, et al. (2000) Prevalence of symptoms of gastroesophageal reflux during childhood. Pediatric Practice Research Group. Arch Pediatr Adolesc Med 154:150–154
5. Schwarz SM, et al. (2001) Diagnosis and treatment of feeding disorders in children with developmental disabilities. Pediatrics 108:671–676
6. Klinkenberg-Knol EC, et al. (2000) Long-term omeprazole treatment in resistant gastroesophageal reflux disease: efficacy, safety and influence on gastric mucosa. Gastroenterol 118: 661–669
7. Rudolph CD, et al (2001) Guidelines for evaluation and treatment of gastroesophageal reflux in infants and children. J Pediatr Gastroenterol Nutr 32(2):S1–S31
8. Berquist W E, et al (1981) Gastroesophageal reflux-associated recurrent pneumonia and asthma in children. Pediatrics 68: 29–25
9. Gonotxategi P, et al (1995) Gastroesophageal reflux disease in association with the Sandifer syndrome. Eur J Pediatr Surg 5: 203–205
10. Herbst JJ, et al (1976) Gastroesophageal reflux with protein losing enteropathy and finger clubbing. Am J Dis Child 130: 1256–1258
11. Orenstein SR, et al (1991) Gastroesophageal reflux. Curr Probl Pediatr 21:193–241

12. Robinson M, et al (1998) Heartburn requiring frequent antacid use may indicate significant illness. Arch Intern Med 158: 2373–2376
13. Hassaall E (1993) Barrett's esophagus: new definitions and approaches in children. J Pediatr Gastroenterol Nutr 16: 345–364
14. Castell OD (2001) Medical, surgical, and endoscopic treatment of gastroesophageal reflux disease and Barrett's esophagus. J Clin Gastroenterol 33(4):262–266
15. Merki HS, et al (1991) The cephalic and gastric phases of gastric acid secretion during H2 antagonist treatment. Gastroenterol 100:599–606
16. Nwokolo CU, et al(1990) Tolerance during 29 days of conventional dosing with cimetidine, nizatidine, famotidine, or ranitidine. Aliment Pharmacol Ther 4 Suppl. 1:29–45
17. Lachman L, Howden C (2000) Twenty-four-hour intragastric pH: tolerance within 5 days of continuous ranitidine administration. Am J Gastroenterol 95:57–61
18. Andersson T, et al (2000) Pharmacokinetics of orally administered omeprazole in children. Am J Gastroenterol 95: 3101–3106
19. Dent J, et al (1994) Omeprazole vs. ranitidine for prevention or relapse in reflux oesophagitis. A controlled double blind trial of their efficacy and safety. Gut 35:590–598
20. Huang J-Q, Hunt RH. (1998) Meta-analysis of comparative trials for healing erosive esophagitis (EE) with proton pump inhibitors (PPIs) and H2-receptor antagonists (H2RAs) (abstract) Gastroenterology 114:A154
21. Abdullaha B, et al (1998) Long-term management of moderate/severe peptic esophagitis in children/adolescents: H2 blockers vs proton pump inhibitor(PPI) (abstract) Gastroenterology 11 114:A51
22. Seiichi Kato, et al (1996) Effect of omeprazole in the treatment of refractory acid relates diseases in childhood: endoscopic healing and twenty-four-hour intragastric acidity. J Pediatr 128:528–532
23. De Giacomo C, et al (2000) Omeprazole for severe reflux esophagitis in children. J Pediatr Gastroenterol Nutr 24: 528–532
24. Hassal E, et al (2000) Omeprazole for treatment of chronic erosive esophagitis in children: a multicenter study of efficacy, safety, tolerability and dose requirements. J Pediatr 137:800–807
25. Franco MT, et al (2000) Lansoprazole in the treatment of gastroesophageal reflux disease in childhood. Dig Liver Dis 32: 660–666
26. Faure C, et al (2001) Lansoprazole in children: pharmacokinetics and efficacy in reflux oesophagitis. Aliment Pharmacol Ther 15:1397–1402.
27. Colletti RB, et al (2001) Use of proton pump inhibitors (PPIs) by pediatric gastroenterologist (abstract) J Pediatr Gastroenterol Nutr 33:414
28. Scott Levin and Associates (2000) IMS American Prescription audit. Scott Levin Audit, Newtown, PA
29. Vandenplas Y, et al (1991) Cisapride decreases prolonged episodes of reflux in infants J Pediatr Gastroenterol Nutr 12: 44–47
30. Scott RB, et al (1997) Cisapride in pediatric gastroesophageal reflux. J Pediatr Gastroenterol Nutr 25:499–506
31. Cohen RC, et al (1999) Cisapride in the control of symptoms in infants with gastroesophageal reflux: a randomized, double blind, placebo-controlled trial. J Pediatr 134:287–292
32. Shulman RJ, et al (1999) The use of cisapride in children. The North American Society for Pediatric Gastroenterology and Nutrition. J Pediatr Gastroenterol Nutr 28:529–533
33. Treem WR, et al (1991) Gastroesophageal reflux in the older children: presentation, response to treatment and long-term follow-up. Clin Pediatr (Phila) 30:435–440
34. Ashorn M, et al (2002) The natural course of gastroesophageal reflux disease in children . Scand J Gastroenterol 37:638–641
35. Gunasekaran TS, Hassal E.(1993) Efficacy and safety of omeprazole for severe gastroesophageal reflux in children. J Pediatr 123:148–154

36. Karjoo M, Kane R (1995) Omeprazole treatment of children with peptic esophagitis refractory to ranitidine therapy. Arch Pediatr Adolesc Med 149:267–271

37. Pashankar D, et al (2001) Omeprazole maintenance therapy for gastroesophageal reflux disease after failure of fundoplication. J Pediatr Gastroenterol Nutr 32:145–149

38. Srinivasan R, et al (2001) Maximal acid reflux control for Barrett's esophagus: feasible and effective. Aliment Pharmacol Ther 15:519–524

39. Peters F, et al (1999) Endoscopic regression of Barrett's esophagus during omeprazole treatment; a randomised double blind study. Gut 45:489–494

40. Israel D M, Hassal E (1998) Omeprazole and other proton pump inhibitors: pharmacology, efficacy and safety with special reference to use in children. J Pediatr Gastroenterol Nutr 27:568–579

41. Hassal E, et al (1985) Barrett's esophagus in childhood. Gastroenterology 89:1331–1337

42. Hassal E, et al (1992) Partial regression of childhood Barrett's esophagus after fundoplication. Am J Gastroenterol 92:1506–1512

43. Sampliner RE, Fass R (1993) Partial regression of Barrett's esophagus: An inadequate endpoint. Am J Gastroenterol 88:2092–2094

44. Freston JW, et al (1995) Effects of hypochlorydia and hypergastrinemia on structure and function of gastrointestinal cells. Dig Dis Sci 40(2):50–62

45. Havu N.(1986) Enterochromaffin-like cell carcinoids of gastric mucosa in rats after life-long inhibition of gastric secretion Digestion 35(Suppl):42–55

46. Mattsson H, et al (1991) Partial gastric corpectomy results in hypergastrinemia and development of gastric enterochromaffin-like cell carcinoids in the rat. Gastroenterol 100:311–319

47. Tolia V, et al (2002) Safety of lansoprazole in the treatment of gastroesophageal reflux disease in children. J Pediatr Gastroenterol Nutr 35:S300–307

48. Kato S, et al (1996) Effect of omeprazole in the treatment of refractory acid-related disease in childhood: endoscopic healing and twenty-four-hour intragastric acidity. J Pediatr 128:415–412

49. Israel DM, et al (1995) Gastric polyps in children on omeprazole (abstract) Gastroenterol 108:A110

50. Pashankar D, Israel DM (1998) Endoscopic gastric change in children on long-term omeprazole therapy. J Pediatr Gastroenterol Nutr 27(4):479

51. Hassal E, et al (1995) Parietal cell hyperplasia in children receiving omeprazole (abstract) Gastroenterol 108:A121

52. Gold BD, Freston JW (2002) Gastroesophageal reflux in children: pathogenesis, prevalence, diagnosis, and role of proton pump inhibitors in treatment. Pediatric Drugs 4(10):673–685

53. Veit F, et al (1995) Trends in the use of fundoplication in children with gastroesophageal reflux. J Pediatr Child Health 31:121–126

54. Rothenberg SS (1998) Experience with 220 consecutive laparoscopic Nissen fundoplications in infants and children. J Pediatr Gastroenterol Nutr 33:274–278

55. Esposito C, et al (2002) Pediatric surgery: laparoscopic treatment of children with GERD. Semin Laparosc Surg 11:177–180

56. Esposito C, et al (2001) Laparoscopic surgery for gastroesophageal disease during the first year of life. J Pediat Surg 36:715–717

57. Tovar JA, et al (1998) Functional results of laparoscopic fundoplication in children. J Pediatr Gatroenterol Nutr 4:457–463

58. Straathof JWA, et al (2001) Provocation of transient lower esophageal relaxations by gastric distention with air. Am J Gastroenterol 96:2317–2323

59. Gremse DA.(2002) Gastroesophageal reflux disease in children: an overview of pathophysiology, diagnosis and treatment. J Pediatr Gastroenterol Nutr 35:S297–299

60. Corbally MI, et al (1992) Nissen fundoplication for gastroesophageal reflux in repaired tracheo-esophageal fistula. Eur J Pediatr Surg 2:332–335

61. Kieffe J, et al (1995) Gastroesophageal reflux after repair of congenital diaphragmatic hernia. J Pediatr Surg 30:1330–1333

62. Beaudoin S, et al (1995) Gastroesophageal reflux after repair of congenital abdominal wall defects. Eur J Pediatr Surg 5:323–326

63. Chung C, et al (1996) Simultaneous correction of malrotation and gastroesophageal reflux in infants Am Surg 62:800–802

64. Fonkalsrud EW, et al(1999) Antireflux surgery in children under 3 months of age. J Pediatr Surg 34:527–531

65. Fonkalsrud EW, et al (1998) Surgical treatment of gastroesophageal reflux in children: a combined hospital study of 7467 patients. Pediatrics 101:419–422

66. Waring JP (1999). Postfundoplication complication: prevention and management. Gastroenterol Clin North Am 28:1007–1019

67. Dall'Oglio L, et al (2000) A new successful change in surgical treatment of gastroesophageal reflux in severely neurologically impaired children: Bianchi's procedure. Eur J Pediatr Surg 10:291–294

68. Dunn JC, et al (1998) Long-term quantitative results following fundoplication and antroplasty for gastroesophageal reflux delayed gastric emptying in children. Am J Surg 175:27–29

69. Allah H, et al (2001) Evaluation of 142 consecutive laparoscopic fundoplication in children: effects of the learning curve and technical choice J Pediatr Surg 36:921–926

70. Esposito C, et al (2002) Complication of laparoscopic antireflux surgery in childhood. Surg Endosc 7:622–624

71. Dalla vecchia LK, et al (1997) Reoperation after Nissen fundoplication in children with gastroesophageal reflux: experience with 130 patients. Ann Surg 226:315–321

72. Spechler SJ (1992). Comparison of medical and surgical therapy for complicated gastroesophageal reflux disease in veterans. N Engl J Med 326:786–792

73. Isolauri J, et al (1997) Long-term comparison of antireflux surgery vs. conservative therapy for reflux esophagitis. Ann Surg 225:295–299

74. Lundell L, et al (2000) Long-term management of gastroesophageal reflux disease with omeprazole or open antireflux surgery: results of a prospective, randomised clinical trial. Eur J Gastroenterol Hepatol 12:879–887

75. Spechler SJ, et al (2001) Long-term outcome of medical and surgical therapies for gastroesophageal reflux disease. JAMA 285:2331–2338

76. Jaroff L Fire in the belly, money in the bank. Time November 6, 1995

77. Myrvold HE, et al (2001) The cost of long-term therapy for gastroesophageal reflux disease: a randomised trial comparing omeprazole and open antireflux surgery Gut 49:488–494

78. Heudebert GR, et al (1997) Choice of long-term strategy for management of patients with severe analysis. Gastroenterology 112:1078–1086

79. Hassal E (1998) Antireflux surgery in children: Time for a harder look. Pediatrics 101(3):467–468

80. Di Lorenzo C, Orenstein S (2001) Fundoplication: friend or foe? J Pediatr Gastroenterol Nutr 34:117–124

Part III
Surgery

Chapter 21

Surgery for Gastroesophageal Reflux?

21

Juan A. Tovar

Gastroesophageal reflux (GER) is so common in children that it is advisable that pediatricians and pediatric surgeons have as clear an understanding of it as currently possible. The problem is that GER is, to a certain extent, a normal phenomenon and that even when it is intense or frequent enough to be considered a disease, its natural history is generally benign and its symptoms tend to alleviate after infancy in most cases. This concept informs both diagnostic and therapeutic attitudes and forms the basis of the current management protocols on both sides of the Atlantic [39, 45]. However, GER disease (GERD) can be disconcerting, and the variety of its clinical presentations and the unpredictable results of treatment in some situations continue to make GERD an ongoing problem.

Looking back at the last 40 or 50 years of the pediatric history of GERD, an oscillatory course with several waves becomes obvious: at first reflux appeared to be a European problem, as it was rarely diagnosed and barely mentioned in the American pediatric literature. At that time the diagnosis was mainly radiologic, often focused on the detection of hiatal hernia or gastric malposition, and the surgical procedures were proposed in some rare cases aimed at reconstructing the anatomy to as normal as possible rather than at correcting a functional disorder [2, 3, 34]. Carre set the rules for conservative treatment after clearly pointing out the favorable natural history of the disease in young infants [8]. Roviralta, a surgeon, called attention to several functional aspects, such as the influence of delayed gastric emptying and the relationship between GER and oropharyngeal infections [37].

In the late 1960s, when I started my surgical training, the Nissen fundoplication, originally designed for the treatment of GERD in adult patients [34] had been already successfully transferred to children, and both my teachers Pellerin in Paris and Monereo in Madrid performed it quite often (completed with drainage procedures) [31] when prolonged diet, antacid, and postural treatment had failed. The results were remarkably good, even to inexperienced eyes like mine, and it was evident even then that a good outcome could be achieved for GERD in children.

When I lived temporarily in the United States as a research fellow in the 1970s, I was amazed by the almost total absence of GER there, although I soon understood that this was rather due to an absence of interest in the disease, probably explained by the elusive diagnosis and by a healthcare system that did not favor either repeated diagnostic tests or relatively long hospitalizations.

However, this situation changed rapidly when the concurrent availability of pH-metry (developed in the U.S.) [22], small-size pediatric fiberscopes [26], and esophageal manometry [19] allowed quantification of acid exposure, inspection, and biopsy of esophageal lesions and detection of some peculiar functional features of GER in children. The advent of these powerful diagnostic tools caused a widening of the scope of GER disease and generated a renewal of our interest in it, attested to by the publication of reports on several series including large numbers of children [12, 13]. However, the frequent inconsistencies of the results of the tests using these tools made the choice of the best treatment so difficult that no one knew for sure which and when one of them should be applied to an individual patient. Therapeutic decisions based on uncertain evidence became more difficult than in the preceding years.

No matter how, GER became a very frequently diagnosed disease among children in the U.S., and pediatricians in many other countries regained interest in its diagnosis and treatment. Although Nissen fundoplication was the first functional operation used for its correction [34], other procedures were adapted to GER in children: the Boerema-pexy to the anterior wall [4], the Thal-Dor anterior plication inspired the Boix-Ochoa [6] and Ashcraft [27] operations, and even the old posterior hemifundoplication proposed by Toupet [24] was adopted by some [5].

In the meantime, several other important developments had taken place: the introduction of H2 receptor blockers [21] and later the development of proton pump inhibitors (PPIs) allowed real control of gastric acid secretion and replaced the old antacids, putting into the hands of pediatricians and pediatric gastroenterologists excellent weapons to control symptoms [18]. Furthermore, the development of prokinetics, particularly cisapride, apparently hastened the natural tendency towards improvement of GER in infants [40]. With a fiberscope in their hands and good drugs on the table, pediatricians became more reluctant to indicate operations, and there was a resurgence of so-called conservative treatment [16, 17].

Then, laparoscopic fundoplication arrived [28] and had a serious impact on the history of GER treatment [15, 20, 30, 35, 44]. Operations similar to those previously performed by the open approach were not only feasible without opening the abdomen, but had apparently the same results [41] with considerable less suffering and with shorter hospital stays [46]. Despite the availability of this new tool, we surgeons (at least many of us) maintained the same indications, the same preventions, and the same limitations for advising surgery. To our surprise, pediatricians and pediatric gastroenterologists began to find that many more patients deserved the benefits of surgery, and some very large series were rapidly collected, particularly in the U.S. [36]. It should be pointed out that the apparently easy laparoscopic fundoplication represented an attractive alternative to months of conservative treatment, that cisapride was found to have some risks, and that the financial burden of prolonged medical treatments could be alleviated by earlier surgery. This had happened before in the field of pediatric urology, with vesico-ureteral reflux and the STING, and the reasons were roughly the same.

However, the problem of GER remains a really complex one, and it is doubtful that a single therapeutic proposal will solve all of the unanswered issues. Increasingly sophisticated functional tests taught us that patients were not all alike, and that a favorable natural history was not to be expected in some children in whom GER is only a part of a spectrum of symptoms and functional disturbances: brain-damaged patients, survivors of neonatal operations for esophageal atresia and tracheoesophageal fistula, those with congenital diaphragmatic hernia, abdominal wall defects, duodenal and jejunal atresia, and others. We also learned that the close relationship between GER and some respiratory diseases such as repeated infection, pneumonia and atelectasis but particularly asthma-like constrictive bronchitis or even real asthma involved new diagnostic difficulties and therapeutic uncertainties: some patients were radically cured after surgery for GER, others improved, but the remaining ones kept their often unbearable symptoms.

Neurologically impaired children are a good example of how our views on the results of surgery were tempered. The antireflux barrier fails and the motility of the esophagus and the stomach can be abnormal in such children, while salivation is disturbed and the gradient of pressures between the abdomen and the thorax is also abnormal. No treatment will change these circumstances, and the best therapeutic weapon in this particular group of patients appeared to be the interposition of a new antireflux barrier, leaving aside all of the contributing factors. Although the results of fundoplication were sometimes excellent, the proportion of long-term wrap failures and the peri-operative morbidity somewhat tempered our enthusiasm about these treatments [1, 7, 9, 29, 33].

Survivors of neonatal operations for malformations such as esophageal atresia with tracheoesophageal fistula had GER so frequently that this soon became another group in which indications for antireflux surgery became frequent. Unfortunately, again the proportion of wrap failures was alarmingly high, which should not come as a surprise since in these cases also the circumstances that contributed to the development of GER remained active despite the use of the new fundoplication: short esophagus with bad angle of His, small stomach, esophageal and gastric dysmotility, and so on [10, 25].

The same limitations also apply to the often refluxing patients previously operated on for congenital diaphragmatic hernia [47] and other neonatal conditions.

The inclusion of many neurologically impaired patients in several large series of patients surgically treated for GER generated some criticism on the pediatric gastroenterologic side about the overall results of surgery, and led to a reinforced tendency to insist on non-operative treatment efforts [17] and also to proposals for other operations such as esophagogastric disconnection with feeding gastrostomy [11]. But again new weapons appeared: the endoscopic modification of the barrier area by radiofrequency coagulation in four quadrants [43, 48] and the endoscopic plication of the gastroesophageal junction [38] offered new perspectives in adults and are currently a matter of some debate [14]. These techniques are not yet applicable to children; they are limited to adult-size patients due to the bulk of the equipment required, but certainly a new wave of approval followed by critical skepticism is to be expected for these techniques too.

I have sought to improve my understanding of GER in children for many years, and I have come to the following conclusions that might serve as an introduction to the surgical part of this book:

1. GER is a complex phenomenon involving gastroesophageal and extradigestive components that change with growth and maturation during infancy and childhood. Several pathologic conditions facilitate reflux because the pathogenic components act more or less strongly in them.
2. It would be naive to believe that a single treatment will be applicable with similar success to all types of refluxing patients. Therapy should be tailored according to the individual circumstances.
3. There is no ideal operation. Nissen fundoplication is, in my opinion, the gold standard, but it can lead to some untoward clinical pictures such as dumping or

gas bloat, reflecting that it overcorrects the problem. All other techniques are less effective, particularly in the long run and more particularly in cases in which GER appears in the context of other conditions such as brain damage, but they may be more bearable in the short run. There is little hope that the new endoluminal procedures might solve the problem in individuals with life expectancies of many decades.

4. Transposition to children of what we have learned from adult refluxers can result in some serious mistakes. Once again, children are not small-sized adults.

5. The pressures exerted by manufacturers and dealers of new equipment or by some healthcare systems should be ignored if the best chances of adequate treatment are to be offered to our refluxing children.

It should be pointed out that many issues remain unresolved, particularly the natural history of the disease in the long term. I am personally convinced that most adult refluxers were refluxing infants and children in whom the leading symptoms that were "cured" or improved over time reappear when age, obesity, pregnancies, tobacco, alcohol, and coffee facilitated the clinical expression [23]. Chronic esophagitis and Barrett's esophagus may lead to cancer, and we do not know whether the current therapeutic choice of options would prevent this dreadful complication. The influence of alkaline reflux in the clinical picture of pediatric reflux is still largely ignored [42], although we suspect that it might be more relevant than previously thought [32].

From a purely surgical standpoint, all diseases for which the choice of operations (or accompanying treatments) is large are basically unsolved problems. If after many years of using a very effective gold standard operation such as Nissen fundoplication the saga continues, we should admit that for some patients we are treating something that can be as elusive as hypospadias, the paradigm of the problem with multiple "ideal" solutions.

References

1. Alexander F, Wyllie R, Jirousek K, Secic M, Porvasnik S (1997) Delayed gastric emptying affects outcome of Nissen fundoplication in neurologically impaired children. Surgery 122:690–697
2. Allison PR (1970) Peptic oesophagitis and oesophageal stricture. Lancet 2:199–202
3. Allison PR (1972) Reflux oesophagitis: its pathology and treatment. Scand J Thorac Cardiovasc Surg 6:318–322
4. Belloli G, Campobasso P, Cappellari F, Bolla G (1994) Treatment of gastroesophageal reflux and hiatal hernia by Boerema anterior gastropexy. Pediatr Surg Int 9:41–46
5. Bensoussan AL, Yazbeck S, Carceller-Blanchard A (1994) Results and complications of Toupet partial posterior wrap: 10 years' experience. J Pediatr Surg 29:1215–1217
6. Boix-Ochoa J (1986) The physiologic approach to the management of gastric esophageal reflux. J Pediatr Surg 21:1032–1039
7. Borgstein ES, Heij HA, Beugelaar JD, Ekkelkamp S, Vos A (1994) Risks and benefits of antireflux operations in neurologically impaired children. Eur J Pediatr 153:248–251
8. Carre IJ (1970) Further on hiatus hernia. Pediatrics 45:341–342
9. Cohen Z, Fishman S, Yulevich A, Kurtzbart E, Mares AJ (1999) Nissen fundoplication and Boix-Ochoa antireflux procedure: comparison between two surgical techniques in the treatment of gastroesophageal reflux in children. Eur J Pediatr Surg 9:289–293
10. Dalla Vecchia LK, Grosfeld JL, West KW, Rescorla FJ, Scherer LR, 3rd, Engum SA (1997) Reoperation after Nissen fundoplication in children with gastroesophageal reflux: experience with 130 patients. Ann Surg 226:315–321
11. Danielson PD, Emmens RW (1999) Esophagogastric disconnection for gastroesophageal reflux in children with severe neurological impairment. J Pediatr Surg 34:84–86
12. Fonkalsrud EW, Ament ME (1996) Gastroesophageal reflux in childhood. Curr Probl Surg 33:1–70
13. Fonkalsrud EW, Ashcraft KW, Coran AG, Ellis DG, Grosfeld JL, Tunell WP, Weber TR (1998) Surgical treatment of gastroesophageal reflux in children: a combined hospital study of 7467 patients. Pediatrics 101:419–422
14. Galmiche JP, Bruley des Varannes S (2003) Endoluminal therapies for gastro-oesophageal reflux disease. Lancet 361:1119–1121
15. Georgeson KE (1998) Laparoscopic fundoplication. Curr Opin Pediatr 10:318–322
16. Hassall E (1995) Wrap session: is the Nissen slipping? Can medical treatment replace surgery for severe gastroesophageal reflux disease in children? Am J Gastroenterol 90:1212–1220
17. Hassall E (1998) Antireflux surgery in children: time for a harder look. Pediatrics 101:467–468
18. Hassall E, Israel D, Shepherd R, Radke M, Dalvag A, Skold B, Junghard O, et al. (2000) Omeprazole for treatment of chronic erosive esophagitis in children: a multicenter study of efficacy, safety, tolerability and dose requirements. International Pediatric Omeprazole Study Group. J Pediatr 137:800–807
19. Hillemeier AG, Grill BB, McCallum R, Gryboski J (1983) Esophageal and gastric motor abnormalities in gastroesophageal reflux during infancy. Gastroenterology 84:741–746
20. Hopkins MA, Stringel G (1999) Laparoscopic Nissen fundoplication in children: a single surgeon's experience. JSLS 3:261–266
21. Inauen W, Emde C, Weber B, Armstrong D, Bettschen HU, Huber T, Scheurer U, et al. (1993) Effects of ranitidine and cisapride on acid reflux and oesophageal motility in patients with reflux oesophagitis–a 24 hour ambulatory combined pH and manometry study. Gut 34:1025–1031
22. Johnson LF, DeMeester T (1974) Twenty-four hour pH monitoring of the distal esophagus: a quantitative measure of gastroesophageal reflux. Am J Gastroenterol 63:325–332
23. Johnston BT, Carre IJ, Thomas PS, Collins BJ (1995) Twenty to 40 year follow up of infantile hiatal hernia. Gut 36:809–812
24. Katkhouda N, Khalil MR, Manhas S, Grant S, Velmahos GC, Umbach TW, Kaiser AM (2002) Andre Toupet: surgeon technician par excellence. Ann Surg 235:591–599
25. Kimber C, Kiely EM, Spitz L (1998) The failure rate of surgery for gastro-oesophageal reflux. J Pediatr Surg 33:64–66
26. Leape LL, Bhan I, Ramenofski ML (1981) Esophageal biopsy in the diagnosis of reflux esophagitis. J Pediatr Surg 16:379–384
27. Lelli JL, Ashcraft KW (1994) Gastroesophageal reflux. Semin Thorac Cardiovasc Surg 6:240–246
28. Lobe TE, Schropp KP, Lunsford K (1993) Laparoscopic Nissen fundoplication in childhood. J Pediatr Surg 28:358–361
29. Martínez DA, Ginnpease ME, Caniano DA, Vinocur C, Golladay S, Martinez DA (1992) Recognition of recurrent gastroesophageal reflux following antireflux surgery in the neurologically disabled child – high index of suspicion and definitive evaluation. J Pediatr Surg 27:983–990
30. Mattioli G, Esposito C, Lima M, Garzi A, Montinaro L, Cobellis G, Mastoianni L, et al. (2002) Italian multicenter survey on

laparoscopic treatment of gastro-esophageal reflux disease in children. Surg Endosc 16:1666–1668

31. Nihoul-Fekete C, Lortat-Jacob S, Jehannin B, Pellerin D (1983) Résultats de l'opération de Nissen avec pyloroplastie et indications chirurgicales du traitement chirurgical du reflux gastroesophagien et de la hernia hiatale chez les enfants. À propos de 267 opérations. Chirurgie 109:875–881

32. Orel R, Markovic S (2003) Bile in the esophagus: a factor in the pathogenesis of reflux esophagitis in children. J Pediatr Gastroenterol Nutr 36:266–273

33. Pimpalwar A, Najmaldin A (2002) Results of laparoscopic antireflux procedures in neurologically impaired children. Semin Laparosc Surg 9:190–196

34. Read RC (2001) The contribution of Allison and Nissen to the evolution of hiatus herniorrhaphy. Hernia 5:200–203

35. Rothenberg SS (1994) Laparoscopic anti-reflux procedures and gastrostomy tubes in infants and children. Int Surg 79:328–331

36. Rothenberg SS (1998) Experience with 220 consecutive laparoscopic Nissen fundoplications in infants and children. J Pediatr Surg 33:274–278

37. Roviralta E (1971) Syndrômes émétisants chez le nourrisson. L'importance des facteurs étiopathogéniques additionels. Ann Pediatr (Paris) 18:399–407

38. Roy-Shapira A, Stein HJ, Scwartz D, Fich A, Sonnenschein E (2002) Endoluminal methods of treating gastroesophageal reflux disease. Dis Esophagus 15:132–136

39. Rudolph CD, Mazur LJ, Liptak GS, Baker RD, Boyle JT, Colletti RB, Gerson WT, et al. (2001) Guidelines for evaluation and treatment of gastroesophageal reflux in infants and children: recommendations of the North American Society for Pediatric Gastroenterology and Nutrition. J Pediatr Gastroenterol Nutr 32(Suppl):S1–S31

40. Saye Z, et al. (1989) Effect of cisapride on esophageal pH monitoring in children with reflux-associated bronchopulmonary disease. J Pediatr Gastroenterol Nutr 8:327–332

41. Tovar JA, Olivares P, Diaz M, Pace RA, Prieto G, Molina M (1998) Functional results of laparoscopic fundoplication in children. J Pediatr Gastroenterol Nutr 26:429–431

42. Tovar JA, Wang W, Eizaguirre I (1993) Simultaneous gastroesophageal pH monitoring and the diagnosis of alkaline reflux. J Pediatr Surg 28:1386–1392

43. Triadafilopoulos G, Utley DS (2001) Temperature-controlled radiofrequency energy delivery for gastroesophageal reflux disease: the Stretta procedure. J Laparoendosc Adv Surg Tech A 11:333–339

44. van der Zee DC, Bax NM (1995) Laparoscopic Thal fundoplication in severely scoliotic children. Surg Endosc 9:1197–1198

45. Vandenplas Y, Ashkenazi A, Belli D, Boige N, Bouquet J, Cadranel S, Cezard JP, et al. (1993) A proposition for the diagnosis and treatment of gastro-oesophageal reflux disease in children: a report from a working group on gastro-oesophageal reflux disease. Working Group of the European Society of Paediatric Gastroenterology and Nutrition (ESPGAN). Eur J Pediatr 152:704–711

46. Viljakka M, Luostarinen M, Isolauri J (1997) Incidence of antireflux surgery in Finland 1988–1993. Influence of proton-pump inhibitors and laparoscopic technique. Scand J Gastroenterol 32:415–418

47. Wakeman C, Bagshaw P, Coulter G, Maoate K (2003) Diaphragmatic herniation of laparoscopic Nissen fundoplication wrap due to forceful post-operative retching: three case reports. N Z Med J 116:U301

48. Wolfsen HC, Richards WO (2002) The Stretta procedure for the treatment of GERD: a registry of 558 patients. J Laparoendosc Adv Surg Tech A 12:395–402

A Retrospective Analysis of Fifty Years of Open Surgery in the Treatment of Gastroesophageal Reflux

22

Jean-Michel Guys · Marco Castagnetti
Fares Benmiloud

Contents

22.1
Introduction

Every evaluation of surgery for gastroesophageal reflux (GER) should address three basic questions. First, is surgery effective in stopping reflux? Second, is surgery able to stop all symptoms and, if symptoms persist, may they be due to coexisting causes? Finally, are morbidity and mortality of surgical treatment lower than those of a medical treatment?

22.1.1
Historical Review of Antireflux Surgery

Historically, early operations for GER aimed to reconstruct the normal anatomy of esophageal hiatus and gastroesophageal junction. Allison described the repair of the phreno-esophageal ligament [1]. Lortat-Jacob advocated a rather similar technique [55]. Hill focused on the fixation of the cardia, suturing the lesser curvature of the stomach to the median arcuate ligament [40]. Similarly, other investigators developed operations to correct what was thought to be only an anatomical disorder [11, 16]. However, in 1973, Allison, reviewing his cases, reported a failure rate of 49% [2], and similar high rates of GER recurrence were reported with different types of cardioplasty and gastropexy proposed in the meantime [11, 16, 41].

Soave proposed a pathophysiologic mechanism for a surgical repair of GER. Withstanding the importance of maintaining cardial continence even during diaphragmatic and gastric contractions, he advised the creation of a positive pressure on the abdominal esophageal segment. Hence, he suggested that an effective operation to prevent reflux should create a valve mechanism and ensure a significant length of intraabdominal esophagus [91]. Both of these goals were achieved by the Nissen technique [69] that, after initial skepticism [86], has gained widespread acceptance in the pediatric setting also, becoming the most-often used procedure [33].

22.1.2
Nissen Fundoplication: The Gold Standard?

Since its first publication, many studies have attested to the efficacy of Nissen fundoplication in ameliorating life-threatening complications of GER, including failure to thrive, aspiration with recurrent pneumonia, apnea, asthma, and esophagitis with pain, bleeding, and stricture formation [46, 52, 57, 67, 103]. Experience with the technique increased with larger and larger series being published. In 1987 Fonkalsrud et al. analyzed the results of a Nissen fundoplication in 340 patients younger than 18 years old. They reported an overall postoperative mortality rate of less than 1%, a morbidity of 12%, and a success rate in controlling reflux of 90% [31]. Similar results were reported in Europe by Bettex and Kuffer [9] and Carcassonne et al. [13] on more than 100 cases. Turnage et al. analyzed a slightly smaller series, but with a mean follow-up longer than 7 years, and still the success rate of the procedure was as high as 88% [103]. Johansson et al. reported "excellent to good results" in 32 of 40 adult patients evaluated 6 months and 5 years after the operation by an independent assessor using endoscopy, esophageal manometry, and 24-h pH monitoring [45]. Bergmeijer et al. reported "excellent or good results" in 22 of 23 patients after a median follow-up of 16 years [7]. Fonkalsrud et al. in an extensive review of 7467 children treated in seven centers over a 20-year period reported a 95% rate of "good or optimal results" in neurologically normal (NN) patients [33].

However, over time, some reports of significant morbidity were published. Spitz et al. analyzing a series of 106 patients found that, although a final success was achieved in 92% of cases, 20% needed secondary surgery due to slippage of the wrap in the thorax, paraesophageal hernia, or bowel obstruction, and 27% developed esophageal strictures. The complication rate was fairly high in neurologically impaired (NI) children: 40% [92]. Hanimann et al. reported similar success (92%) and reoperation (22%) rates, but also underlined that 40% of their patients experienced early or late complications [38].

Negre reported an incidence of postoperative symptoms such as dumping syndrome, increased abdominal meteorism, modifications of swallowing habit, dysphagia. or inability to vomit and belch in 76% of 226 adult patients after a mean follow-up of 5–6 years. All patients experienced a transient postoperative dysphagia lasting on average 3–5 months [67]. These troublesome symptoms persisted after 10 years in more than 10% of the patients [68].

In the extensive review of Fonkalsrud et al., results were better: 3.6% of patients had a gas bloat syndrome, 2.4% dysphagia, 2.6% a bowel obstruction. Considering the status of the patient, major complications occurred in 4.2% of NN and 12.8% of NI patients [33].

These data warrant three considerations. First, the complication rate and the success rate are closely related to the criteria considered. Second, complications vary with time. Third, some subsets of patients are at increased risk of complications.

And what is the role of the surgeon? Might technical choices affect the outcome?

22.2
Surgery for Gastroesophageal Reflux

22.2.1
From Original Nissen to Modified Nissen Procedures

Several modifications to the original Nissen procedure have been proposed in an attempt to reduce associated complications such as dysphagia, gas-bloat, dumping syndrome, wrap disruption or dislocation, and paraesophageal hernia.

In the original procedure, proposed by Nissen in 1956, the distal esophagus was mobilized, through a laparotomy, in order to obtain a good length of intra-abdominal segment that was subsequently wrapped with the posterior aspect of the gastric fundus passed behind. The wrap was closed with 4–5 interrupted silk stitches, one or more also incorporating the anterior wall of the esophagus. A large-bore esophageal stent was left during the procedure. Section of the triangular ligament of the liver was advised. Gastropexy was restricted only to patients with hiatal hernia. Short gastric vessels were always preserved. The diaphragmatic crura were left untouched [69].

Major modifications could be grouped as follows:

1. Use of the anterior aspect of stomach for the wrap
2. Extensive dissection of the gastric fundus
3. Fixation of the wrap to avoid its dislocation
4. Association of cruroplasty
5. Reduction of the length of the wrap
6. Creation of less than complete wrap
7. Association of pyloroplasty and/or gastrostomy in subsets of patients

Use of the anterior aspect of the stomach was first proposed by Rossetti in 1968 [81]. This modification is theoretically advantageous, as it allows a more precise tailoring of the wrap, and since its introduction it became the technique of choice in Nissen's clinic [82]. However, the anterior surface of the stomach provides less tissue, increasing the risk of wrap tightness. The tension produced on the esophagus by the tethered stomach may cause the creation of a spiral-narrowed lumen impairing food progression but refractory to dilatations, since it is not properly stenotic [42]. To overcome this problem, a wide fundus mobilization by section of short gastric vessels was proposed [83, 87]. Different studies addressed this issue comparing Nissen procedures performed with or without mobilization [58, 59]. Results showed that this maneuver does not reduce the risk of wrap disruption or the incidence of postoperative dysphagia. In contrast, Luostarinen et al. et al. reported an abnormally prolonged esophageal transit time in patients undergoing fundus mobilization, suggesting the risk of partial denervation of the stomach during dissection [59]. Furthermore, fundus mobilization increased the recurrence rate of diaphragmatic hernia due to a slipping up of the wrap, the telescope phenomenon [58, 59]. This phenomenon can be prevented by the inclusion of the anterior wall of the esophagus in the wrap. Fixation of the wrap to the crura [77] and the so-called Rossetti stitch, anchoring the wrap to the gastric body [84] are further proposed solutions to avoid a wrap dislocation. A downward sliding of the wrap is less common, but a possible modification to avoid it consists of the preservation of the hepatic branch of the anterior vagus so that the wrap would be in between this and the crura [15].

Wideness of the hiatal opening is another risk factor for recurrence of hiatal hernia. Moreover, research on animal models and humans has shown the relevance of the crura itself as an antireflux mechanism [64, 65]. Therefore it is not surprising that closure of the crura is generally agreed upon [17]. Cruroplasty is usually accomplished by a posterior suturing of the hiatus, but an anterior suture may be good as well, and easier [105]. It should be noted that the precise visualization of the hiatus by laparoscopy has shown that reflux may occur even in the presence of a normal hiatus [62]. Moreover, excellent results and no increase in the rate of paraesophageal hernias have been reported by authors not performing any crural repair [13, 53].

In the mid-1980s, Donahue et al. [23] and DeMeester et al. [20] proposed a modified Nissen procedure called the "short floppy Nissen." This procedure consisted of a wide mobilization of the gastric fundus by short gastric vessel section, abdominalization of the lower esophagus, cruroplasty, and the fashioning of a short wrap (about 2 cm) anchored to the encircled esophagus. The wrap was calibrated around a large intraesophageal bougie. In De Meester et al.'s experience, this technique allowed a drop in the incidence of temporary and persistent dysphagia from 83% to 39% and 21% to 3%, respectively. Most patients preserved the ability to belch. Therefore the authors concluded that the operation remained effective in controlling pathologic gastroesophageal reflux, even if the fundoplication was performed with a loose and short wrap. Cross-matching the results of this modified Nissen with the aforementioned regarding fundus mobilization, it could be assumed that the reduced length of the wrap was the cornerstone of their success. Furthermore it is of note that Levy et al. reported excellent comparable results with a technique involving a short wrap but without section of the gastric vessels and cruroplasty [53].

The other point stressed by DeMeester et al., in order to prevent wrap tension, was its calibration by an indwelling bougie and/or by passing an instrument or a finger between the esophagus and the wrap after accomplishment of the latter [20]. Although general agreement has existed on this principle since the first procedure performed by Nissen, the ideal size of the bougie is still debated. In adults, gastric sounds of a diameter variable between 32 and 60 Fr have been used [20, 23, 59, 73, 87], while in children a criterion based on patient weight has been suggested. Recommended size varied from 20–24 Fr for patients of 2.5–4 kg of weight to 36–40 Fr for those of 36–40 kg [72]. Nevertheless, surgeons have also achieved good results performing Nissen without any indwelling esophageal bougie [29, 31]. In contrast, others have proposed the use of more complex devices such as intra-operative esophageal manometry [43].

Suture materials used to fix wrap edges are another potentially important factor for the success of a fundoplication. In his original technique Nissen used silk sutures. Nowadays nonabsorbable sutures seem the standard in order to avoid a wrap disruption [7, 17]. The suture line can be either single or double.

Even on suture technique DeMeester et al. described an interesting detail; they advised closing the wrap with a horizontal mattress suture tied on Teflon pledgets to minimize the cutting effect of the stitch on the tissues [20]. The effectiveness of such a detail has also been described in children [79]

The Nissen procedure has been performed by both an abdominal and a transthoracic route. In 1965 Nissen and Rossetti underlined that the thoracic approach was justified only in exceptional cases [70]. Among the indications for a thoracotomy, they mentioned chronic ulcer of the cardia, esophageal stenosis, and carcinoma, all scenarios almost nonexistent in children. Even in children, therefore, the transabdominal Nissen fundoplication is technically easier and less traumatic [30]. A transthoracic approach could be necessary in cases of long-gap esophageal atresia, in which a primary anastomosis may result in a brachyesophagus with severe reflux.

22.2.2
Other Wrap Configurations

Other wrap configurations have been proposed in order to prevent some of the disadvantages associated with a 360° fundoplication. They mainly consist of 180° to 270° wraps, either anterior (Thal [96], Boix-Ochoa [12], Dor [24]) or posterior (Toupet [99]). Looking at the published series, great confusion exists about the denomination of the different procedures [73], but overall results of total and partial wraps seem to be comparable, and various fundoplication procedures extensively used in clinical practice result in similar long-term control of reflux and reoperation rates [53, 85, 97, 106]. We believe that, if the goal of stopping GER and associated symptoms is achieved ensuring a low morbidity meantime, these operations should be justified.

Thal initially proposed his technique as a unified strategy and approach to the surgical problem of the esophagogastric junction [96]. In the U.S., Aschcraft has been a very active promoter of this type of fundoplication in children [4, 85]. According to his data, this technique is as effective as the Nissen technique in controlling reflux, but with a lower complication rate. In a series of 355 children followed from 1 to 8 years, he reported no mortality, 5% recurrence, and an overall reoperation rate of 9% [4]. Van der Zee et al. compared the two wraps in a series of 44 patients and reported a lower reflux recurrence in the Thal group, 4% versus 37%. In addition, the rate of children experiencing an uneventful postoperative course was better after Thal fundoplication (87% vs. 30%) [104].

The Boix-Ochoa technique is basically a modification of Thal wrap [12]. The author reported results comparable to those of major series of Nissen fundoplications. Two recent series have compared the two types of wrap. Surprisingly, Choen et al, concluded that the two techniques are equally effective but that the Boix-Ochoa is associated with a lower complication rate [14], while in Subramaniam et al.'s experience the Nissen fundoplication was more effective and associated with less complications [95].

The Dor fundoplication is another 180° anterior wrap [24]; its use is nowadays generally restricted to a prophylactic procedure after Heller myotomy for megaesophagus [74]. In principle it allows the surgeon to cover the exposed esophageal mucosa, ensure an antireflux barrier, and minimize the risk of dysphagia in an esophagus at high suspicion of intrinsic dysmotility.

The posterior 270° wrap described by Toupet in 1963 [99] has been analyzed in many pediatric series [6, 106]. In the beginning of the 1980s, Bensoussan et al., based on a series of 112 patients followed over a 10-year period, concluded that the results of the Toupet procedure compared favorably with those of Nissen fundoplication. Functional complications were reported in 7%, with a general optimal outcome in 90% of all patients. Interestingly, the series also included 30% neurological impaired patients and 41% children under 1 year of age [6]. Lundell et al. addressed the questions of whether encircling more than half of the esophagus is necessary to control reflux and whether comparable results with lower mortality may be achieved using semifundoplication. They showed that the partial Toupet wrap controlled reflux equally well and durably when assessed objectively by an independent clinical observer with endoscopy and 24-h pH monitoring [56].

22.2.3
Other Surgical Solutions to Treat GER

A surgical procedure proposed for the treatment of reflux, as an alternative to a wrap, is the so-called Angelchik prosthesis: a ring-shaped silicon prosthesis positioned subdiaphragmatically around the esophagus [3]. Rossetti was critical of this device as challenging the dynamic physiology of the lower esophageal sphincter [82]. However Gourley et al., in a prospective randomized trial in disabled patients undergoing either a prosthesis placement or a Nissen fundoplication, reported no significant differences in the outcome. Nevertheless, the authors themselves pointed out the importance of a long-term follow-up, since the prosthesis is a foreign body [37]. No recent publications have further developed this procedure.

In 1997 Bianchi introduced the esophagogastric dissociation for the treatment of reflux in children with profound NI. The procedure consists of an end to end anastomosis between the terminal esophagus, detached from the stomach at the esophagogastric junction, and a bowel loop in Roux-en-Y fashion. Feeding is allowed by a gastrostomy, either continent or not [10]. Results of this technique are still under evaluation [19, 21, 35]. Gatti et al. prospectively compared 12 patients undergoing a Nissen fundoplication and gastrostomy with 14 patients undergoing an esophagogastric dissociation. In their experience the latter allowed a significant improvement in many anthropometric and biochemical parameters and in quality of life when assessed by a standardized parental questionnaire [35]. In our opinion, this technique can be taken into account in cases of repeated failure of conventional surgery or of severe pharyngeal incoordination.

22.2.4
Are Results Comparable?

A complete understanding of the relevance of each single technique or modification is difficult. Studies are often retrospective and, if two successive periods are compared, a learning curve effect is unavoidable. Clinical trials often enroll a limited number of patients, allowing a significant risk of type II error. More than one modification has been introduced at the same time, and the techniques are often not described in enough detail. Differences in case selection, data acquisition, and definitions may all influence the results. Postoperative follow-up is usually not carried out by an independent assessor, not using objective criteria, and at variable intervals after the procedure, thus misjudging possible improvement due to patient adaptation to the new anatomy. Clinical examination or patients interviewing may only show persistence of symptoms but not of reflux, and symptoms may be unrelated to reflux persistence [94]. Of greatest importance is the lack of objective, standardized criteria of assessment to define success, since with the present standard comparison within results is almost impossible. It should be noted, however, that no general agreement exists regarding the need for objective measurements of reflux to define success. Pope withstood that, since subjective symptoms are the principal problem affecting patients' quality of life, subjective symptoms should be considered the criteria for evaluation of a technique [76]. Nevertheless, even in this view an effort should be made to establish standardized questionnaires and clinical scores to allow comparisons among series [27, 71, 76].

The extensive review of Fonkalsrud et al. is, in light of all of these pitfalls, an example, not enabling meaningful conclusions [39]. Nevertheless, awareness of these problems is increasing among pediatric surgeons [71, 94, 102].

22.3
The Surgical Patient with GER

Patient selection is one of the principal issues affecting many studies. Some subsets of patients have, in fact, an increased risk of unsatisfactory outcome. Major patient-related factors are: respiratory symptoms, delayed gastric emptying (DGE), esophageal dysmotility, neurological impairment (NI), previous story of esophageal atresia (EA) or congenital diaphragmatic hernia (CDH), and age at surgery under 4 months. Often these conditions are associated with each other; for example, DGE and esophageal dysmotility are more frequent in NI children, and most patients with a history of CDH have respiratory symptoms, and almost all with a history of EA have esophageal dysmotility, at least in the distal esophagus. These factors may affect the postoperative outcome and identify subsets of patients at increased risk of unsatisfactory outcome.

22.3.1
Infants Under Four Months of Age

Need of antireflux surgery in early infancy may not be a risk factor per se. The outcome in these patients may be poor solely because children needing such a precocious intervention usually have extremely severe reflux or severe associated conditions or have already experienced an adverse life-threatening event. In light of this, Fonkalsrud et al., reviewing their experience with fundoplications performed before 3 months of age, found that antireflux surgery performed in this period of life allowed symptom resolution in only 79% of cases and was associated with a relatively high mortality of 9%. However, deaths were mostly related to the underlying disease more rather than to the procedure itself [34]. Similarly Kubiak et al., in a series of 66 patients undergoing antireflux surgery under 4 months of life, reported presence of isolated GER in only 10 cases, whereas the remaining 56 had an associated pathological condition leading or not to GER: 19 EA, 14 CDH, and 26 more-complex syndromes. Surgery was successful in 90% of children with isolated GER, and in only 64% of those with associated anomalies [51].

22.3.2
Neurologically Impaired Children

Rice et al., in a comparative series of 52 children with and without neurological problems undergoing Nissen fundoplication, concluded that antireflux surgery could be performed safely in both patient groups; nevertheless, perioperative mortality was 0% in normal children versus 6% in the NI children [78]. Smith et al. reported a high rate of recurrent pneumonia (40%) and vomiting (31%) after antireflux surgery in children with profound neurologic disability [89]. Similarly, Martinez et al., in a series of 240 children with profound NI undergoing antireflux surgery, reported GER recurrence in 46% of cases and an astonishing 75% of their patients presenting symptoms postoperatively. Therefore those authors advised a high index of suspicion of GER recurrence in the postoperative follow-up of NI children [61]. Kimber et al., in a study of 66 patients requiring redo fundoplication during a 15-year period, reported that herniation or disruption of the wrap were the major causes of failure, and that failure was more frequent in children with hypertonic cerebral palsy [50]. Presence of increased risk of morbidity in this population was well shown by Spitz et al. in a 1993 study in which an extensive review of the literature was also carried out [93]. Based on their findings, those authors recommended a gastrostomy placement in all NI patients (although only 38% of their patients had one) and the correction of any suspected gastric outlet obstruction in children with neurological impairment needing antireflux surgery. Although such a policy also remains controversial in NI children, the tendency nowadays is to place a gastrostomy whenever a pathological swallowing pattern and/or feeding problem is present.

22.3.3
Patients with Delayed Gastric Emptying and Esophageal Dysmotility

Delayed gastric emptying (DGE) plays a potentially important role in postoperative symptoms [75]. Approximately 50% of patients with symptomatic GER are believed to have abnormal gastric emptying, with a higher percentage reported in children with NI [32]. Moderate DGE has been suggested to be the cause of most of the gas bloat syndrome [60]. Fonkalsrud et al. advised pyloroplasty in all patients with more than 60% gastric retention of technetium-99m sulfur colloid in semisolid feeding at 90 min, and using this cut-off they performed a gastric emptying procedure in 20% of their patients. [32]. Conversely, Maxson et al. did not find any difference in the incidence of recurrent symptoms, readmissions, or reoperations comparing NI patients undergoing Nissen with or without an associated pyloroplasty. Children undergoing both procedures instead had a higher complication rate (23.8% vs. 5%) and needed more days to return to full oral feeding (14.6% vs. 3.9%) [63]. Bias et al. reached the same conclusion in NN patients [5]. According to the multicentric audit of Fonkalsrud et al., a gastric emptying procedure is performed in association with antireflux surgery in 11.5% of NN and in 40% of NI children [33].

The role of esophageal dysmotility is even more debated. Fonkalsrud et al. reported an incidence of esophageal dysmotility approaching 40% and therefore advised as imperative the creation of a loose wrap not constricting the gastroesophageal junction [31, 32]. On the other hand, Godoy et al. showed in a group of patients the persistence of the same dysmotility esophageal pattern before and after fundoplication regardless of the presence of symptoms, and therefore they concluded that esophageal dysmotility does not affect the outcome [36].

2.3.4
Patients with a Previous History of EA or CDH

Esophageal dysmotility is a major problem in patients with a previous history of EA [101]. It reduces the esophageal clearance, therefore increasing the risk of respiratory infection and peptic anastomotic stricture if surgery is not performed. On the other hand, it potentially increases the risk of postoperative dysphagia. It is not surprising therefore that while some authors advised an aggressive treatment [8, 28], others suggested that surgery should be delayed as much as possible [18, 107]. The risk of dysphagia has also been used as an argument in favor of partial fundoplication in this group of patients, but in fact no supporting evidence exists, and the choice is based only on the personal wisdom of the surgeon [22].

Esophageal dysmotility is not the only problem in EA children. A failure rate of antireflux surgery (30%) [90, 107] and an incidence of delayed gastric emptying [47, 80] higher than in the general population have also been reported. A long-term, close follow-up of these patients should be considered mandatory [54].

GER is present in about 60% of patients with a CDH [26, 44, 49, 66], and fundoplication will be necessary in 20% of these cases [48]. Although controversy exists regarding the relation between GER and CDH, all of the authors point out the need for a careful follow-up of GER/CDH patients, who should be managed with early surgery if medical treatment is ineffective [88].

22.3.5
Patients with Supraesophageal Symptoms

A further debated group is that of patients with supraesophageal symptoms. The existence of a relation between GER and such symptoms is still debated, but even more uncertain are diagnostic criteria, indications for surgery, and type of surgical repair [98]. In these children symptoms may be due both to a chronic aspiration of refluxing acid gastric contents and to a vagal reflex elicited by stimulation of nerves ending in the distal esophagus. This means that even minimal reflux in the presence of a normal anatomy of the gastroesophageal junction, without any objective evidence, may cause symptoms. Tovar et al. reported 14 patients operated on for a suspicion of GER despite normal pH monitoring. Surgery was performed after an average period of 24 months of unsuccessful medical treatment and was effective in 13 of the 14 patients [100]. The term "silent reflux" has been suggested, and the problem of its clinical definition is evident. New criteria have been tested to indicate surgery in this population. Eizaquirre pointed out the importance of the mean duration of nocturnal episodes of reflux at pH monitoring [25]. Theoretically, the goal of a surgical procedure in these patients should be to avoid any reflux at all. But again it is difficult to say whether a 360° wrap could be more effective than a partial one and whether it increases the risk of postoperative symptoms.

22.4
Conclusions

Surgical management of GER has improved over the years due to technical modifications, and to improvements in perioperative investigations, medical treatment, anesthesia, and intensive care. The latter have led to an increase in the number of children with neurological disability eligible for the procedure, whereas the reduced morbidity associated with surgery has facilitated parents' and pediatricians' acceptance. Hence, the number of NN children referred to surgery has also increased. Interestingly, comparable results are obtained with different techniques or modified procedures, while results widely divergent are reported in series apparently using a similar technique. Meticulous surgery and surgical experience should probably be still considered the keys to success. Nevertheless, the factor of utmost importance remains the indications for surgery. The need for reflux prevention is not the same among children with gastroenterologic or respiratory symptoms, neurological patients, and children without neurological disabilities. Factors other than technical details of the wrap should be kept in mind regarding the choice of procedure. Postoperative symptoms may be in fact unrelated to the technique, may improve with time, and may be subjective. Efforts should be made to establish standardized criteria to define success as well as possible complications, thus making results of different studies comparable.

The introduction of laparoscopic fundoplication in the mid1990s has broadened our armamentarium for the care of GER. If we recall and take advantage of what has already been done in open surgery and if we improve collaboration among surgeons, pediatricians, anesthetists, and gastroenterologists, long-term results of surgery for the treatment of GER will surely continue to improve in the years to come.

References

1. Allison PR (1951) Reflux esophagitis, sliding hiatal hernia and anatomy of repair. Surg Gynecol Obstet 92:419
2. Allison PR (1973) Hiatus hernia. A 20-year retrospective survey. Ann Surg 178:273–276
3. Angelchik J, Choen R (1979) A new surgical procedure for the treatment of gastroesophageal reflux and hiatal hernia. Surg Gynecol Obstet 148:246–248
4. Aschcraft KW, Holder TM, Amoury RA (1981) Treatment of gastroesophageal reflux in children by Thal fundoplication. J Thorac Cardiovasc Surg 82:706–712
5. Bais JE, Samsom M, Boudesteijn EAJ et al (2001) Impact of delayed gastric emptying on the outcome of antireflux surgery. Ann Surg 234:139–146
6. Bensoussan AL, Yazbeck S, Carceller-Blanchard A (1994) Results and complications of Toupet partial posterior wrap: 10 years' experience. J Pediatr Surg 29:1215–1217
7. Bergmeijer JHLJ, Harbers JS, Molenaar JC (1997) Function of pediatric Nissen-Rossetti fundoplication followed up into adolescence and adulthood. J Am Coll Surg 184:259–261
8. Bergmeijer JH, Tibboel D, Hazebroek FW (2000) Nissen fundoplication in the management of gastroesophageal reflux occurring after repair of esophageal atresia. J Pediatr Surg 35:573–576
9. Bettex M, Kuffer F (1969) Long-term results of fundoplication in hiatus hernia and cardio-esophageal chalasia in infants and children. Report of 112 consecutive cases. J Pediatr Surg 4:526–530
10. Bianchi A (1997) Total esophagogastric dissociation: an alternative approach. J Pediatr Surg 32:1291–1294
11. Boerema I, Germs R (1955) Fixation of the lesser curvature of the stomach to the anterior wall after reposition of the hernia through the esophageal hiatus. Arch Chir Neerl 7:351–354
12. Boix-Ochoa J, Rowe MI (1998) Gastroesophageal reflux. In: O'Neill, Rowe MI, Grosfeld JL, Fonkalsrud EW, Coran AG (eds) Pediatric surgery. Mosby, St. Louis, pp 1007–1017
13. Carcassonne M, Guys JM, Delarue A et al (1985) Surgery of gastroesophageal reflux. World J Surg 9:269–276
14. Choen Z, Fishman S, Yulevich A et al (1999) Nissen fundoplication and Boix-Ochoa antireflux procedure: comparison between two surgical techniques in the treatment of gastroesophageal reflux in children. Eur J Pediatr Surg 9:289–293
15. Chrysos E, Tzortzinis A, Tsiaoussis J et al (2001) Prospective randomised trial comparing Nissen to Nissen-Rossetti technique for laparoscopic fundoplication. Am J Surg 182:215–221
16. Collis JL (1957) An operation for hiatus hernia with short esophagus. Thorax 12:181–184
17. Consensus statement (1997) Laparoscopic antireflux surgery for gastroesophageal reflux disease (GERD). Surg Endosc 11:413–426
18. Curci MR, Dibbins AW (1988) Problems associated with a Nissen fundoplication following tracheoesophageal fistula and esophageal atresia repair. Arch Surg 123:618–620
19. Danielson PD, Emmens RW (1999) Esophagogastric dissociation for gastroesophageal reflux in children with severe neurological impairment. J Pediatr Surg 34:84–86
20. De Meester TR, Bonavina L, Albertucci M (1986) Nissen fundoplication for gastroesophageal reflux disease. Evaluation of primary repair in 100 consecutive patients. Ann Surg 204:9–20
21. Dell'Oglio L, Gatti C, Villa M et al (2000) A new rapid chance in surgical treatment of gastroesophageal reflux in severely neurologically impaired children: Bianchi's procedure. Eur J Pediatr Surg 10:291–294
22. Di Lorenzo C, Orenstein S (2002) Fundoplication: friend or foe? J Pediatr Gastroenterol Nutr 34:117–124
23. Donahue PE, Samelson S, Nyhus LM et al (1985) The floppy Nissen fundoplication. Effective long-term control of pathologic reflux. Arch Surg 120:663–668
24. Dor J (1962) L'interet de la technique de Nissen modifiee dans la prevention du reflux. Mem Acad Chir 88:877–878
25. Eizaguirre I, Tovar JA (1992) Predicting preoperatively the outcome of respiratory symptoms of gastroesophageal reflux. J Pediatr Surg 27:848–851
26. Fasching G, Huber A, Uray E et al (2000) Gastroesophageal reflux and diaphragmatic motility after repair of congenital diaphragmatic hernia. Eur J Pediatr Surg 10:360–364
27. Feussner H, Petri A, Walker S et al (1991) The modified ASP score: an attempt to make the results of anti-reflux surgery comparable. Br J Surg 78:942–946
28. Fonkalsrud EW (1979) Gastroesophageal reflux following repair of esophageal atresia. Experience with nine patients. Arch Surg 114:48–51
29. Fonkalsrud EW, Ament ME (1996) Gastroesophageal reflux in childhood. Curr Prob Surg 33:1–70
30. Fonkalsrud EW, Ament ME, Byrne WJ et al (1978) Gastroesophageal fundoplication for the management of reflux in infants and children. J Thorac Cardiovasc Surg 1978:655–664
31. Fonkalsrud EW, Berquist W, Vargas J et al (1987) Surgical treatment of gastroesophageal reflux syndrome in infants and children. Am J Surg 154:11–18
32. Fonkalsrud EW, Foglia RP, Ament ME et al (1989) Operative treatment for the gastroesophageal reflux syndrome in children. J Pediatr Surg 24:525–529
33. Fonkalsrud EW, Ashcraft KW, Coran AG et al (1998) Surgical treatment of gastroesophageal reflux in children: A combined hospital study of 7467 patients. Pediatrics 101:419–422
34. Fonkalsrud EW, Bustorff-Silva J, Perez CA, et al (1999) Antireflux surgery in children under 3 months of age. J Pediatr Surg 34:527–531
35. Gatti C, Federici di Abriola G, Villa M et al (2001) Esophagogastric dissociation versus fundoplication: which is the best for severely neurologically impaired children? J Pediatr Surg 36:677–680
36. Godoy J, Tovar JA, Vicente Y et al (2001) Esophageal motor dysfunction persists in children after surgical cure of reflux: an ambulatory manometric study. J Pediatr Surg 36:1405–1411
37. Goureley GR, Pellett JR, Li BUK et al (1986) A prospective randomised double blinded study of gastroesophageal reflux surgery in pediatric-sized developmentally disabled patients: Nissen fundoplication versus Angelchik prosthesis. J Pediatr Gastroenterol Nutr 5:52–61
38. Hanimann B, Sacher P, Stauffer UG (1993) Complications and long-term results of the Nissen fundoplication. Eur J Pediatr Surg 3:12–14
39. Hassall E (1998) Antireflux surgery in children. Time for a harder look. (Commentary) Pediatrics 101:467
40. Hill LD (1967) An effective operation for hiatal hernia: an eight-year appraisal. Ann Surg 166:681–692
41. Hill LD (1972) Surgery and gastroesophageal reflux. Gastroenterology 63:183–185
42. Hunter JG, Swanstrom L Waring JP (1996) Dysphagia after laparoscopic antireflux surgery. The impact of operative technique. Ann Surg 224:51–57
43. Inge TH, Carmeci C, Ohara LJ et al (1998) Outcome of Nissen fundoplication using intraoperative manometry in children. J Pediatr Surg 33:1614–1617
44. Jaillard SM, Pierrat V, Dubois A et al (2003) Outcome at 2 years of infants with congenital diaphragmatic hernia: a population based study. Ann Thorac Surg 75:250–256
45. Johansson J, Johnsson F, Joelsson B, Florén CH, Walther B (1993) Outcome 5 years after 360° fundoplication for gastrooesophageal reflux disease. Br J Surg 80:46–49
46. Johnson DG, Herbst JJ, Oliveros MA, Stewart DR (1977) Evaluation of gastroesophageal reflux surgery in children. Pediatrics 59:62–69

47. Jolley SG, Johnson DG, Roberts CC et al (1980) Patterns of gastroesophageal reflux in children following repair of esophageal atresia and distal tracheoesophageal fistula. J Pediatr Surg 15:857–862

48. Kamiyama M, Kawahara H, Okuyama H et al (2002) Gastroesophageal reflux after repair of congenital diaphragmatic hernia. J Pediatr Surg 37:1681–1684

49. Kieffer J, Spain E, Berg A et al (1995) Gastroesophageal reflux after repair of congenital diaphragmatic hernia. J Pediatr Surg 30:1330–1333

50. Kimber C, Kiely EM, Spitz L (1998) The failure rate of surgery for gastro-oesophageal reflux. J Pediatr Surg 33:64–66

51. Kubiak R, Spitz L, Kiely EM et al (1999) Effectiveness of fundoplication in early infancy. J Pediatr Surg 34:295–299

52. Leape LL, Ramenofsky (1980) Surgical treatment of gastroesophageal reflux in children. Results of Nissen's fundoplication in 100 children. Am J Dis Child 134:935–938

53. Levy MS, Sorrels CW, Wagner CW, Jackson RJ, Barnes RW, Smith SD (1999) Evolution of the modified Rossetti fundoplication in children: Surgical technique and results. Ann Surg 229(6):774–780

54. Lindahl H, Rintala R, Louhimo I (1989) Failure of Nissen fundoplication to control gastroesophageal reflux in esophageal atresia patients. J Pediatr Surg 24:985–987

55. Lortat-Jacob JL (1967) Resultats du traitement chirurgical du reflux gastroesophagien Congres Français de chirurgie infantile. Ann Chir Pediatr 4:345

56. Lundell L, Abrahamsson H, Ruth M, Rydberg L, Lönroth H, Olbe L (1996) Long-term results of a prospective randomized comparison of total fundic wrap (Nissen-Rossetti) or semifundoplication (Toupet) for gastroesophageal reflux. Br J Surg 83:830–835

57. Luostarinen MES (1993) Nissen fundoplication for reflux esophagitis. Long-term clinical and endoscopic results in 109 of 127 consecutive patients. Ann Surg 217:329–337

58. Luostarinen MES, Isolauri JO (1999) Randomized trial to study the effect of fundic mobilization on long-term results of Nissen fundoplication. Br J Surg 86:614–618

59. Luostarinen MES, Koskinen MO, Isolauri JO (1996) Effect of fundal mobilisation in Nissen-Rossetti fundoplication on oesophageal transit and dysphagia (a prospective, randomised trial). Eur J Surg 162:37–42

60. Maddern GJ, Jamieson GG, Chatterton BE, Collins PJ (1985) Is there an association between failed antireflux procedures and delayed gastric emptying? Ann Surg 202:162–165

61. Martinez DA, Ginn-Pease ME, Caniano DA (1992) Recognition of recurrent gastroesophageal reflux following antireflux surgery in the neurologically disabled child: high index of suspicion and definitive evaluation. J Pediatr Surg 27:983–990

62. Mattioli G, Repetto P, Leggio S et al (2002) Laparoscopic Nissen-Rossetti fundoplication in children. Semin Lap Surg 9:153–162

63. Maxson RT, Harp S, Jackson RJ, Smith SD, Wagner CW (1994) Delayed gastric emptying in neurologically impaired children with gastroesophageal reflux: the role of pyloroplasty. J Pediatr Surg 29:726–729

64. Mittal RK, Rochester RW (1987) Effect of the diaphragmatic contraction on lower esophageal sphincter pressure in man. Gut 28:1564–1568

65. Montedonico S, Diez-Prado JA, Tovar JA (1999) Gastroesophageal reflux after combined lower esophageal sphincter and diaphragmatic crura sling inactivation in the rat. Dig Dis Sci 44:2283–2289

66. Muratore CS, Utter S, Jakis T Lund DP, Wilson JM (2001) Nutritional morbidity in survivors of congenital diaphragmatic hernia. J Pediatr Surg 36:1171–1176

67. Negre JB (1983) Post-fundoplication symptoms. Do they restrict the success of Nissen fundoplication? Ann Surg 198:698–700

68. Negre JB, Markkula HT, Keyrilainen O, Matikainen (1983) Nissen fundoplication. Results at 10 year follow-up. Am J Surg 146:635–637

69. Nissen R (1956) Eine einfache Operation zur Beeinflussung der Reflux Oesophagitis. Schweiz Med Wochenschr 86:590–592

70. Nissen R, Rossetti M (1965) Surgery of hiatal and other diaphragmatic hernias. J Int Coll Surg 43:663–674

71. O'Neill JK, O'Neill JP, Goth-Owens T et al (1996) Care-giver evaluation of anti-gastroesophageal reflux procedure in neurologically impaired children: what is the real life outcome? J Pediatr Surg 31:375–380

72. Ostlie DJ, Miller KA, Holcomb III GW (2002) Effective Nissen fundoplication length and bougie diameter size in young children undergoing laparoscopic Nissen fundoplication. J Pediatr Surg 37:1664–1666

73. Patti JM, Arcerito M, Feo CV, De Pinto M, Tong J, Gantert W, Tyrell D, Way LW (1998) An analysis of operations for gastroesophageal reflux disease. Arch Surg 133:600–607

74. Patti MG, Albanese CT, Holcomb GW III et al (2001) Laparoscopic Heller myotomy and Dor fundoplication for esophageal achalasia in children. J Pediatr Surg 36:1248–1251

75. Pellegrini CA (2001) Delayed gastric emptying in patients with abnormal gastroesophageal reflux (editorial). Ann Surg 234:147–148

76. Pope CE (1992) The quality of life following antireflux surgery. World J Surg 16:355–358

77. Price MR, Janik JS, Wayne ER, Janik JE, Martinez LA, Burrington JD (1997) Modified Nissen fundoplication for reduction of fundoplication failure. J Pediatr Surg 32:324–326

78. Rice H, Seashore JH, Touloukian RJ (1991) Evaluation of Nissen fundoplication in neurologically impaired children. J Pediatr Surg 26:697–701

79. Robie DK, Pearl RH (1991) Modified Nissen fundoplication: improved results in high-risk children. J Pediatr Surg 11:1268–1272

80. Romeo C, Baldari S, Centorrino A et al (2000) Gastric motility disorders in patients operated on for esophageal atresia and tracheoesophageal fistula: long-term evaluation. J Pediatr Surg 35:740–744

81. Rossetti M (1968) Zur Technic der fundoplication. Aktuelle Chir 3:29–31

82. Rossetti M (1993) Una vita con ernie iatali e malatti da ra riflusso. Sintesi storica e attualità. Ann Ital Chir 64:249–254

83. Rossetti M, Hell K (1977) Fundoplication for the treatment of gastroesophageal reflux disease in hiatal hernia. World J Surg 1:439–443

84. Rossetti M, Hell K, Rothlisbergher PA (1976) La fundoplication, intervention de choix dans la maladie du reflux gastro-oesophagien. Praxis 65:799

85. Roy-Choudhurby S, Ashcraft KW (1998) Thal fundoplication for pediatric gastroesophageal reflux disease. Semin Pediatr Surg 7:115–120

86. Scharli AF (1985) To Nissen or not to Nissen. Prog Pediatr Surg 18:96–100

87. Siewert R, Feussner H (1989) Surgical considerations for antireflux therapy. Scand J Gastroenterol 24:50–59

88. Sigalet DL, Nguyen LT, Adolph V, Laberge JM, Hong AR, Guttman FM (1994) Gastroesophageal reflux associated with large diaphragmatic hernias. J Pediatr Surg 29:1262–1265

89. Smith CD, Othersen HB, Grogan NJ, Walker JD (1992) Nissen fundoplication in children with profound neurologic disability. High risks and unmet goals. Ann Surg 215:654–659

90. Snyder CL, Ramchandran V, Kennedy AP, Gittes GK, Ashcraft KW, Holder TM (1997) Efficacy of partial wrap fundoplication for gastroesophageal reflux after repair of esophageal atresia. J Pediatr Surg 32:1089–1091

91. Soave F (1967) Hernies hiatales de l'enfant. Physiopathologie. Ann Chir Infant 4:270–278

92. Spitz L, Kirtkane J (1985) Results and complications of surgery for gastro-oesophageal reflux. Arch Dis Child 60:743–747

93. Spitz L, Roth E, Kiely EM, Brereton RJ, Drake DP, Milla PJ (1993) Operation for gastroesophagal reflux associated with severe mental retardation. Arch Dis Child 68:347–351

94. Strecker-Mc Graw MK, Lorenz ML, Hendrickson M, Jolley SG, Tunell WP (1998) Persistent gastroesophageal reflux disease after antireflux surgery in children. 1. Immediate postoperative evaluation using extended esophageal pH monitoring. J Pediatr Surg 33:1623–1627

95. Subramaniam R Dikinson AP (2000) Long-term outcome of Boix-Ochoa and Nissen fundoplication in normal and neurologically impaired children. J Pediatr Surg 53:1214–1216

96. Thal AP (1968) A unified approach to surgical problems of the esophagogastric junction. Ann Surg 168:542–549

97. Thor KBA, Silander T (1989) A long-term randomized prospective trial of the Nissen procedure versus a modified Toupet technique. Ann Surg 210(6):719–724

98. Tolia V (2002) Gastroesophageal reflux and supraesophageal complications: really true or ballyhoo? J Pediatr Gastroenterol Nutr 34:269–273

99. Toupet A (1963) Technique d'oesophago-gastroplastie avec phrenogastropexie applique dans la cure radicale des hernies hiatales et comme complement de l'operation de heller dans le cardiospasmes. Mem Acad Chir 89:394–398

100. Tovar JA, Angulo JA, Gorostiaga L et al (1991) Surgery for gastroesophageal reflux in children with normal pH studies. J Pediatr Surg 26:541–545

101. Tovar JA, Diaz Pardo JA, Murcia JA et al (1995) Ambulatory 24-hours manometric and pH metric evidence of permanent impairment of clearance capacity in patients with esophageal atresia. J Pediatr Surg 30:1224–1231

102. Tovar JA, Olivares P, Diaz M et al (1998) Functional results of laparoscopic fundoplication in children. J Pediatr Gastroenterol Nutr 26:429–431

103. Turnage RH, Oldham KT, Coran AG, Blane CE (1989) Late results of fundoplication for gastroesophageal reflux in infants and children. Surgery 105:457–464

104. Van der Zee DC, Röverkamp MH, Pull ter Gunne AJ, Bax NMA (1994) Surgical treatment for reflux esophagitis: Nissen versus Thal procedure. Pediatr Surg Int 9:334–337

105. Watson Di, Jamieson GG, Devit PG et al (2001) A prospective randomised trial of laparoscopic Nissen fundoplication with anterior vs posterior hiatal repair. Arch Surg 136:745–751

106. Weber TR (1998) Toupet fundoplication for pediatric gastroesophageal reflux disease. Semin Pediatr Surg 7:121–124

107. Wheatley MJ, Coran AG Wesley JR (1993) Efficacy of Nissen fundoplication in the management of gastroesophageal reflux following esophageal atresia repair. J Pediatr Surg 28:53–55

Can Laparoscopy Be Considered the "Gold Standard" in the Management of Children with GERD?

23

Ciro Esposito · Steven Rothenberg · Philippe Montupet · Craig T. Albanese

Contents

23.1
Introduction

Laparoscopic antireflux surgery (LARS) in adults has seemingly replaced the open approach worldwide [6, 11, 12, 63]. Findings show it to be an established treatment option for chronic gastroesophageal reflux disease, with an excellent clinical outcome and success rates ranging between 90% and 100% [6].

Laparoscopic surgery for gastroesophageal reflux disease (GERD) was first reported in children in 1993 [37]. Laparoscopic surgery has recently become increasingly common, particularly in children, and is presently the third most common pediatric surgical procedure [55, 59]. Although the outcomes of LARS in the adult population have been published extensively, only recently have large studies in children also become available [1, 20, 42, 48, 54]. Although no randomized control trials in children exist to date, many retrospective studies have been published [19, 24, 25, 38].

In addition, in children the problem of the management of GERD is more complicated than in adults. In fact, almost 30–50% of the indications for surgery in children are presented by children with neurological impairment, whose management is extremely difficult and who represent a true challenge for the surgeon [22, 27, 31]. For this reason this aspect will be treated in different chapters.

In contrast, in terms of results, the management of neurologically normal children can be considered comparable to that of adults, with a success rate above 90% [17, 48, 55].

The aim of this article is to analyze the surgical literature to try to assess whether LARS may be considered the gold standard in the management of neurologically normal children with GERD. We analyzed the various aspects of the procedure on the basis of our experience and based on the findings reported in the international literature.

23.2
Surgical Considerations

During recent years, LARS has become the standard procedure in surgical centers worldwide for treating children with severe GERD. In fact with the laparoscopic approach to the treatment of GERD, there are a variety of technical advantages that are not possible with the open surgery procedure. With proper ergonomic positioning of the patient, utilizing in-line video monitoring and the use of an angled (e.g. 30°) telescope, precise dissection is facilitated due to enhanced visualization and magnification. This is perhaps the greatest advantage of this technique compared to open surgery. Additionally, with the use of gravity (e.g. the reversed Trendelenburg position), the bowel need not be manipulated, thus decreasing postoperative adhesions. This was clearly noted in children who underwent upper abdominal reoperation. Short (20-cm) instruments with a small diameter (3 mm) require smaller skin incisions and allow these procedures to be performed on neonates as small as 1–2 kg. This leads to smaller and less conspicuous scars, with obvious cosmetic and possible psychological benefits to the child and parents. Laparoscopic robotic surgery has also been proven possible and may provide additional advantages in the future [3, 46]. The summation of all of these technical advances allows laparoscopic fundoplication to be performed safely and effectively in the most difficult pediatric populations: children less than 5 kg, children with previous abdominal operations, children in the first year of life, and in disabled infants and children [21, 35, 36, 41]. Should the primary operation fail for any reason, reoperation may be readily performed laparoscopically.

23.3
The Surgeon's Experience

The surgeon's experience is a crucial factor in the success of the laparoscopic intervention, for two main reasons. First of all, each year in every country there is a limited number of children referred for a laparoscopic fundoplication, and therefore not all pediatric surgical units can develop adequate experience in the management of this pathology. For this reason in each country there are only a few centers with sound experience in this field.

The second reason is that the small abdominal region and decreased abdominal wall compliance may complicate the laparoscopic procedures in children. While the application of minimal access surgery was initially limited to small children with symptomatic GERD, size-appropriate instrumentation has allowed this procedure to be performed safely and effectively. However, the learning curve – particularly to perform intracorporeal sutures and tie knots within a small space – affects operating time, complications, and long-term outcome. In one center, a learning curve of 25 to 50 cases was needed to achieve efficient operating times (comparable to open surgery) and led to decreased intraoperative complications [7, 8, 15, 18]. Operative time in each case varied widely but usually decreased on average from 100–200 min in the first group of procedures to 45–100 min after experience aggregated. In the latter cases, there was a reduced number of complications, including conversions to open procedures, and decreased costs. It is difficult to actually assess the factor responsible for this improvement. In many cases, technical skill with the instruments, familiarity with the proper placement of trocars, optimized dissection, retraction, and knot-tying, and lastly the presence of a dedicated minimal-access operating-room team appeared to be vital components in this improvement.

23.4
Correct Indications for Surgery

It is important to underline the importance of a correct indication for surgery in children with GERD, in order to achieve good surgical results [17]. As a matter of fact, several papers report that in the majority of cases the failure of LARS is related to a wrong indication for surgery.

Indeed, an accurate pre-operative evaluation of the patient (pH-metry, endoscopy, barium swallow, manometry, and echographic control of gastric emptying) is extremely important; for instance, if a child has delayed gastric emptying after surgery, chances are the problem was already there before surgery, and this information is fundamental preoperatively to choose the surgical procedure to adopt [23, 26, 30].

The results of LARS depend also on the collaboration between pediatric gastroenterologists and pediatric surgeons; for this reason the indications for surgery must be decided together after an accurate analysis of a patient's data.

23.5
The Antireflux Procedure

Most authors generally agree that the results of laparoscopic antireflux procedures depend on the surgical experience with this pathology, and for this reason, since antireflux procedures are generally scheduled procedures, children with GERD should be referred only to centers with adequate experience in this field [9, 14, 45].

Moreover, every author prefers to adopt in laparoscopy the same technique adopted previously in open surgery (antireflux procedures are the same in both open surgery and laparoscopy; what changes is the way they are performed) [16, 28, 43, 62].

Regarding the surgical procedure to adopt, considering that laparoscopy is now considered the approach of choice to perform an antireflux procedure in children with GERD, three techniques seem to give comparable results, provided that they are performed by expert pediatric surgeons: Nissen's, Toupet's, and Thal's procedures [48, 55, 62]. However, a few centers perform other antireflux procedures such as Boix-Ochoa, Lortat-Jacob, or other techniques [40, 58].

Concerning neurologically impaired (NI) children with GERD, there is now strong debate among pediatric surgeons as to whether it is preferable to perform a jejunostomy or a gastrostomy alone, or an additional antireflux procedure, considering these patients' limited life expectancy [5, 22, 31, 32].

23.6
Hemodynamic and Respiratory Considerations

Some articles report that the increase in intraabdominal pressure during pneumoperitoneum can create hemodynamic instability during laparoscopy. Theoretically, gas insufflation at 8–12 mmHg pressure with positioning in steep reverse Trendelenburg and concomitant carbon dioxide resorption may lead to impaired ventilation. However, hypooxygenation and hypercarbia with resultant acidosis due to cephalad diaphragmatic displacement and decreased lung volumes has not been significant and may be reversed by increasing minute ventilation by 20–25% [56]. When studied postoperatively, laparoscopic fundoplication results in little to no physiologic alteration in respiration, and since no large painful upper abdominal incision is present, the approach translates to postoperative benefits. There is little postoperative atelectasis and pneumonia, findings which may be linked to increased vital and total lung capacity [55, 64]. Meehan reported a 1.8% rate of postoperative pneumonia in neurologically impaired children compared to a historical incidence of postoperative pneumonia after open surgery of 14–40% in a similar patient population [43–45].

23.7
Complications of LARS

Several reports have demonstrated that LARS can be performed safely and effectively in children with lower morbidity and fewer complications than typically seen with the traditional open approach. It seems that intraoperative complications during pediatric laparoscopic fundoplication occur in about 5% of cases [20]. Mortality is almost never reported and, when present, is a complication of an underlying disease. In a study on adults published in 1997, the rate of complications in one series of 2453 patients demonstrated viscus perforation in 1%, transfusion in 1%, pneumothorax in 2%, splenectomy in 0.1%, and conversion to open procedures in 6% [50]. Reoperation was rarely necessary and was due to persistent bleeding, missed perforation, crural disruption, or paraesophageal hernia. Death occurred in 0.2% of cases [27, 54]. Intraoperative complications in large series of children are just as infrequent.

Recent studies do show a trend toward increased complications in the open surgery group (25% vs. 10%) [29, 60, 64]. In these studies, the greatest benefit of laparoscopic fundoplication appears to be in lowered rates of wound complication that can occur in up to 20% of open procedures [13, 16]. The mechanism behind this may be linked to a transient suppression of cell-mediated immunity in open procedures compared to laparoscopic procedures, and the presence of a larger incision. Other complications more likely to be seen with open procedures include adhesive bowel obstruction and postoperative pulmonary impairment. Estimated blood loss appears to be significantly reduced in laparoscopic procedures.

Intraoperative complications that are more common and/or more difficult to manage in laparoscopic procedures include bowel/vessel injury during trocar insertion, pneumothorax from diaphragmatic injury, trocar site hernia, and bleeding [20, 49]. Many of these, if recognized, can be treated laparoscopically. Evidence suggests that the majority of complications in large series occur early in the surgeon's experience (first 50 cases) and thereafter are significantly reduced [45].

Conversions from laparoscopic to open cases are infrequent and decrease as experience improves. Rates vary from 0.9% to 7.5% due to a combination of equipment problems, inadequate visualization, and dense adhesions. Some series have reported 0% conversion rates [18, 44, 55]. Overall, conversions to open procedures in children can be expected in 2% of cases [27]. Two-thirds are due to technical reasons and one-third to complications.

23.8
Hospitalization

Probably the main advantages of LARS are the short hospital stay and, especially, the patient's attainment of a normal level of function. This has been evaluated in two different ways: patients who go home following their operation are evaluated simply according to the length of their hospital stay; those who have prolonged hospitalizations not related to their antireflux surgery are evaluated by time to full feeds [8, 10, 54]. Using either of these methods, there has been a significant decrease in length of stay with the minimal-access approach. Length of stay in children can be as low as 1–3 days in large series. This is of utmost importance, in terms of the considerable decrease in cost not only in terms of hospital charges but for the shorter work leave for the parents and days of school and regular activities missed for the children. Several factors may be responsible for this, among which is an earlier normalization of bowel function and decreased pain requiring less narcotic use.

Over 50% of children undergoing minimal-access procedures are feeding by postoperative day 1 and 85% by day 2 [4, 48, 51]. Patients are then kept on a soft diet for the first 15–30 days following surgery to avoid early complaints of dysphagia associated with postoperative edema [19]. Patients undergoing concomitant gastrostomy placement are usually kept in hospital a day longer because their feeds are not started until the first postoperative day [22, 44].

This normalization of function translates into improved quality of life and improved patient satisfaction, variables that have been well studied in adults. In followup questionnaires in adults, the laparoscopy group experienced an earlier return to "general health" and an earlier return to work. Another study showed significant improvements in disease-specific reflux symptom scores in both open and laparoscopic surgery, but laparoscopy was associated with better postoperative scores in terms of physical functioning.

23.9
Cost

There is the misconception that LARS is more expensive than open surgery. Historically, this was mostly related to the use of mechanically complex, fragile, and often expensive disposable instruments, retractors and trocars, as well as the longer operating time required for laparoscopic procedures. However, when considered within the setting of offset expenses by shorter hospitalization and faster return to function, the costs may in fact be reduced [2]. In addition, the routine use of reusable instruments and trocars and decreased operative times as experience increases will further increase savings [33, 53, 61]. Several studies performed in both adults and children have shown lower total hospital costs for laparoscopic fundoplication compared to open surgery. In some instances, cost savings in adults ranged from $1276 to $6721, all in favor of laparoscopy, with none of these studies taking into account productivity gain from an earlier return to work [2, 33, 39]. In a randomized control trial in adults, laparoscopic and open fundoplication showed similar hospital costs, but total costs were lower ($7506 versus $13,118) in the laparos-

copic group as a result of an earlier return to work [33, 39, 47]. Luks et al. compared 16 laparoscopic and 18 open fundoplications in a series of children and found excess operating costs equal to $634 for the laparoscopic group, but a shorter hospital stay that resulted in an overall savings of $5390 for the laparoscopic group [39].

23.10
Long-Term Outcome

Several short- and midterm studies were recently published reporting good to excellent results after LARS, with healing rates from of 90% to 100% [34, 61]. Failure rates for adults undergoing fundoplication, in terms of persistent or recurrent symptoms, are approximately 1% per year with both techniques [6, 52].

In children, the recurrence rates with open procedures are well known. These are somewhat increased compared to the adult population, since neurologically impaired children comprise a large percentage of operated patients and experience a higher percentage of recurrence. The largest experience to date with over 7400 cases noted a recurrence rate of 7.1% [24, 25]. When stratified, this rate was 5% in normal and 15% in neurologically impaired children [20, 44]. Higher rates of recurrence have also been seen in children with chronic lung disease, in children less than 3 months old [4], and in series with smaller numbers of patients. In the latter studies, this number was sometimes as high as 19% [32]. The failure rate with laparoscopy varies but can be

Table 1. Large studies of LARS in children (>50 patients)

Author (year)	Number of patients	Conversion rate	Complication rate	Rate of recurrent GERD	Comment
Steyaert (2003)	53	3.7%	NA	6.6%	Long-term followup (4.5 years)
Van der Zee (2002)	157	NA	NA	19.4%	48% neurologically impaired children
Mattioli (2002)	288	NA	1.4%	3.2%	Multicenter study
Montupet (2001)	284	NA	1%	2%	Four-trocar technique
Allal (2001)	142	2.1%	Intraoperative 0.5%, postoperative 2%	NA	91% good results (no symptoms)
Iglesias (2001)	104	1%	11.5%	2.9%	Multicenter series in infants <3 months of age
Esposito (2000)	289	1.3%	Intraoperative 5.1%, postoperative 3.4%	2.1%	Detailed analysis of complications following laparoscopic intervention
Georgeson (1998)	389	3.3%	NA	5%	Two deaths in this large series, one related to operative complication
Rothenberg (1998)	220	1%	Intraoperative 2.6%, postoperative 7.3%	3.4%	Good demonstration of steep learning curve
Meehan (1996)	160	7.5%	7.4%	1.4%	1 death due to error in gastrostomy placement

NA, not available; GERD, gastroesophageal reflux disease

as low as 2–14% when evaluated from a physiological point of view [61]. The largest series in pediatric literature demonstrate wrap failure rates of 2–5%, a number lower than that reported for traditional open fundoplication [1, 20].

23.11
Conclusion

The past 10 years have witnessed a significant change in the role of surgery for GERD in children, thanks to the advent of LARS. In fact, antireflux surgery was initially reserved only for patients who had failed every kind of medical therapy. Currently LARS is a common and regular part of the treatment algorithm. In recent years the indications for LARS in children have steadily increased, always respecting a correct indication for surgery . Our analysis of pediatric cases has shown that after LARS the complication rate is lower, the recovery period is quicker, and the failure rate appears to be lower than for open fundoplication. Although the learning curve is steep because of the advanced laparoscopic skills needed, the procedure can be performed quickly and effectively once the technique is mastered. The dramatic decrease in hospital stay appears to result in overall cost reduction. We have summarized in Table 1 the results of some of larger studies published in recent years on the application of LARS in children with GERD. Analyzing these data we have identified only two criticisms concerning the role of LARS in children with GERD: the first one is that no randomized controlled trials are available in children, and the second point is that the management of neurologically impaired children with GERD remains unclear considering the several pathologies that affect these patients.

The role of LARS in neurologically normal children, in contrast, is extremely clear. In fact, on the basis of our analysis and of the data of the international literature, LARS can be considered the "gold standard" in children with GERD when medical therapy fails. However two crucial points must be respected to obtain excellent results with LARS: a correct indication for surgery, and sound experience of the operative team with laparoscopic procedures.

The results of LARS depend also on the collaboration of pediatric gastroenterologists and surgeons, who should work together to provide the most appropriate and correct treatment for children with GERD.

References

1. Allal H, Captier G, Lopez M, et al (2001) Evaluation of 142 consecutive laparoscopic fundoplications in children: effects of the learning curve and technical choice. J Pediatr Surg 36: 921–926

2. Blewett CJ, Hollenbeak CS, Cilley RE, et al (2002) Economic implications of current surgical management of gastroesophageal reflux disease. J Pediatr Surg 37:427–430

3. Cadiere GB, Himpens J, Vertruyen M, et al (2001) Evaluation of telesurgical (robotic) Nissen fundoplication. Surg Endosc 15: 918–923

4. Campos GM, Peters JH, DeMeester TR, et al (1999) Multivariate analysis of factors predicting outcome after laparoscopic Nissen fundoplication. J Gastrointest Surg 3:292–300

5. Caniano DA, Ginn-Pease ME, King DR (1990) The failed antireflux procedure: analysis of risk factors and morbidity. J Pediatr Surg 25:1022–1026

6. Champault GG, Barrat C, Rozon RC, et al (1999) The effect of the learning curve on the outcome of laparoscopic treatment for gastroesophageal reflux. Surg Laparosc Endosc Percutan Tech 9:375–381

7. Chen MK, Schropp KP, Lobe TE (1996) Complications of minimal-access surgery in children. J Pediatr Surg 31:1161–1165

8. Collins JB, III, Georgeson KE, Vicente Y, et al (1995) Comparison of open and laparoscopic gastrostomy and fundoplication in 120 patients. J Pediatr Surg 30:1065–1071

9. Coster DD, Bower WH, Wilson VT, et al (1995) Laparoscopic Nissen fundoplication–a curative, safe, and cost-effective procedure for complicated gastroesophageal reflux disease. Surg Laparosc Endosc 5:111–117

10. Cunniffe MG, McAnena OJ, Dar MA, et al (1998) A prospective randomized trial of intraoperative bupivacaine irrigation for management of shoulder-tip pain following laparoscopy. Am J Surg 176:258–261

11. Dallemagne B, Weerts JM, Jehaes C, et al (1991) Laparoscopic Nissen fundoplication: preliminary report. Surg Laparosc Endosc 1:138–143

12. DeMeester TR, Bonavina L, Albertucci M (1986) Nissen fundoplication for gastroesophageal reflux disease. Evaluation of primary repair in 100 consecutive patients. Ann Surg 204:9–20

13. Dick AC, Coulter P, Hainsworth AM, et al (1998) A comparative study of the analgesia requirements following laparoscopic and open fundoplication in children. J Laparoendosc Adv Surg Tech A 8:425–429

14. Dick AC, Potts SR (1999) Laparoscopic fundoplication in children–an audit of fifty cases. Eur J Pediatr Surg 9:286–288

15. Di Lorenzo C, Orenstein S (2002) Fundoplication: friend or foe? J Pediatr Gastroenterol Nutr 34:117–124

16. Eshraghi N, Farahmand M, Soot SJ, et al (1998) Comparison of outcomes of open versus laparoscopic Nissen fundoplication performed in a single practice. Am J Surg 175:371–374

17. Esposito C (2003) Fundoplication: certainly a friend for children with GERD if the indication for surgery is correct. J Pediatr Gastroenterol Nutr 7:118–119

18. Esposito C, Ascione G, Garipoli V, et al (1997) Complications of pediatric laparoscopic surgery. Surg Endosc 11:655–657

19. Esposito C, Garipoli V, De Pasquale M, et al (1997) Laparoscopic versus traditional fundoplication in the treatment of children with refractory gastro-oesophageal reflux. Ital J Gastroenterol Hepatol 29:399–402

20. Esposito C, Montupet P, Amici G, et al (2000) Complications of laparoscopic antireflux surgery in childhood. Surg Endosc 14: 622–624

21. Esposito C, Montupet P, Reinberg O (2001) Laparoscopic surgery for gastroesophageal reflux disease during the first year of life. J Pediatr Surg 36:715–717

22. Esposito C, Van Der Zee DC, Settimi A, Doldo P, Staiano A, Bax NM. (2003) Risks and benefits of surgical management of gastroesophageal reflux in neurologically impaired children. Surg Endosc 17:708–710

23. Fonkalsrud EW, Ament ME (1996) Gastroesophageal reflux in childhood. Curr Probl Surg 33:1–70

24. Fonkalsrud EW, Ashcraft KW, Coran AG, et al (1998) Surgical treatment of gastroesophageal reflux in children: a combined hospital study of 7467 patients. Pediatrics 101:419–422

25. Fonkalsrud EW, Bustorff-Silva J, Perez CA, et al (1999) Antireflux surgery in children under 3 months of age. J Pediatr Surg 34:527–531

26. Fung KP, Seagram G, Pasieka J, et al (1990) Investigation and outcome of 121 infants and children requiring Nissen fundoplication for the management of gastroesophageal reflux. Clin Invest Med 13:237–246

27. Georgeson KE (1998) Laparoscopic fundoplication and gastrostomy. Semin Laparosc Surg 5:25–30

28. Heikkinen TJ, Haukipuro K, Bringman S, et al (2000) Comparison of laparoscopic and open Nissen fundoplication 2 years after operation. A prospective randomized trial. Surg Endosc 14:1019–1023

29. Heikkinen TJ, Haukipuro K, Koivukangas P, et al (1999) Comparison of costs between laparoscopic and open Nissen fundoplication: a prospective randomized study with a 3-month followup. J Am Coll Surg 188:368–376

30. Hopkins MA, Stringel G (1999) Laparoscopic Nissen fundoplication in children: a single surgeon's experience. JSLS 3:261–266

31. Humphrey GM, Najmaldin AS (1996) Laparoscopic Nissen fundoplication in disabled infants and children. J Pediatr Surg 31:596–599

32. Iglesias JL, Kogut K, Owings E, et al (2001) Safety and efficacy of laparoscopic Nissen fundoplication in early infancy. Ped Endosurg Innov Tech 5:379–384

33. Incarbone R, Peters JH, Heimbucher J, et al (1995) A contemporaneous comparison of hospital charges for laparoscopic and open Nissen fundoplication. Surg Endosc 9:151–155

34. Kawahara H, Imura K, Nakajima K, et al (2000) Motor function of the esophagus and the lower esophageal sphincter in children who undergo laparoscopic Nissen fundoplication. J Pediatr Surg 35:1666–1671

35. Kawahara H, Imura K, Yagi M, et al (1998) Mechanisms underlying the antireflux effect of Nissen fundoplication in children. J Pediatr Surg 33:1618–1622

36. Liu DC, Flattmann GJ, Karam MT, et al (2000) Laparoscopic fundoplication in children with previous abdominal surgery. J Pediatr Surg 35:334–337

37. Lobe TE, Schropp KP, Lunsford K (1993) Laparoscopic Nissen fundoplication in childhood. J Pediatr Surg 28:358–361

38. Longis B, Grousseau D, Alain JL, et al (1996) Laparoscopic fundoplication in children: our first 30 cases. J Laparoendosc Surg 6 (Suppl):S21–29

39. Luks FI, Logan J, Breuer CK, et al (1999) Cost-effectiveness of laparoscopy in children. Arch Pediatr Adolesc Med 153:965–968

40. Martinez DA, Ginn-Pease ME, Caniano DA (1992) Recognition of recurrent gastroesophageal reflux following antireflux surgery in the neurologically disabled child: high index of suspicion and definitive evaluation. J Pediatr Surg 27:983–990

41. Martinez DA, Ginn-Pease ME, Caniano DA (1992) Sequelae of antireflux surgery in profoundly disabled children. J Pediatr Surg 27:267–273

42. Mattioli G, Esposito C, Lima M, Garzi A, Montinaro L, Cobellis G, Mastoianni L, Aceti MG, Falchetti D, Repetto P, Pini Prato A, Leggio S, Torri F, Ruggeri G, Settimi A, Messina M, Martino A, Amici G, Riccipetitoni G, Jasonni V (2002) Italian multicenter survey on laparoscopic treatment of gastro-esophageal reflux disease in children. Surg Endosc. 16:1666–1668

43. Meehan JJ, Georgeson KE (1996) Laparoscopic fundoplication in infants and children. Surg Endosc 10:1154–1157

44. Meehan JJ, Georgeson KE (1997) Laparoscopic fundoplication yields low postoperative pulmonary complications in neurologically impaired children. Ped Endosurg Innov Tech 1:11–14

45. Meehan JJ, Georgeson KE (1997) The learning curve associated with laparoscopic antireflux surgery in infants and children. J Pediatr Surg 32:426–429

46. Meininger DD, Byhahn C, Heller K, et al (2001) Totally endoscopic Nissen fundoplication with a robotic system in a child. Surg Endosc 15:1360

47. Mendoza-Sagaon M, Hanly EJ, Talamini MA, et al (2000) Comparison of the stress response after laparoscopic and open cholecystectomy. Surg Endosc 14:1136–1141

48. Montupet P, Mendoza-Sagaon M, De Dreuzy O, et al (2001) Laparoscopic Toupet fundoplication in children. Ped Endosurg Innov Tech 5:305–308

49. Pearl RH, Robie DK, Ein SH, et al (1990) Complications of gastroesophageal antireflux surgery in neurologically impaired versus neurologically normal children. J Pediatr Surg 25:1169–1173

50. Perdikis G, Hinder RA, Lund RJ, et al (1997) Laparoscopic Nissen fundoplication: where do we stand? Surg Laparosc Endosc 7:17–21

51. Peters JH, Heimbucher J, Kauer WK, et al (1995) Clinical and physiologic comparison of laparoscopic and open Nissen fundoplication. J Am Coll Surg 180:385–393

52. Rattner DW, Brooks DC (1995) Patient satisfaction following laparoscopic and open antireflux surgery. Arch Surg 130:289–294

53. Richards KF, Fisher KS, Flores JH, et al (1996) Laparoscopic Nissen fundoplication: cost, morbidity, and outcome compared with open surgery. Surg Laparosc Endosc 6:140–143

54. Rothenberg SS, Chang J (1997) Experience with advanced endosurgical procedures in neonates and infants. Ped Endosurg Innov Tech 1:107–110

55. Rothenberg SS (1998) Experience with 220 consecutive laparoscopic Nissen fundoplications in infants and children. J Pediatr Surg 33:274–278

56. Rowney DA, Aldridge LM (2000) Laparoscopic fundoplication in children: anaesthetic experience of 51 cases. Paediatr Anaesth 10:291–296

57. Smith CD, Othersen HB, Jr., Gogan NJ, et al (1992) Nissen fundoplication in children with profound neurologic disability. High risks and unmet goals. Ann Surg 215:654–659

58. Steyaert H, Al Mohaidly M, Lembo MA, Carfagna L, Tursini S, Valla JS (2003) Long-term outcome of laparoscopic Nissen and Toupet fundoplication in normal and neurologically impaired children. Surg Endosc 17(4):543–546

59. Sydorak RM, Albanese CT (2002) Laparoscopic antireflux procedures in children: evaluating the evidence. Semin Laparosc Surg 9(3):133–138

60. Taylor LA, Weiner T, Lacey SR, et al (1994) Chronic lung disease is the leading risk factor correlating with the failure (wrap disruption) of antireflux procedures in children. J Pediatr Surg 29:161–166

61. Tovar JA, Olivares P, Diaz M, et al (1998) Functional results of laparoscopic fundoplication in children. J Pediatr Gastroenterol Nutr 26:429–431

62. Van der Zee DC, Bax NMA, Ure MGH (2002) Long-term results after laparoscopic Thal procedure in children Semin Laparosc Surg 9(3):143–146

63. Velanovich V (1999) Comparison of symptomatic and quality of life outcomes of laparoscopic versus open antireflux surgery. Surgery 126:782–789

64. Viljakka MT, Luostarinen ME, Isolauri JO (1997) Complications of open and laparoscopic antireflux surgery: 32-year audit at a teaching hospital. J Am Coll Surg 185:446–450

Chapter 24

Nissen's Procedure

24

Steven Rothenberg

Contents

24.1
Introduction

Esophageal-gastric fundoplication is one of the most common procedures performed by pediatrics surgeons today [1–3]. A recent report of over 7000 cases from seven major U.S. institutions concluded that fundoplication was a safe and effective procedure in the pediatric population [4], but failed to make any mention of a laparoscopic approach. The type of fundoplication varies by physician preference, but most agree that a Nissen fundoplication, a full 360° wrap, is the most competent of the antireflux procedures. The Nissen fundoplication was first described in 1959 and has been one of the standards for antireflux surgery for the last 40 years. The choice of which procedure to perform therefore often lies with the surgeon's experience, perceived technical difficulties, and the incidence of postoperative complications including dysphagia and gas bloat. However, the incidence and severity of these complications is directly related to formation of the wrap, and a new understanding of the anatomy of the fundoplication and new laparoscopic techniques may be changing previous biases.

Indications for antireflux procedures in children include respiratory compromise, neurologic impairment, failure to thrive, and esophagitis and stricture formation. An increasing incidence of Barrett's esophagitis is also being documented in children. Another common association has been with the placement of a gastrostomy tube for feeding and a significantly increased risk of gastroesophageal reflux (GER). Ten to fifty percent of these patients will eventually require fundoplications.

Recent studies have also indicated that GER may have a more important role in respiratory problems including the development of apnea and bradycardia, sudden death spells, recurrent lung infections, and even reactive airway disease. All of the factors have resulted in a large increase in the number of fundoplications being performed [5–8].

The choice of fundoplications performed has varied greatly with surgeon preference, but the most common procedure performed in children is a Nissen fundoplication. In general, most surgeons agree that a Nissen (360°) wrap is the most effective antireflux valve. However, some feel that the complete wrap is associated with a higher incidence of dysphagia, gas bloat, and retching. Newer studies suggest that these symptoms may be diminished by paying careful attention to the geometry of the wrap, limiting the length of the fundoplication (2 cm), and ensuring that the wrap is loose. This is generally referred to as a short, floppy fundoplication.

Nissen fundoplications have routinely been performed through large upper abdominal incisions and required an extensive hospital stay and recovery period. These procedures were associated with a relatively high complication rate, especially postoperative pulmonary complications, wound infections, wrap failure, hiatal hernia development, and bowel obstruction. The laparoscopic approach appears to have changed this.

Numerous current reports in the adult surgical literature have shown that laparoscopic fundoplications can be performed safely with lower morbidity, shortened hospital stays, and recurrence rates at 5-year follow-up better than that achieved with traditional open surgery [9, 10] . Initial reports by pediatric surgeons have also shown that laparoscopic fundoplications can be performed safely and effectively in the smallest neonate as well as larger infants and children [11, 12].

4.2
Preoperative Work-up

As with any disease process, a thorough history and physical is the essential initial stage of any work-up for gastroesophageal reflux disease (GERD). After that a number of different tests can be extremely useful. Most children should have a barium swallow. This is not so much to demonstrate reflux as to look for an anatomic abnormality. Because it is a single point in time study, the presence or absence of reflux during the study does not quantify the degree of the problem. This study is necessary in children to rule out mechanical causes of reflux such as a gastric outlet obstruction from pyloric stenosis, a duodenal web, or malrotation. If gross reflux is seen to the thoracic inlet in a child with recurrent aspiration, then no other studies may be necessary.

The most helpful test is a 24-h pH probe study. This test not only quantifies the incidence and degree of reflux but may also show a correlation with symptoms of apnea, cough, wheezing, or discomfort. It measures the total length of acid reflux (pH<4) as well as the number and duration of episodes. This test gives the surgeon the best evidence of the magnitude of the problem and is very helpful in determining when surgical intervention is appropriate. The only disadvantage of this study is that it does not measure nonacid reflux events, which may play a significant role in some of the symptoms in patients with significant GERD. A new probe which measures impedance rather then changes in pH may provide a new way to evaluate these patients, especially those with a significant reactive airway component.

Gastric emptying studies are another test that many surgeons feel is important, but may be of little true value in the patient with significant GER. A radionuclide-labeled Tc sulfur colloid is used to quantitatively assess gastric emptying. It measures the time at which the isotope leaves the stomach. Approximately half of the isotope should be expected to have left the stomach at 60 min. Many have advocated that a gastric outlet procedure be performed if significantly delayed gastric emptying is present, but more recent data suggests that this may not be true. A recent report by Johnson et al. showed that preoperative studies showing delayed gastric emptying do not correlate with postfundoplication studies. In other words, postfundoplication emptying cannot be determined based on a preoperative study. This was further documented by Farrell et al., who showed that a Nissen fundoplication actually improves gastric motility in patients with delayed gastric emptying [13]. These findings would suggest that it may be better to evaluate gastric emptying only in those patients who appear to have problems following fundoplication.

Esophagoscopy is becoming more widely used preoperatively to assess the extent and degree of esophageal inflammation. This information helps the surgeon determine the severity of the disease and the effectiveness of medical therapy. Esophagoscopy may also help in the diagnosis of hiatal hernia and Barrett's esophagus, both of which should be considered absolute indications for surgical intervention.

24.3
Surgical Technique

Depending on the size of the child, the patient is supine or in a modified dorsal lithotomy position at the end of the table. The surgeon stands at the foot of the table at the infant's feet or between the legs in a larger child. The monitor should be placed over the child's chest if possible to allow for the best ergonomic set-up for the procedure (Fig. 1). The assistant is on the surgeon's left and controls the camera and the stomach retractor. A five-trocar technique is routinely used. Trocars are placed in the umbilicus (camera port), the right and left mid-quadrants (the working ports), the right upper-quadrant (liver retractor), and the left upper quadrant (stomach retractor and gastrostomy tube site) (Fig. 2). The abdomen is insufflated through the infra-umbilical ring incision using a veres needle and a closed technique. If there was a previous incision in this area, an alternate site is used to avoid adhesions. Insufflation pressures between 10 and 15 mmHg are used depending on the size and respiratory status of the patient. Oxygen saturation and end tidal CO_2 should be monitored in each case.

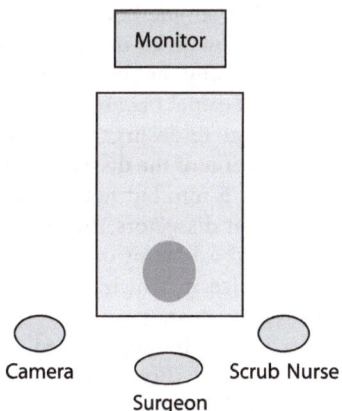

Fig. 1. Room set-up and patient positioning for a Nissen fundoplication

Trocar Placement

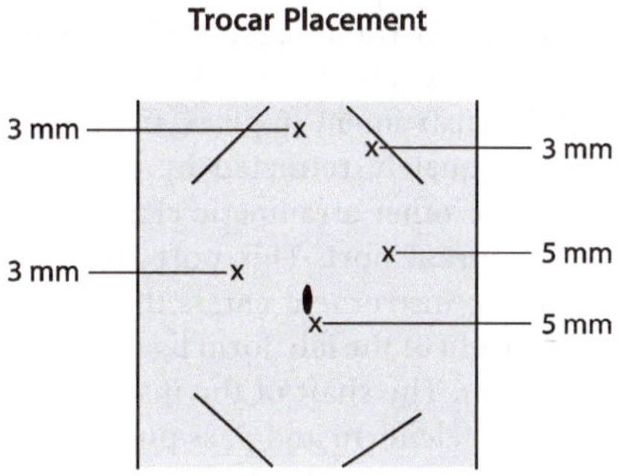

Fig. 2. Trocar placement for a fundoplication in a child

Selection of instruments and trocar size is also dependent on the size of the child. In general for infants and children less then 10 kg, 3-mm instruments of 18-to 20-cm length are appropriate. These shorter, smaller instruments are much more ergonomic and greatly facilitate the procedure. For children over 10 kg, standard-length 3- or 5-mm instruments are appropriate. The choice of endoscopes also varies based on patient size. For larger children, standard-length 5-mm 30° scopes are used. For smaller infants, short (20-cm) wide-angle 4-mm and 2.7-mm scopes work well. The new optics, imaging systems, and digital cameras now available make the visualization with these smaller scopes comparable to that previously only obtained with a 5- or 10-mm lens. A 30° angled scope is preferentially used, as it greatly enhance the surgeon's ability to view the area of the hiatus, upper short gastric vessels, and the retro-esophageal space. It also limits instrument dueling, as it allows the surgeon to place the telescope above the shafts of the right and left working ports and enables the surgeon to look down on his working tips.

The choice of energy source used is surgeon-dependent. In small infants and children, monopolar cautery is usually sufficient to perform the needed dissection as well as divide the short gastric vessels. This can be achieved either with a simple hook or the tips of the scissors. In larger patients with more fat in the greater omentum and surrounding the short gastric vessels, the use of the Harmonic Scalpel Laparoscopic Coagulating Shears (LCS) (Ethicon Endosurgery, Cincinnati, OH) greatly eases this portion of the dissection. This instrument is available in a 5-mm but not 3-mm size. Other options include bipolar dissectors, the Ligasure (Valleylab, Boulder, CO), and a host of other sealer/dividers. Limitations are the size in which each instrument is available and its relative cost.

The operation should be approached in the same fashion in each case, as the success of the procedure depends on meticulous dissection and creating the correct geometry of the wrap. The left lobe of the liver is retracted superiorly to expose the G-E junction. This was initially accomplished by the use of a fan retractor through a right lateral port. The problem was that the fan often caused liver trauma, especially in smaller patients, and that it required someone or a mechanical arm to hold the instrument in place. In most cases the liver can be adequately retracted by using a locking Babcock clamp or other atraumatic clamp through the right upper quadrant port. This port should be positioned so that the instrument enters the abdomen just to the patient's right of the falciform ligament just below the tip of the liver. The shaft of the instrument is then used to hook the falciform and pass under the left lobe of the liver up towards the diaphragm. This aids in elevating the left lobe. The diaphragm is then grasped above the esophageal hiatus, thus allowing the shaft of

the instrument to act as a self-retaining retractor. Alternatively a snake or fan retractor can be used and attached to a self-retaining arm.

A second Babcock or atraumatic clamp is placed through the left upper quadrant port to retract the stomach as necessary. When working at the hiatus, the stomach is retracted inferiorly and laterally to help expose the esophagus. While mobilizing the short gastric vessels, the stomach is grasped near the greater curve and retracted medially to better expose the vessels for ligation. Ideally the surgeon's right hand operating port is placed directly below the upper port so that there is no instrument dueling. The procedure is started by dividing the gastrohepatic ligament. The hepatic branches of the vagus nerve may be taken without untoward effects. In about 25% of cases, an aberrant left hepatic artery arises off the left gastric artery and is present and should be left intact. Dissection is started here because it is an avascular plain and allows the surgeon to get oriented and test the chosen energy source. The peritoneum overlying the right and left crus is cleared to allow for adequate mobilization of the intra-abdominal esophagus. The stomach is then retracted medially, and the upper short gastric vessels and posterior attachments of the stomach are divided. This allows clear delineation of the left crus and makes development of the retro-esophageal window much safer. Division of the short gastrics also ensures the formation of a tension-free wrap. It is true that the wrap can be constructed in most cases without the division of the short gastrics (Nissen-Rosetti), but it is very difficult to ensure the correct geometry of the wrap without it.

A retro-esophageal window is then developed from the patient's right side, taking care not to injure the posterior vagus nerve. Dissection should proceed along the right crus, not the esophagus. This combined with the previous mobilization of the left crus helps prevent injury to the back wall of the esophagus and stomach. Mobilization of a good length of intra-abdominal esophagus (4 to 6 cm depending on the size of the child) is critical to ensure the formation of an adequate wrap. Once the esophageal mobilization is complete, the clamp in the left upper quadrant port is placed behind the esophagus and used to expose the esophageal hiatus. At least one crural stitch should be placed in all cases using a strong nonabsorbable suture, even if the hiatus looks to be of normal size (Fig. 3). It is important not to strip the peritoneal lining off the crural fibers, as this will weaken the repair. Routine closure of the crus will help prevent development of a hiatal hernia, one of the most common complications following a Nissen.

The mobilized portion of the posterior fundus is then brought around behind the esophagus to form a 360° wrap. The anterior wall of the fundus is brought anterior to the esophagus to complete the fundal wrap. The geometry of the fundoplication is extremely impor-

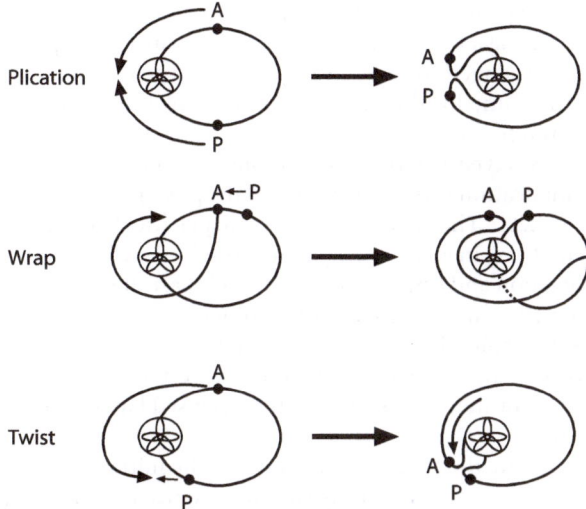

Fig. 3. Schematic drawing representing the desired geometry of the fundoplication (from Peters et al 1995)

tant in creating a tension-free wrap which does not twist or torque the stomach or esophagus (Fig. 4). The idea is basically to plicate the esophagus with the stomach. The wrap should be formed around an intraesophageal stent, the size of which is dependent on the size of the patient. The wraps is made 2–3 cm in length and consists of three to four sutures going from stomach, to anterior wall of the esophagus, to the wrapped portion of the stomach (Fig. 4). It is important to include the esophagus in each suture in order to prevent a slipped Nissen. The top stitch may also include the anterior diaphragmatic rim, a step which may aid in preventing the wrap from herniating up into the mediastinum. A properly positioned wrap should be sutured at approximately at the 10:00 to 11:00 position on the esophagus (just to

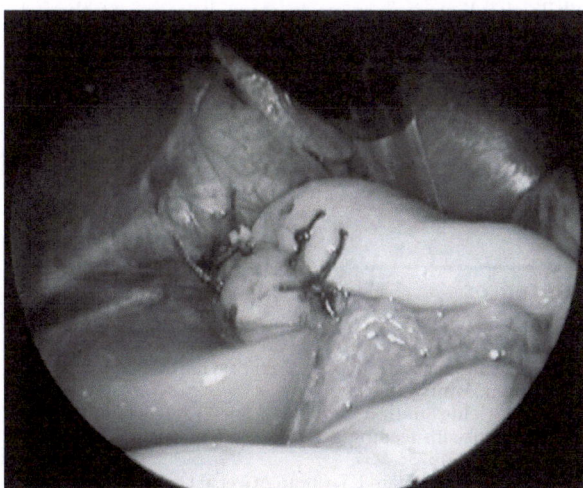

Fig. 4. The completed fundoplication

the surgeon's left of midline). Additional stitches (collar stitches) may be placed between the wrap and the right and left crus to help secure the wrap in the abdomen. Previous reports with open fundoplications suggest this may help prevent the occurrence of hiatal hernia formation, especially in the neurologically impaired. A gastrostomy tube may also be placed if needed, utilizing the left upper quadrant port. Gastrostomy tubes should not be placed unless they are needed for feeding; it is not necessary to place one simply to vent the stomach. In general it is not necessary to leave a nasogastric tube in postoperatively, and the majority of patients can be started on liquids just a few hours after surgery. Most patients can be discharged from the hospital in under 24 h.

24.4
Discussion

Fundoplications for GER continue to be one of the most commonly performed operations in the United States in the pediatric population. A recent report by Fonkalsrud et al. of over 7,000 fundoplications performed via laparotomy at seven major children's hospitals in the U.S. has shown this operation to be safe and effective in treating medically refractory or life-threatening GERD in infants and children. They reported a wrap disruption rate of 7.1% and a respiratory complication rate of 4.4%, figures that are better than most of the large series previously reported. Unfortunately it is often necessary to do these procedures in patients with significant neurologic or respiratory compromise, and major complications occurred in nearly 13% of this group of patients in their study. Others have also demonstrated a relatively high surgical morbidity in this group of patients [14, 15]. Peters, Hunter, and others have demonstrated that laparoscopic fundoplications (LFs) can be safely and effectively performed in adults with relatively little morbidity, significantly decreased hospital stay, and good clinical control of the patients' reflux symptoms [16, 17]. They also recently reported follow-up data with LF failure rates of between 2% and 8%, a rate favorable to that of open fundoplications.

There have now also been a number of initial reports from pediatric centers confirming the feasibility and efficacy of performing LF in the pediatric population [18]. Georgeson et al., with one of the largest series reported in pediatric patients, compared the operative time, complication rate, and hospital stay between a laparoscopic group and a retrospective control group who had undergone an open fundoplication (OF) and/or gastrostomy tube placement. He found a slightly lower complication rate and a significant decrease in hospitalization in the LF group compared to the OF group. More recently this group reported on a larger series of 390 fundoplications, 55% of which were Toupet procedures and the rest Nissen fundoplication. In looking at postoperative complications, the authors found that the rate of recurrent reflux in the Toupet group was twice that of the Nissen fundoplication group, and the rate of re-operation was three times that of the Nissen group[19]. More surprisingly, they found the incidence of postoperative dysphagia was over twice that of the Nissen group.

The single largest series of Nissen fundoplications in children to date was reported by us in 1998 [18]. Our initial report of a series of just over 200 LFs also showed promising early results with significantly decreased morbidity and hospital stays, but long-term follow-up was relatively limited. However a similar low dysphagia rate of less then 1.5% was documented. It is likely that the lack of this complication, which is thought to be the Achilles heel of the Nissen wrap, is because of the dedication by the authors to the geometry of the wrap, and the formation of a loose floppy Nissen. While a great deal of debate remains about the cause of dysphagia, most authors agree that a short floppy Nissen fundoplication is one of the keys to eliminating this complication. The previously discussed anatomy of the wrap would seem to be best achieved after complete fundal mobilization, which requires division of the short gastric vessels and posterior attachments. However even this point is debatable, as a number of authors have reported a low incidence of dysphagia while performing the Nissen without division of the short gastric vessels [20]. What is clear is that the retro-esophageal dissection and mobilization is much easier and safer if the left crus and fundus have been mobilized prior to performing this part of the operation.

There is now significant experience with the Nissen procedure in infants under 5 kg, documenting the safety and efficacy of the Nissen in this age group [21, 22]. Because of the minimal morbidity associated with the procedure including low rates of dysphagia, the procedure is being sought out earlier to prevent the long- and short-term complications of significant reflux. Early intervention in this age group may prevent many of the chronic respiratory problems and nutritional issues experienced by many of these infants.

24.5
The Author's Experience

Between 1992 and 2003 I performed over 1000 laparoscopic Nissen fundoplications. The most common indications were for medically refractory GERD (43%), significant failure to thrive (28%), and severe respiratory compromise or reactive airway disease (22%). Six percent of the procedures were redo fundoplications of failed previous open and laparoscopic procedures. Pa-

tient weights ranged from 1.2 kg to 120 kg and ages from 5 days to 18 years. The operative time for the procedure ranged from 20 to 240 minutes. The average operative time for the first 30 cases was 109 min, and was 38 min for the last 30. Thirty-eight percent of patients also received gastrostomy buttons. The intraoperative complication rate was 0.32%, and the postoperative rate was 4.2%. The incidence of dysphagia was 0.8%, and symptoms in all of these patients resolved with a single dilatation and time. There was a single case of postoperative pneumonia and almost no other respiratory problems, despite the significant respiratory compromise of many of the patients. The wrap failure rate was 2.8%, and all of these patients have been revised laparoscopically.

Despite the favorable outcomes of the initial reports, there has been a relatively slow acceptance and significant criticism of use of the LF in the pediatric population. Part of this resistance has been secondary to the advanced laparoscopic skills required to perform fundoplications. However as therapeutic pediatric laparoscopic procedures become more common and as more pediatric surgical trainees enter their fellowship with significant laparoscopic experience, this has become less of a barrier.

The other major limiting factor has been the belief that a fundoplication performed laparoscopically would not be as good as the open procedure at preventing GERD and would show limited, long-term success. However the initial reports and now up to 10-year follow-up seem to support that laparoscopic Nissen fundoplication has better clinical results and perhaps a lower failure rate than the same procedure done open.

This series shows that laparoscopic fundoplication can be safely performed in infants and children with the same expected advantages as those seen in adult patients. The complication rate is lower, the recovery period is quicker, and the failure rate appears to be lower. While the learning curve is steep because of the advanced laparoscopic techniques required to perform a fundoplication, the procedure can be performed quickly and effectively once these skills are mastered. Based on current reports, the laparoscopic Nissen fundoplication is clearly becoming the technique of choice for antireflux procedures in children.

References

1. Fonkalsrud EW, Berquist W, Vargas J, et al (1987) Surgical treatment of gastroesophageal reflux syndrome in infants and children. Am J Surg 154:11–18
2. Jolley SG, Ide Smith E, Tunnel WP (1987) Protective antireflux operation with feeding gastrostomy. Experience in children. Ann Surg 201:736–739
3. Turnage RH, Oldham KT, Coran AG, et al (1989) Late results of fundoplication for gastroesophageal reflux in infants and children. Surgery 105:457–463

4. Fonkalsrud EW, Ashcraft KW, Coran AG, et al (1998) Surgical treatment of gastroesophageal reflux in children: a combined hospital study of 7467 patients. Pediatrics 101:419–422
5. Coben RM, Weintrsub A, Dimarino AJ, et al (1994) Gastroesophageal reflux during gastrostomy feeding. Gastroenterology 106:13–18
6. Grunow JE, Al-Hafidh, Tunnel WP (1989) Gastroesophageal reflux following percutaneous gastrostomy in children. J Pediatr Surg 24:42–45
7. Berquest WE, Rachelefsky GS, Kadden M (1981) Gastroesophageal reflux associated with recurrent pneumonia and chronic asthma in children. Pediatrics 68:1225–1228
8. Herbst JJ, Hillman BC (1993) Gastroesophageal reflux and respiratory sequelae in Pediatric respiratory disease: diagnosis and treatment. WB Saunders, Philadelphia, pp 521–532
9. Hinder RA, Filipi CJ, Wetscher G, et al (1994) Laparoscopic Nissen fundoplication is an effective treatment for gastroesophageal reflux disease. Ann Surg 220:472–481
10. Weerts JM, Dallemagne B, Hamoir E, Demarche M, et al (1993) Laparoscopic Nissen fundoplication: Detailed analysis of 132 patients. Surg Laparosc Endosc 3:359–364
11. Collins JB, Georgeson KE, Vicente Y, et al (1995) Comparison of open and laparoscopic gastrostomy and fundoplication in 120 patients. J Pediatr Surg 3:1065–1071
12. Rothenberg SS Experience with laparoscopic Nissen fundoplication in infants and children less then 10 kg. Presented at the Society of American Gastrointestinal Endoscopic Surgeons, San Diego, CA, March 1997
13. Farrell TM, Richardson WS, Halker R, et al (2001) Nissen fundoplication improves gastric motility in patients with delayed gastric emptying. Surg Endosc 15:271–274
14. Smith CD, Otherson HB, Grogan NJ, et al (1992) Nissen fundoplication in children with profound neurologic disability. High risks and unmet goals. Ann Surg 215:654–659
15. Stringel G, Delgado M, Guertin L, et al (1989) Gastrostomy and fundoplication in neurologically impaired children. J Pediatr Surg 24:1044–1048
16. Peters JH, Heimbucher J, Kauer WK, et al (1995) Clinical and physiologic comparison of laparoscopic and open Nissen fundoplication. J Am Coll Surg 180:385–393
17. Richardson WS, Hunter JG (1997) The floppy Nissen is a completely competent antireflux valve (abstract). Surg Endosc 11:179
18. Rothenberg SS (1998) Experience with 220 consecutive laparoscopic Nissen fundoplications in infants and children. J Pediatr Surg 33:274–278
19. Chung DH, Georgeson KE (1998) Fundoplication and gastrostomy. Semin Ped Surg 7:213–219
20. Anvari M, Allen CJ (1996) Prospective evaluation of dysphagia before and after laparoscopic Nissen fundoplication without routine division of short gastrics. Surg Laparosc Endosc 6:424–429
21. Iglesias JL, Kogut K, Rothenberg SS (2001) Safety and efficacy of laparoscopic Nissen fundoplication in early infancy. Pediatr Endosurg Innovative Tech (5):379–383
22. Esposito C, Montupet P, Reinberg O (2001) Laparoscopic surgery for gastroesophageal reflux disease during the first year of life. J Pediatr Surg 36:715–717

Chapter 25

Nissen-Rossetti Procedure 25

Girolamo Mattioli · Vincenzo Jasonni

Contents

25.1
Introduction

Rossetti modified the Nissen fundoplication by wrapping only the anterior wall of the stomach, used to encircle the distal esophagus in extremely obese patients. This technique was described in detail by Rossetti in 1968 and became the procedure of choice in Nissen's clinic. Although the original Nissen procedure did not involve division of short gastric vessels and posterior gastric vessels, complete mobilization of the fundus by division of these vessels was proposed to provide as loose a wrap as possible in an effort to avoid complications [1–22]. Donahue and DeMeester modified the original Nissen fundoplication creating the so-called short "floppy" Nissen, which included:

1. Abdominalization of the esophageal sphincter
2. Hiatoplasty to restore a somewhat anatomic hiatus
3. Mobilization of the gastric fundus by dividing the short gastric vessels
4. Sutures including the anterior wall of the esophagus to prevent the stomach from slipping up through the wrap, thus preventing the so-called telescope phenomenon

The earliest description of a Nissen fundoplication in children was by Bettex and Kuffer in 1969. However, this procedure was largely debated, and Scharli published a famous article in 1985 entitled "To Nissen or not to Nissen". He underlined that Nissen fundoplication would not be the treatment of choice in children and that it was indicated only in cases where a total absence of reflux was tolerable. Several authors have underlined that

many successful reflux-preventing operations have evolved over the years but not every exponent of a technique is satisfied with the results of the originator. Ideally, follow-up after these procedures should be carried out by an independent assessor, thus offering objective data.

In pediatric patients, the first publication on the minimal invasive approach to the treatment of gastro-esophageal reflux disease appeared in 1993 when Lobe presented his first experience. After that paper, many similar studies were carried out [23–36].

25.2
Preoperative Work-Up

Esophageal pH monitoring, X-ray upper-GI barium meal, esophageal endoscopy, and manometry are performed in all cases. Patients with atypical respiratory symptoms have bronchoalveolar lavage and CT scan of the thorax in case of suspected focal lung lesions.

Patients are operated only in case of unsuccessful prolonged conservative treatment (e.g., postural and dietetic modifications, enteral feeding in infants, PPIs, and prokinetics) or in case of complications.

25.3
Technique

The procedure is performed with the patient under general anesthesia and tracheal mechanical ventilation. A large tube is positioned in the stomach through the mouth; it is moved during the procedure and removed soon after awakening.

The surgeon works at the end of the bed between the patient's legs or in frog-leg position, the cameraman seated on the right of the patient and the scrub nurse on the left. The endoscopic system column is near the left shoulder of the patient and the anesthesiologic column near the right shoulder. The patient is positioned in a 30-degree reverse-Trendelenburg supine position. Pneumoperitoneum is done until a pressure of 8–10 mmHg and five ports are introduced under direct vision.

In children smaller than 10 kg, a 30° 5-mm telescope is inserted through the navel and in larger patients 1–2 cm proximally to the navel. This position allows a better view of the back wall of the esophagus and stomach during dissection. The liver is retracted through an epigastric or a subcostal 5-mm port in relationship with the dimension of the left liver lobe. The stomach is grabbed and retracted downward using a 5-mm port in the left iliac region. Two 5-mm operative ports are inserted high in the upper abdomen with a sufficient distance between them in order to have a good triangulation. The right port (surgeon's left hand) is positioned higher than the left port (surgeon's right hand). In children smaller than 10 kg, the ports for the retracting instruments (liver and stomach) and the right operating port are 3 mm in diameter. The other two ports, for the telescope and for the needle holder, are generally 5-mm in diameter, also in infants.

Three atraumatic graspers, a monopolar hook, a curved klemmer clamp, a suction-irrigation tube, and one needle holder are required. A 2/00 nonreabsorbable suture with intracorporeal knotting is used. We do not use a Babcock clamp to retract the stomach because we are afraid of the risk of gastric perforation during retraction with this instrument that is, in our experience, traumatic.

The procedure starts by cutting, using scissors, the lesser omentum just above the liver vagal branches and the left gastric hepatic vascular branches, which are always preserved. After the caudatus segment of the liver is identified, the peritoneum is widely opened, using scissors, from right-to-left just in front of the esophagus, following the arch of the crus, and identifying and sparing the anterior vagus.

The gastric fundus and the left crura are completely released from the posterior and anterior peritoneal attachments. The phrenoesophageal and phrenogastric attachments are posteriorly cleared off the crura as far as possible. Then the right crus is identified and released from peritoneal attachment, and the esophagus is pushed upward, using atraumatic instruments. The retroesophageal window is bluntly created. In the retroesophageal space, we prefer blunt dissection and never coagulate but grab the tissue and pull it in a safer position.

Dissection of the right crura is very limited, the so-called "minimal hiatal dissection," and it is principally directed toward the esophagus and stomach more than to the diaphragm. The posterior vagal nerve is always identified first but never dissected and always left close to the esophagus.

The window is again cleared from the gastric attachment on the left side where a phrenic vein sometimes comes in the field and must be coagulated or ligated if too large. A rigorous technique of dissection should prevent the most severe complications, including perforation of the posterior esophageal wall, vagal injury, and pneumothorax.

When the window is completed and the gastric fundus is completely released from anterior and posterior peritoneal attachments, hiatoplasty is performed, usually using a single simple nonreabsorbable suture. The wrap must be prepared with extreme attention because it is possible to twist the esophagus or the stomach itself. The fundus is not grabbed at the dome; rather it is grabbed at the level of the esophagus close to but not on the large curvature (Fig. 1). An atraumatic grasper is

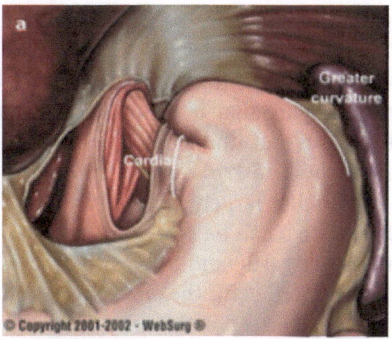

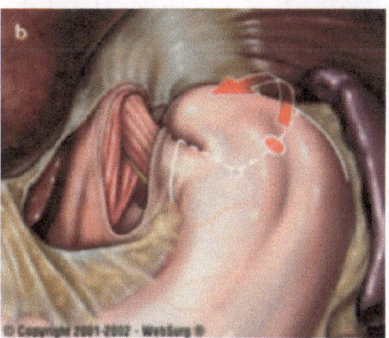

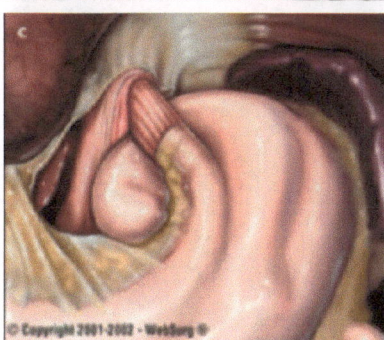

Fig. 1. Dissection of the right crura is very limited, the so-called minimal hiatal dissection, and the gastric fundus is completely released from anterior and posterior peritoneal attachments. The fundus is grabbed not at the dome but rather at the level of esophagus close to but not on the large curvature. The anterior wall of the fundus is pushed and pulled exactly to the chosen position. The retroesophageal grasper pulls the stomach behind the esophagus to the right side. The wrap is created by pulling and pushing the stomach in the correct position, making sure that it is not under tension and that the esophagus and stomach are not twisted. (From [44])

passed right-to-left behind the esophagus, through the right operative port. The esophagus is pushed downward, left-to-right, with a second grasper inserted through the left iliac port, to enable the surgeon to see the retroesophageal instrument near the diaphragm up to the stomach. The fundus is pushed upward, with the third grasper inserted through the left operative port, and with the retroesophageal grasper grabbing the fundus, exactly in the chosen position of the anterior wall, near the great curvature, at the level of the esophageal junction. The retroesophageal grasper pulls the stomach behind the esophagus to the right side. The other two instruments are released.

The flap is maintained in position, without tension, using the right grasper. The wrap is created pulling and pushing the stomach in the correct position, with the surgeon making sure that it is not under tension and that the esophagus and stomach are not twisted (Fig. 2).

Division of short gastric vessels is not always necessary if the stomach is largely released and can be easily handled. However, it can be necessary in order to move the stomach more easily and to be sure that a tension-free wrap is achieved, with the spleen not coming over the wrap. If the spleen is positioned too high, division of short gastric vessels is mandatory, also if the wrap is floppy, because the spleen can come down after surgery, modifying the wrap location and creating stricture on the esophagus due to wrap tension or esophageal twisting. Occasionally, short gastric vessel division must be enlarged if it causes wrap tension. This is performed using a coagulating hook or bipolar instruments. In older children, the ultrasound-activated scissors or sutures could be safer. We do not generally use clips because they can slip during gastric handling.

During preparation of the wrap, the esophageal sound is moved up and down to be sure the esophagus is not angled. Before definitive suturing, many attempts are made to find the best position of the wrap (Fig. 3). After evaluating the "optimal" position (no spontaneous retraction, no tension, no twisting, no stricture on the esophagus, and no angled position of the esophagus), the wrap is done by suturing the two margins of the anterior wall of the stomach in front of the esophagus.

Two or three nonreabsorbable sutures for a length of 1 cm are used. The sutures include only the stomach and no other structures. At the end of suturing, a grasper is passed and opened between the wrap and the esophagus to be sure of its looseness. If any doubt is present regarding the wrap, the procedure must be repeated and other short gastric vessels divided if necessary.

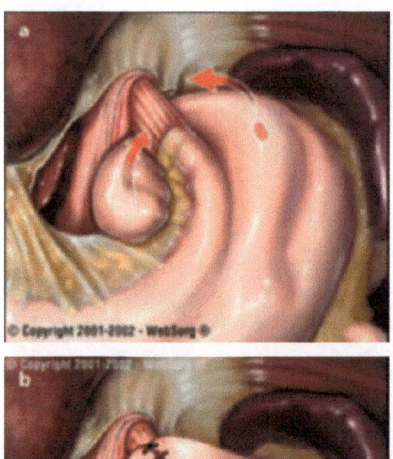
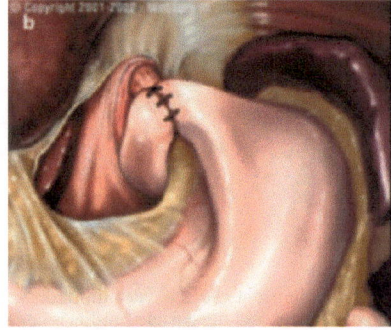

Fig. 2. After evaluating the "optimal" position (no spontaneous retraction, no tension, no twisting, no stricture or angled position of the esophagus), the wrap is done by suturing the two margins of the anterior wall of the stomach in front of the esophagus. Two nonreabsorbable sutures for a length of 1 cm are used. The sutures pick only the stomach and no other structures. One more suture can be used to fix the wrap to the gastric body at the level of the gastroesophageal junction. (From [44])

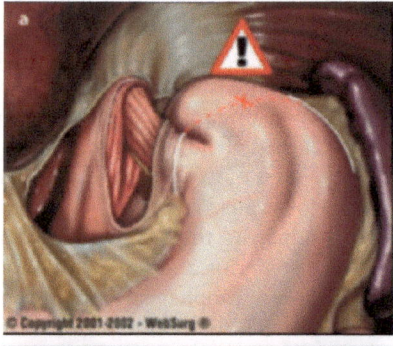
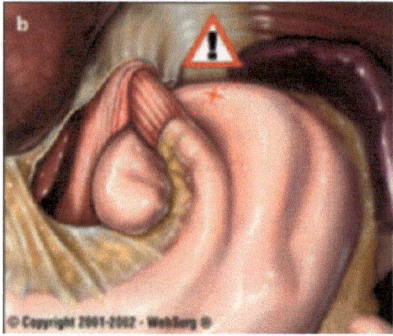

Fig. 3. The common mistake is to grab the stomach in an erroneous position, creating a too tight or a twisted wrap. Twisting of the wrap is a main cause of postoperative dysphagia, which will require re-operation because endoscopic dilation is not useful due to absence of stricture. (From [44])

One more suture can be used to fix the wrap to the gastric body at the level of the gastroesophageal junction. A gastrostomy tube is inserted, if required, at the end of the procedure using a PEG technique or through a port site. It is not generally necessary to remove the gastrostomy tube, if correctly positioned, to perform a correct operation. The nasogastric tube is removed soon after the tracheal tube is taken out and the child spontaneously breaths. In case of gastric distension, it can be inserted again in the postoperative period.

The patient is fed by mouth or by gastric tube soon after peristalsis appears, normally 7–10 h after end of anesthesia. Feeding starts with clear fluids and then with semisolid meals. The patient is sent home on post-operative day 2. Short-term antibiotic prophylaxis is administered for 24 h. PPI and prokinetic therapy is continued for 4 weeks after surgery [37–42].

25.4
Discussion

The use of the stomach anterior surface has many advantages and risks. It is simple to handle and to decide the exact position of the wrap, which can have a precise size, because the surgeon can see the anterior surface very well. It is impossible to create a too-loose or wandering wrap, reducing the risk of herniation or slipping. This is the reason why it is useless to fix the wrap to the esophagus or diaphragm. The telescope phenomenon is impossible.

Sparing the vagal branches to the liver and the distal part of the lesser omentum has two main advantages. The first is the prevention of downward slipping of the wrap, which could create an incompetent valve on the stomach and not on the esophagus. The second advantage is that, because the vagal branches go to the caudatum segment and then to the duodenum, they can have an effect not only on the liver but also on duodenal motility. In our opinion, a minimal trauma to the involved structures cannot be avoided, to assure the best functional outcome in a growing patient.

Moreover, the use of only the anterior surface of the stomach can contribute to a more stable long-term outcome, because the anterior and posterior walls of the stomach are thought to grow at different speeds. This is particularly important in infants and young children, where fundoplication may change during growth [43].

In our experience, the risk of tension and stricture after a Nissen-Rossetti or a Nissen wrap is the same with the use of only the anterior wall or both the anterior and posterior walls without short gastric vessel division. We absolutely agree that, in order to reduce postoperative dysphagia, the wrap must be short and floppy. The use of the anterior surface of the stomach, that is, the modification that Rossetti did to the Nissen fundoplication, does not interfere with this concept, which does not come from Nissen but from Donahue and Demeester.

In our opinion, the esophagus must be free from the wrap in order to let it move in a functionally good position, reducing the risk of twisting and of consequent functional obstruction that cannot be dilated. The nasogastric tube's upward and downward movements during wrap creation are important to check that it is tension-free and that the esophagus is not twisted; this must also be checked after the nasogastric tube's removal.

The same risk is present for hiatoplasty. We contend that the esophagus must always fit freely inside the diaphragmatic hiatus. Hiatoplasty must be done mainly if it is enlarged. We do not know for certain whether minimal invasive access surgery can modify this concept. We are doing a prospective randomized study in children with gastroesophageal reflux and no hernia, without hiatal repair and only minimal hiatal dissection. Follow-up is as yet too short to show definitive results.

It is sure that hiatoplasty can cause dysphagia if it is too tight or if it causes an esophageal distortion. In this case a different procedure should be suggested.

To conclude, it is important to underline that the use of the anterior wall of the stomach as described by Rossetti is not feasible in all pediatric patients. When the fundus is not large enough, the stomach has been previously operated, or a gastrostomy tube is in place, it can be necessary to perform a different type of antireflux procedure.

References

1. Nissen R (1937) Die transpleurale Resektion der Kardia. Dtsch Chir 249:311–316
2. Nissen R (1956) Eine einfache Operation zur Beeinflussung der Reflux Oesophagitis. Schweiz Med Wochenschr 86:590
3. Ellis FH (1992) The Nissen fundoplication. Ann Thorac Surg 54:1229–1230
4. Nissen R, Rossetti M (1965) Surgery of hiatal and other diaphragmatic hernias. J Int Coll Surg 43:663–674
5. Rossetti M (1968) Zur Technik der Fundoplication. Actuelle Chir 3:29
6. Rossetti M, Allgower M (1973) Fundoplication for the treatment of hiatal hernia. Progr Surg 12:1
7. Rossetti M, Hell K (1977) Fundoplication for the treatment of gastro-esophageal reflux disease in hiatal hernia. World J Surg 1:439–443
8. Rossetti M (1993) Life with hiatal hernias and reflux disease. An historical synthesis and an update. Ann Ital Chir 64:249–254
9. Rossetti M (1995) Antireflux surgery: from Nissen to mini-invasive technics. Minerva Chirurgica 50:104–108
10. Donahue PE, Samelson S, Nyhus LM, Bombeck CT (1985) The floppy Nissen fundoplication: effective long term control of pathologic reflux. Arch Surg 120:663–667
11. DeMeester TR, Bonavina L, Albertucci M (1986) Nissen fundoplication for gastroesophageal reflux disease. Ann Surg 204:9–20
12. Cuschieri A, Hunter J, Swanstrom L, Hutson W (1993) Multicenter prospective evaluation of laparoscopic antireflux surgery: preliminary report. Surg Endosc 7:505–510

13. Hunter JG, Swanstrom L, Waring JP (1996) Dysphagia after laparoscopic antireflux surgery. The impact of operative technique. Ann Surg 224:51–57
14. Dallemagne B, Weerts JM, Jehaes C, Markiewicz S (1996) Causes of failures of laparoscopic antireflux operations. Surg Endosc 10:305–310
15. Luostarienen MES, Isolauri JO (1999) Randomized trial to study the effect of fundic mobilization on long-term results of Nissen fundoplication. Br J Surg 86:614–618
16. Luostarinen ME, Koskinen MO, Isolauri JO (1996) Effect of fundal mobilisation in Nissen-Rossetti fundoplication on oesophageal transit and dysphagia. A prospective, randomised trial. Eur J Surg 162:37–42
17. Blomqvist A, Dalenback F, Hagedorn C, Lonroth H, Hyltander A, Lundell L (2000) Impact of complete gastric fundus mobilization on outcome after laparoscopic total fundoplication. J Gastroint Surg 4:493–500
18. Watson DL, Pike GK, Baigrie RJ (1997) Prospective double blind randomized trial of laparoscopic Nissen fundoplication with division and without division of short gastric vessels. Ann Surg 226:642–652
19. Pessaux P, Arnaud JP, Ghavami B, Flament JB, Trebuchet B, Meyer C, Huten N, Champault G (2000) Laparoscopic antireflux surgery: comparative study of Nissen, Nissen-Rossetti, and Toupet fundoplication. Surg Endosc 14:1024–1027
20. Chrysos E, Tzortzinis A, Tsiaoussis J, Athanasakis H, Vassilakis J, Xynos E (2001) Prospective randomized trial comparing Nissen to Nissen-Rossetti technique for laparoscopic fundoplication. Am J Surg 182:215–221
21. Zaninotto G, Molena D, Ancona E (2000) A prospective multicenter study on laparoscopic treatment of gastroesophageal reflux disease in Italy Type of surgery, conversions, complications, and early results. Surg Endosc 14:282–288
22. Rydberg L, Ruth M, Abrahamsson H, Lundell L (1999) Tailoring antireflux surgery: a randomized clinical trial. World J Surg 23:612–618
23. Bettex M, Kuffer F (1969) Long-term results of fundoplication in hiatus hernia and cardio-esophageal chalasia in infants and children. J Pediatr Surg 4:526–530
24. Scharli AF (1985) To Nissen or not to Nissen. Prog Pediatr Surg 18:96–100
25. Levy MS, Sorrels CW, Wagner CW, Jackson RJ, Barnes RW, Smith SD (1999) Evolution of the modified Rossetti fundoplication in children: surgical technique and results. Ann Surg 229:774–779
26. Bergmeijer JHLJ, Harbers JS, Molenaar JC (1997) Function of pediatric Nissen-Rossetti fundoplication followed up into adolescence and adulthood. J Am Coll Surg 184:259–261
27. Visick AH (1948) Measured radical gastrectomy. Review of 505 operations for peptic ulcer. Lancet 254:505–511
28. Lundell L, Abrahamsson H, Ruth M, Rydberg L, Lonroth H, Olbe L (1996) Long-term results of a prospective randomized comparison of total fundic wrap (Nissen-Rossetti) or semi-fundoplication (Toupet) for gastro-esophageal reflux. Br J Surg 83:830–835
29. Bais JE, Bertelsman JFWM, Bonjer HJ, Cuesta MA, Go PMNYH, Klinkenberg-Knol EC, Van Lanschot JJB, Nadorp JHSM, Smout AJPM, Van der Graaf Y, Gooszen HG (2000) The Netherlands Antireflux Surgery Study Group: Laparoscopic or conventional Nissen fundoplication for gastro-esophageal reflux disease: randomised clinical trial. Lancet 355:170–174
30. Herron DM, Swanstrom LL, Ramzi N, Hansen PD (1999) Factors predictive of dysphagia after laparoscopic Nissen fundoplication. Surg Endosc 13:1180–1183
31. Lobe-TE, Schropp KP, Lunsford K (1993) Laparoscopic Nissen fundoplication in childhood. J Pediatr Surg 28:358–360
32. Lobe TE (1993) Laparoscopic fundoplication. Semin Pediatr Surg 2:178–181
33. Longis B, Grousseau D, Alain JL, Terrier G (1996) Laparoscopic fundoplication in children: our first 30 cases. J Laparoendosc Surg 6:S21–S29
34. Allal H, Captier G, Lopez M, Forgues D, Galifer RB (2001) Evaluation of 142 consecutive laparoscopic fundoplications in children: effects of the learning curve and technical choice. J Ped Surg 36:921–926
35. Esposito C, Montupet P, Amici G, Desruelle P (2000) Complications of laparoscopic antireflux surgery in childhood. Surg Endosc 14:622–624
36. Liu DC, Wynn A, Rodriguez JA, Hill C, Loe W (2001) Laparoscopic Nissen-Rossetti fundoplication in children. Ped Endosurg Innov Tech 5:19–22
37. Jasonni V, Cagnazzo A, Caffarena PE, Granata C, Bisio G, Ivani G, Mattioli G (1993) La plastica secondo Nissen-Rossetti laparoscopica nel bambino. In: Chirurgia endo-laparoscopica e mini-invasiva. L'Antologia, Napoli, pp 103–105
38. Jasonni V, Cagnazzo A, Mattioli G, Granata C, Caffarena PE, Ivani G (1994) Nissen fundoplication in children: laparoscopic technique. III International Congress on Endoscopy-Laparoscopy in Children. Münster, p 15
39. Mattioli G, Cagnazzo A, Repetto P, Carlini C, Granata C, Lampugnani E, Montobbio G, Jasonni V (2000) Lap-Nissen fundoplication: technical aspects. Ped Endosurg 4(1):80
40. Mattioli G, Repetto P, Carlini C, Torre M, PiniPrato A, Mazzola C, Leggio S, Montobbio G, Gandulli P, Barabino A, Cagnazzo A, Sacco O, Jasonni V (2002) Laparoscopic vs open approach for the treatment of gastroesophageal reflux in children. Surg Endosc 16(5):750–752
41. Mattioli G, Repetto P, Leggio S, Castagnetti M, Jasonni V (2002) Laparoscopic Nissen-Rossetti fundoplication in children. Semin Laparosc Surg 9(3):153–162.
42. Mattioli G, Esposito C, Lima M, Garzi A, Montinaro L, Cobellis G, Mastoianni L, Aceti MG, Falchetti D, Repetto P, Pini Prato A, Leggio S, Torri F, Ruggeri P, Settimi A, Messina M, Martino A, Amici G, Riccipetitoni G, Jasonni V (2002) Italian multicenter survey on laparoscopic treatment of gastro-esophageal reflux disease in children. Surg Endosc 16(12):1666–1668
43. Nebot-Cegarra J, Maraculla-Sanz E, Reina-De la Torre F (1999) Factors involved in the "rotation" of the human embryonic stomach around its longitudinal axis: computer-assisted morphometric analysis. J Anat 194:61–69
44. Marescaux Francois, Nissen-Rossetti wrap. With permission from Websurg.com. IRCAD CENTER, Strasbourg, France

Chapter 26

Toupet's Procedure

26

Philippe Montupet

Contents

Among various procedures to restore the function of the gastroesophageal sphincter, our choice of the Toupet procedure (Fig. 1) is driven by the following two priorities: to respect the anatomical features and to prevent side effects. For many years, the partial posterior wrap seemed to fulfill these priorities, and numerous experts in adult surgery reported its usefulness [1].

Before the decision for surgical correction, all of the attachments of a patient's abdominal esophagus have been stretched by repetitive episodes of coughing, vomiting, and edema due to the periesophagitis. The surgery has only to stabilize the lower part of the esophagus in its correct position below the hiatus, so that the physiology of the internal sphincter will be efficient again; then the external sphincter consisting of both crura will be reinforced in the same way. Nothing else is necessary.

André Toupet, who described in 1963 his original procedure [2], adapted the most conservative refashioning of the cardial area, and the Toupet technique gained many adherents during the 1980s.

However in children, and especially before the development of minimally invasive surgery, the arguments to delay operative treatment remained strong; thus, if sur-

Fig. 1.
A schema of a Toupet's procedure. The "x" marks the position of the seven stitches necessary to fix the Toupet's valve

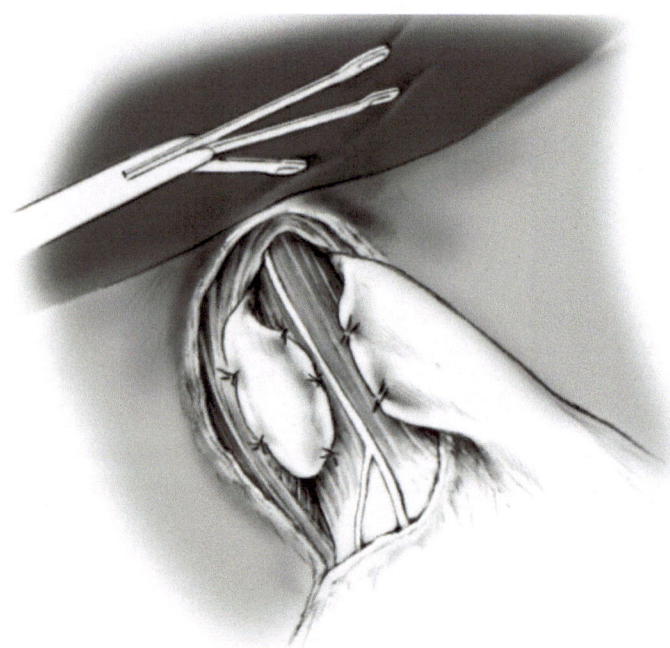

gery was to be considered the only remaining option, it would essentially be to prevent major esophagitis with stricture or life-threatening conditions such as repetitive apnea due to the acid reflux towards the trachea. The Nissen technique was attractive in this regard because the full wrap around the esophagus seemed to create a very strong antireflux procedure, despite the rates of secondary dysphagia, gas bloat syndromes, and intrathoracic valve migrations.

Toupet's procedure avoids the latter side effects, and now performed by a laparoscopic approach, it should be considered earlier as an alternative to medical treatment in cases of incomplete success of prolonged medical treatment and after suitable investigations.

We have learned several laparoscopic antireflux techniques, including the Nissen, Thal, and Boix-Ochoa, also as laparoscopic antireflux surgery (LARS). Today our series of laparoscopic Toupet's is more than 700 children, with a failure rate of 1.2%. All of these children are submitted to a close follow-up: manometric study after 6 months, UGI series after 6, 24, and 60 months. However, the most telling information regarding the procedures' success is the parents' reports of the new way of life for their child and for them.

26.1
Investigations

Routinely, we receive parents and patients for a long discussion where the surgery is only an alternative versus continuing medical treatment. Pediatricians, then often gastroenterologists, have already described the problem of gastroesophageal reflux disease (GERD) to the parents, and all investigations or the beginnings of them have been performed.

The clinical history is obvious, although it has sometimes gone on far too long. Endoscopy, 24-h pH-metry, and manometric studies are required before discussing surgery (Fig. 2). If any two parts of this check-up are discordant, prolonged medical treatment is advised, as a UGI series is required anyway before a surgery is scheduled.

Usually, pH-metric studies are considered to be the main test, and they are probably accurate. However, in terms of toxicity of a reflux, numerous short refluxes (pH<4) can also be more significant than a rate over 5% during a 24-h test.

We pay very much attention to the results of the manometric studies, because they are the most reliable index of failure of the lower esophageal sphincter (LES). Concerning the endoscopy, some evidence may appear, but no studies provide a comparison between this exam performed with or without general anesthesia. Obviously, the level of esophagitis is considered. In case of obvious evidence of toxic reflux despite prolonged med-

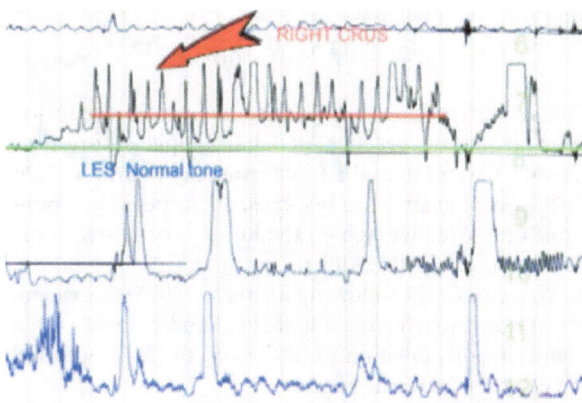

Fig. 2. A correct manometric evaluation is a fundamental exam to perform before each laparoscopic antireflux procedure

ical treatment, we propose the surgical alternative: a minimally invasive surgery (conversion to a laparotomy must stay exceptional). We illustrate for the parents the causes leading to sphincter failure, and describe the repairing technique.

26.2
Technique

All of the LARS (laparoscopic antireflux surgery) include two steps: dissection of the lower esophagus and reconstruction of hiatal area.

26.2.1
Dissection of the Lower Esophagus, Reconstruction of Hiatal Area

The dissection is probably the step that most depends on the experience of the surgeon. We used to approach the hiatal area on the right side of it: the liver is retracted, as is the caudate lobe, the small omentum is opened, and the right crus is easily identified. The latter goes down the esophagogastric junction, so it is easy to push an instrument into the angle between the right crus and the esophagus and at this level to start the dissection. Now an essential landmark appears or must be identified: the posterior vagus nerve. It must be preserved, and it also serves as a main landmark to find the relief of the left crus. When the fascia of the left crus has been found, a large window towards the splenic area is opened, as a way to easily grasp the gastric fundus.

Then, the low esophagus is freed on its right side, its anterior wall, and on its left side, including the division of the gastrophrenic ligament. A 30° telescope helps especially with this step. This completes the dissection.

26.2.2
The Reconstruction Step

The reconstruction step is also demanding, because apart from the practice in laparoscopic sutures, we must be careful to pull a large wrap, to obtain the right thickness of gastric fundus, crus, and especially esophagus; moreover, we tighten the knots very gently in order to avoid a cutting suture.

To facilitate the following fixation of the wrap, we put the fundus around the esophagus, and a loose stitch maintains this position until the end of the procedure. We call this the frame stitch.

Three rows of sutures can now ensure the Toupet's: first between the fundus wrap and the right crus, second between the right esophagus and the fundus wrap, and third between the fundus wrap and the left esophagus.

When the frame stitch is removed, a true partial posterior wrap encircles the esophagus on three-quarters of its girth, without tension.

Each port entry is closed by a suture. Suitable analgesia is provided in the recovery room; the anti-GERD drugs are stopped but the nasogastric tube is left until the day after the surgery.

26.2.3
Postoperative Care

Three days of hospitalization are scheduled: the nasogastric tube is removed on the morning following the surgery; liquid oral feeding is resumed 2 h later; the second day, normal diet is provided. On the third day, the patient is advised to eat slowly, and an appointment to remove the small dressing and to check the feeding is made for 5–7 days in the future.

A UGI series will be performed at 6 months, 2 years, and 5 years postoperatively, with a manometric study to check the LES at 6 months.

26.3
Results

Between February 1992 and June 2003, we performed 754 Toupet's procedures. The patients' ages ranged from 3 months to 16 years (mean 3.6 years). It is interesting that the mean age at surgery moved downward year after year, reaching 3 years in 1998, while the majority of our indications moved to otolaryngologic (ORL) and bronchopulmonary diseases. The mean duration of the procedure is routinely 1 h, including anesthesia and setting-up. A gastrostomy was added in 16 cases of neurologic impaired patients (NI).

There were no anesthetic complications, and no conversions to laparotomy. Peri-operatively, three right

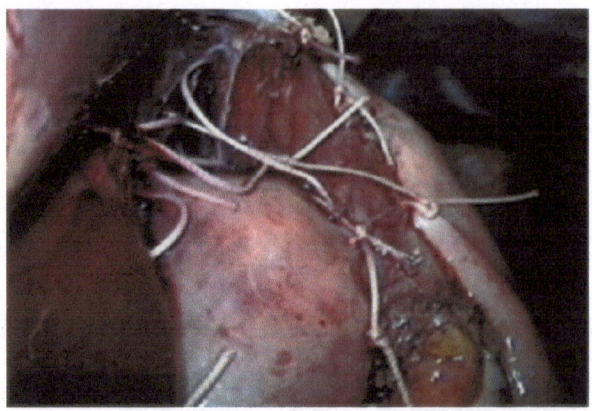

Fig. 3. An operative picture of the completed Toupet's valve

pneumothorax resolved without drainage, two injuries of the vagus nerve caused a transient diarrhea, and some slight bleeding stopped spontaneously.

During the three-day postoperative period, four omentum protrusions occurred through the port orifices, due to a lack of closure; short-term anesthesia was necessary. Two other peri-operative complications consisted of a shot through the nasogastric tube by a suture: one could be removed under endoscopic vision, the other required a redo procedure.

Including the 11 operative and peri-operative complications (1.4%), the mean hospital stay was 3 days. During the first 3 weeks, some patients transiently complained of moderate dysphagia or back pain, which never persisted. Two patients aged 2 and 3 years unexpectedly any feeding after 7 and 5 days, and a short reperfusion restored the status.

All patients were clinically improved, and closely controlled after 6 months: on the manometric studies, the LES pressure was over 12 mm H_2O, and it was located 70% at least under the hiatus; on the UGI series, the appearance of the valve was clear, without stricture of the esophagus, or reflux (Fig. 3).

However, seven recurrences (0.9%) occurred, one after 5 months, five between 2 and 5 years, and one after 5 years. Among them, there were some associated pathologies such as spastic crisis and a mucoviscidosis; otherwise the close follow-up allowed the identification of early episodes of bronchitis after the surgery.

These seven children underwent a redo Toupet. The operative observations were only a slippage of the valve behind the cardia, due to a disruption of the right crus attachment, easy to correct. No conversions were necessary. There were no intrathoracic slipped wraps. Therefore, three rows of three sutures were placed, again without tension. A third procedure was performed 4 years later for the child suffering a mucoviscidosis, with a good follow-up after 4 years.

26.4
Discussion

The physiopathology of the gastroesophageal junction has been described by several major authors in the field [3–5]. Their conclusions reinforce an fundamental point: the intraabdominal segment of esophagus is the key to the whole system for preventing GERD. Thus, several techniques converge at the same goal, and each includes essential factors to be considered: (1) the rate of good and reproducible results, (2) the avoidance of side effects, and (3) the skill level of the surgeon. Usually any surgeon using the same technique for a long time is confident due to his high rate of success, and is concerned to reduce the side effects. The routine for LARS is therefore not unique, and we have a true respect for the Nissen, Thal, and Boix-Ochoa procedures.

Toupet's technique has won over many surgeons worldwide [6, 7]. We were among the practitioners who agreed with this technique early on [8], and since the laparoscopic era began our experience has increased, improving some technical details. Our results are gratifying in terms of safety, easy surgery, and early comfort for the patients. We no longer select any other techniques when clinical investigations demonstrate a toxicity of GERD despite medical treatment. We are reluctant to operate only in children under 6 months of age, except when the medical circumstances are life-threatening.

Medical treatment always must be applied for 8 - months at least.

We have progressively changed some details of the original technique: we start by the valve fixation, we increase the surface of the valve on the right side, we use a frame stitch to stabilize the valve during sutures, and we add some stitches to secure the sutures. Intracorporeal knotting appears to improve the skill of surgeons better than extracorporeal knotting.

We have had to reoperate on children after a Thal or Nissen procedure. Either the valve was too tight in front of the esophagus, or it was slipping towards the mediastinum. In these cases the redo appeared to be slightly more difficult.

Regarding the complications [9], very few have to be considered (0.9%) with respect to a dissection which is not specific to the Toupet. We describe conversion to the parents as exceptional, and we inform them about the possibility of the necessity of a redo in 1–2% of the cases. Our failures for NI patients improved from 15% to 6%.

The results, in terms of repairing surgery, obviously do not depend on the technique only: GERD investigations must be completed to check the motility and the LES, to differentiate multiple short reflux and prolonged ones, and to study the gastric emptying. Barrett's esophagus will require a more prolonged follow-up. The follow-up should be scheduled at the first appointment with the parents. Five years are a minimum; and as a UGI series is systematically requested and checked, this close follow-up would display a possible failure of the valve, if it occurs.

LARS is a very satisfying surgery in terms of a truly notable change of the family's way of life. The relationship among pediatricians, gastroenterologists and ORL has progressively become more confident, due to patient satisfaction.

26.5
Conclusion

After one decade of experience with Toupet's procedure, the LARS technique has been improved to a high level of good results. The technique is simple, without side effects, and long-term follow-up is routine. We present a large series, but we did not select the patients ourselves, and the mean age for the radical treatment has moved downward due to the ages of the referred patients. The satisfaction indices of patients and family has encouraged us to continue to perform minimally invasive and safe surgery.

References

1. Mc Kerman JB (1994) Laparoscopic repair of gastro-esophageal reflux disease. Toupet partial fundoplication versus Nissen fundoplication. Surg Endosc 8:851–856
2. Toupet A (1963) La technique d'oesophagoplastie avec phrenoplastie appliquée dans la cure radicale des hernies hiatales et comme complement de l'opération de Heller dans les cardoispames. Mem Acad Chir 89:394–399
3. Cargill G, Goutet JM, Vargas J (1983) Gastroesophageal reflux in infants and children. Manometric analysis: Possible relation with chronic bronchopulmonary disease. Gut 24:357–361
4. Tovar JA, Morras I, Arana J, Garay J, Tapia I (1986) Etude fonctionnelle du reflux gastro-oesophagien chez les enfants encéphalopathes. Chir Pédiatr 27:134–137
5. Boix-Ochoa J (1986) Address of honored guest: the physiologic approach of the management of gastric esophageal reflux. J Pediatr Surg 21:1032–1039
6. De Meester TR, Stein HJ (1992) Minimizing the side effects of antireflux surgery. World J Surg 16:335–336
7. Bensoussan AL, Yazbeck S, Carceller-Blanchard A (1994) Results and complication of Toupet's partial posterior wrap: 10 years experience. J Pediatr Surg 29:1215–1217
8. Montupet P (2002) Toupet's fundoplication in children. Semin Laparosc Surg 9:163–167
9. Esposito C, Montupet P, Amici G, Desruelle P (2000) Complications of laparoscopic antireflux surgery in childhood. Surg Endosc 14:658–660

Chapter 27

Jaubert De Beaujeu's Procedure 27

Jean Stephane Valla

Contents

There is no perfect operation for gastroesophageal reflux; many procedures have been described [1]. The goals of the ideal procedure are to correct the incompetence of the lower esophageal sphincter, to maintain this result during the growth of the child and during the entire life, and to avoid side effects. Anterior partial fundoplication offers theoretically a more anatomical reconstruction and a more physiological antireflux procedure. It is now our preferred technique for use in neurologically normal children.

Jaubert de Beaujeu's procedure [2] combines various techniques:
1. Reconstruction of a good His angle as described by Lortat-Jacob [3]
2. Anterior fundoplication as described by Thal and Dor
3. And the most important point, the first step: pulling the esophagus down as far as possible into the abdomen and anchoring it to crus and diaphragm, because (probably) the main antireflux factor is the length of the intra-abdominal esophagus

27.1
Preoperative Work-Up

Routine preoperative assessment has no specificity and includes in most cases 24-h pH-metry, upper gastrointestinal series, and fiberoptic examination. Manometry is indicated if dyskinetic anomalies of the esophagus are suspected.

27.2
Anesthesia

The patient is anesthetized with endotracheal intubation and full muscle relaxation. A nasogastric tube with a diameter of 10–16 French, depending on the size of the child, is inserted. No vesical catheter is needed. Prolonged mask ventilation during induction should be avoided due to its tendency to induce gastric and small bowel dilatation. Nitrous oxide should be avoided due to its tendency to induce dilatation of transverse colon, particularly in infants.

27.3
Position of Patient, Crew, and Equipment

The child lies supine; the operating table is tilted head-up to allow the stomach and other organs to fall away from the esophageal hiatus. If the patient is less than 5 years old, the legs are folded up at the end of the table (frog position). If he is older, the patient is in the lithotomy position and the surgeon stands between the legs. The monitor is positioned on the right of the patient at the head of the table. All the cables and tubes are fastened to his right thigh. The cameraman is on the right, and the assistant on the left of the child (Fig. 1).

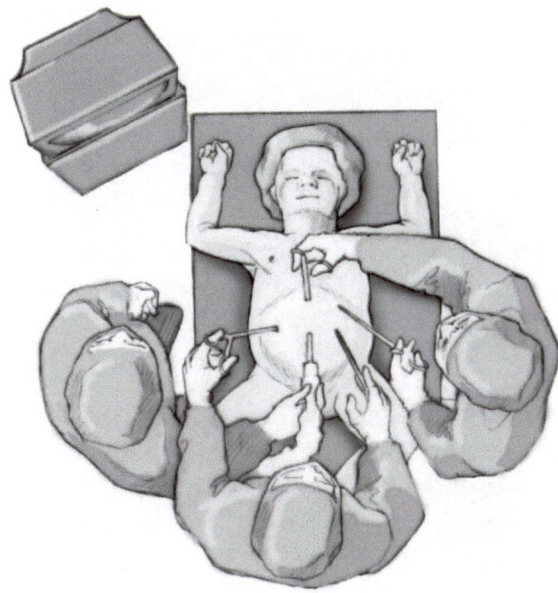

Fig. 1. Position of the patient and team

27.4
Position of Trocars

A five-port technique is used. Local anesthesia could be injected intradermally at each trocar site. The position of these trocars varies depending on the size of the child: in children the scope (5–10 mm, 30° or 45°) is inserted through the umbilicus, but in infants it is sometimes better to introduce the scope (5 mm 30°) a few centimeters above the umbilical. For this first trocar, the peritoneal cavity is entered under direct vision (open technique).

The pneumoperitoneum is induced with CO2 via the first cannula. Pressure is maintained between 6 and 12 - mmHg depending the age of the child.

Under laparoscopic visualization, four additional trocars are inserted: two for the surgeon (5–3 mm, depending on the size of the child); in the left upper quadrant and right upper quadrant and two 3-mm trocars for the assistant in the xiphoid area for liver retractor and on the left subcostal area for gastric retractor. Sometimes, especially in infants an abdominal wall suspensor – designed by MOURET – is used to reduce intra-abdominal CO_2 pressure, to allow good visualization even during aspiration, and to retract the left lobe and hepato-umbilical ligament. This 2-mm suspensor is introduced in the xiphoid area instead of the 3-mm trocar.

The surgeon's trocars are sealed with simple silicone caps in order to facilitate needle passage and must be secured to the abdominal wall to avoid any dislodgment.

27.5
Technique

27.5.1
Extensive Mobilization of Esophagus and Dissection of the Crus (Figs. 2, 3)

The liver left lobe is gently retracted through the epigastric port (right hand of the assistant) and the stomach is pulled downward using an atraumatic forceps through the subcostal port (left hand of the assistant); during retraction, care must be taken not to tear the liver or the stomach. The hepatogastric ligament is divided from the lesser curve up to the diaphragm, allowing the caudate lobe and the right crus to come into view and taking care to preserve a possible sizable neurovascular branch heading for the left lobe. Usually the right crus and the esophagus are clearly identified; both anatomical structures are separated by blunt dissection, all the way down to the point where the right crus joins the left crus. Then the esophagus is cleared of its attachments on the anterior aspects. The stomach is pulled downwards and to the right to expose and dissect the left border of the esophagus free from the left crus.

A window is created behind the esophagus from the right. During manipulation behind the esophagus, care must be taken to avoid damage to the esophagus, posterior vagus, left pleural membrane, and spleen. Blunt-tip palpators are useful.

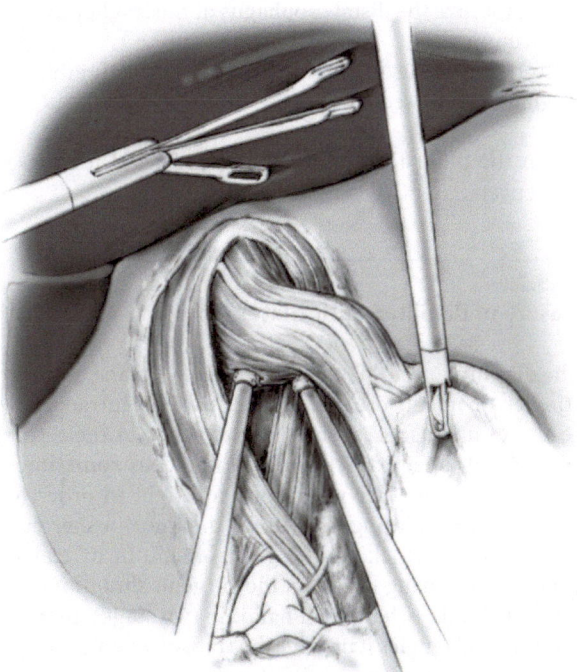

Fig. 2. Dissection of the crus and mobilization of the esophagus; the left grasper pulls down the stomach

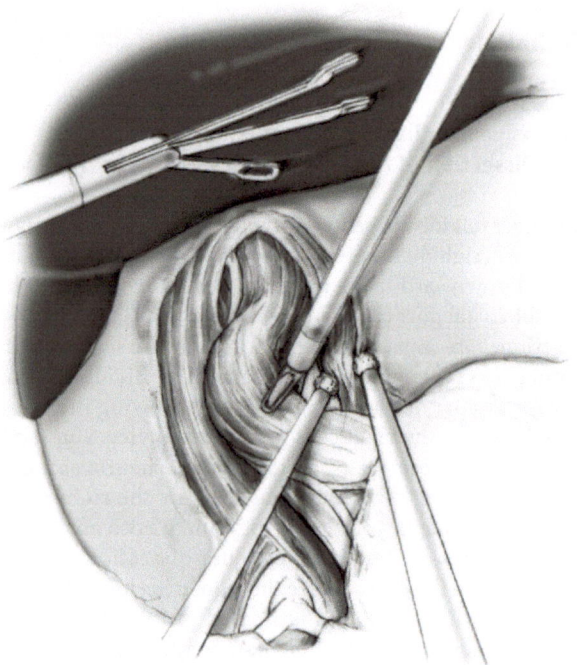

Fig. 3. Dissection of the left pilar

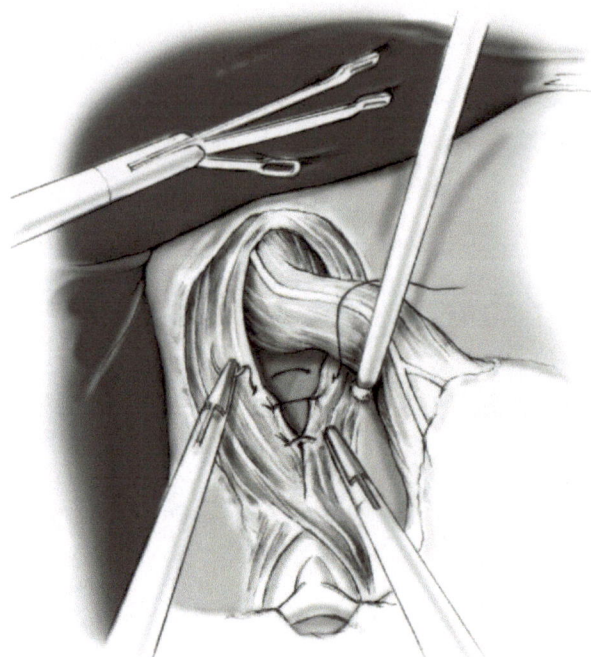

Fig. 4. Narrowing of the hiatus, the left atraumatic endopeanut retracts the esophagus on the left

There is no need to divide short vessels. To achieve an adequate abdominal length of esophagus and to fix it, (at least 3 to 6 cm according to age and size) it is mandatory:

1 to mobilize the distal esophagus at the level of mediastinum.
2 to free the crus on the left side until the left adrenal gland can be seen.

Again the blunt-tip dissection is very useful for these maneuvers.

27.5.2
Closure of Diaphragmatic Hiatus (Fig. 4)

The diaphragmatic hiatus is narrowed with one to three stitches of nonabsorbable 2/0 sutures tied intracorporeally; in infants, because of lack of space in the retroesophageal area, extracorporeal knots can sometimes be useful, taking care not to pull too tight in order to avoid muscle splitting. The tip of the knot pusher can easily become stuck on the great omentum or transverse colon during this step; the surgeon should introduce the knot pusher (right hand) in two stages: first he intentionally angles it up over the transverse colon, then he points the tip down to the crural knots.

While suturing the crura, care must be taken not to cause damage, with the long needle, the liver and vena

cava to the right, spleen behind, and aorta underneath. To allow better visualization of the right crus while suturing, the surgeon should use his atraumatic instrument (left hand) to gently push the caudate lobe of the liver to the right.

27.5.3
Intra-Abdominal Fixation of the Esophagus Around the Hiatus (Fig. 5)

This is the main step of the procedure. The right border of the esophagus is sutured to the right crus, the left border to the left crus, and the anterior part of the esophagus to the diaphragma. Seven stitches are needed: three on each side and one at the top.

27.5.4
Recreating the His Angle Is the Next Step (Figs. 6, 7)

This is performed by suturing (2/0 non-absorbable separated stitches) the anterior gastric wall to the left crus and the left border of the esophagus. It is important to secure these three anatomical elements together; it is easier to begin at the lower part of the field (at the level of the left adrenal gland) and to go up to the hiatus. Three or four stitches with extracorporeal knots are used.

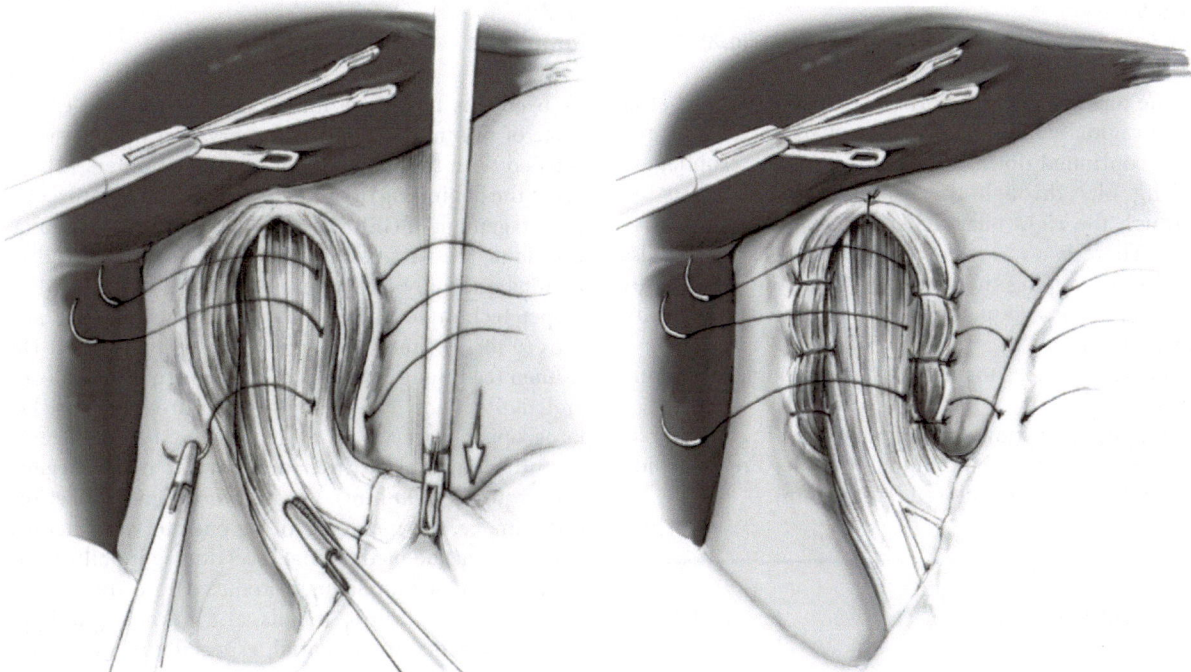

Fig. 5. The left border of the esophagus is sutured to the left crus

Fig. 6. The entire intraabdominal esophagus is already fixed to the hiatus (7 stitches) then the His angle is recreated by suturing together anterior gastric wall, left crus, left border of the esophagus (3 stitches)

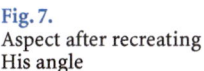

Fig. 7.
Aspect after recreating
His angle

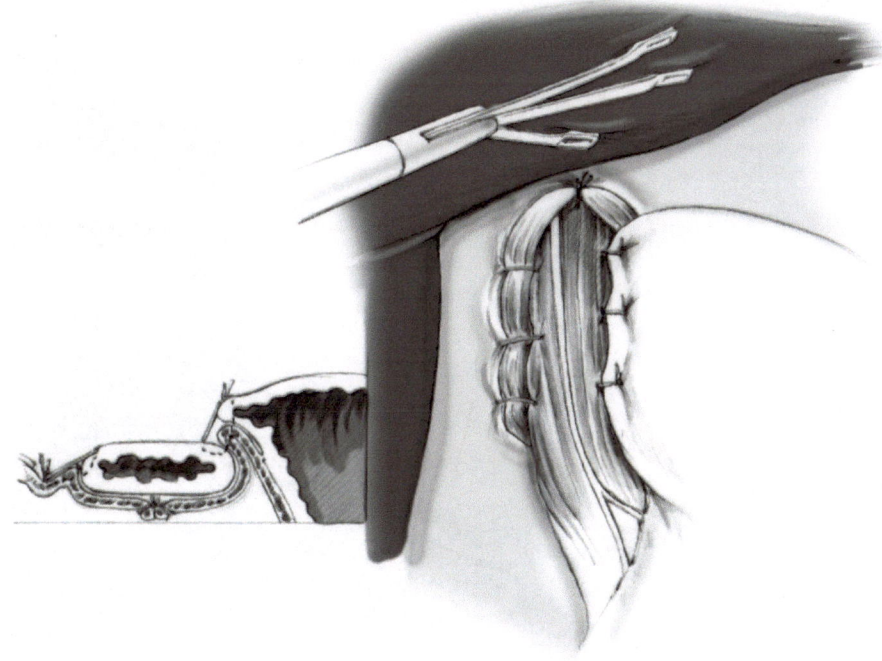

27.5.5
The Last Step is Anterior Fundoplication (Fig. 8)

At the top, the suture incorporates bits of stomach, the diaphragmatic hiatus, and the esophagus. The suture is then continued down the right side of the esophagus, taking bits through the esophageal muscularis or through the right pilar depending the traction of tissues. There is no need to cut the short gastric vessels; this suture applies the anterior wall of the stomach to the esophagus as a patch more or less over 180° of its circumference.

There is no need to push a bougie through the esophagus.

Trocars are removed under laparoscopic guidance so that any inadvertent abdominal wall bleeding is avoided. Each trocar site is closed (even 3 mm).

27.6
Postoperative Care

The nasogastric tube is removed intraoperatively or within 2 h postoperatively. Liquid feeding is restarted within 24 h.

27.7
Comments

We used this technique for 15 years before the emergence of minimally invasive surgery, and we were very satisfied with the results, as were its promoters [2]. In fact at the beginning of our experience with laparoscopic management of GER (1994–1996,) we chose a simpler technique, the Nissen procedure, which needs few dissections and only five sutures. Then we moved to the Toupet technique (1996–2000) which needs more sutures (9 to 11). Since 2001 we have used the Jaubert De Beaujeu technique, which is slightly more complex (extended dissection up and down–15 sutures). Because laparoscopic surgery is now well mastered in our team, this procedure takes the same time as open surgery (mean duration 90 mm). Because of the magnification of the image, the incidence of damage to vagal nerves and pleura at the mediastinal level during mobilization of the terminal esophagus is reduced to a minimum. Meticulous attention to details, and proper technique and instruments are essential, especially in newborns and infants.

This technique is particularly well adapted to manage mega-esophagus. It allows a surgeon to recreate an antireflux mechanism after myotomy and to cover the esophageal mucosa.

Fig. 8.
Partial anterior fundoplication

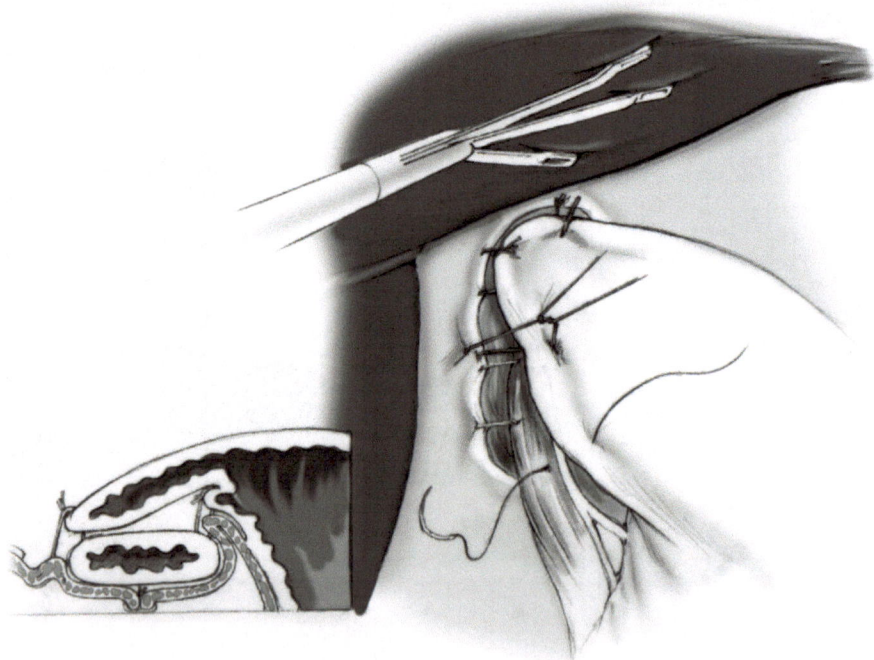

References

1. Chardot C, Montupet P, Duquesne B, Gauthier F (1996) Hernies diaphragmatiques de l'enfant. In: Encycl. Med. Chir. Techniques Chirurgicales – Appareil Digestif. Elsevier, Paris, pp 1–14, 40–255
2. Gounot E, Louis D, Zabot JM, Mollard P (1989) La technique de Jaubert de Beaujeu pour le traitement des hernies hiatales du nourrisson et de l'enfant. Chir Pediatr 30:203–208
3. Montinaro L, Paradies G, Leggio S (2002) The Lortat-Jacob operation by laparoscopic access to treat gastro-esophageal reflux in pediatric patients. Surg Endosc 16:1438–1440

Chapter 28

Laparoscopic Anterior Fundoplication of the Stomach According to Thal

28

Nicholas M. A. Bax · David C. van der Zee

Contents

28.1 Introduction

Gastro-esophageal reflux (GER) is a major health problem, in adults as well as children [4]. The incidence is difficult to estimate due to the different definitions and evaluations used in many centers. In a number of children's hospitals, procedures related to GER are the most common intraabdominal operations. The incidence of GER is much higher in the mentally retarded population than in the general population [3], and in many pediatric surgical series, 40% or more of the patients are mentally retarded [7–9].

Proton pump inhibitors (PPIs) have dramatically changed the treatment of GER, but life-long use of these drugs is not advisable, certainly not in children because of concerns of toxicity in the long run and of compliance [5]. Moreover, these drugs do not resolve the problem of non-acid reflux [13].

With the introduction of minimal-access surgical techniques in the early 1990s, many patients have opted for surgical treatment of GER. There is not much discussion anymore as to the superiority of these minimal-access techniques; they have proven to be as good as the classic open techniques as far as treatment results are concerned but with shorter hospital stays, quicker recovery, and a better cosmetic result [20].

In contrast, the discussion regarding the most optimal surgical technique is still a matter of debate. It leaves little doubt that the experience of the surgeon with one particular technique is of utmost importance. In Utrecht we changed in 1988 from the open Nissen fundoplication to the open anterior fundoplication as described by Ashcraft and Holder, because of a relatively high complication rate with the former technique [1, 2]. We were more satisfied with the results of the Thal procedure, especially in mentally retarded patients [14, 16].

With the explosive development of minimally invasive techniques, many surgeons went back to the Nissen because of its relative simplicity. As we believed that the Thal was superior, we started to do laparoscopic Thal procedures in 1994. We have reported on the technique and on the early and long-term results [14–17, 19]. This chapter focuses on the laparoscopic anterior fundoplication technique according to Thal.

28.2 Preoperative Work-Up

All patients undergo initial contrast studies of the esophagus, stomach, and duodenum in order demonstrate concomitant hiatal herniation and to exclude distal obstruction. A preoperative pH study is performed on all patients for quantitative evaluation of GER. An enema is given the evening before the operation in order to avoid a feces-loaded transverse colon obscuring the laparoscopic view.

28.3
Technique

28.3.1
Anesthesia

General anesthesia is used in all patients, often in combination with a regional anesthesia. During the procedure full muscle relaxation is maintained. A urine catheter is only inserted when epidural anesthesia is given as well. No nasogastric tube is inserted. An 8–10 mm diameter stent is kept at hand to be inserted through the distal esophagus during the narrowing of the posterior hiatus.

28.3.2
Positioning of Patient, Crew, and Equipment

The patient is placed in the supine head-up position at the lower end of the operating table. In smaller children, the legs are put in a frog-like position (Fig. 1). The lower table sheet is folded as an envelope over the legs and clipped together on both sides in order to prevent slipping of the patient. In older children, the legs are placed in slight flexion and abduction on the leg rests of the operating table and fixed with bandage. In younger children, the surgeon stands at the lower end of the table, in the older child in between the legs. In severely scoliotic children, the position is adapted to the possibilities. It may be necessary to operate entirely from the right in these children. Limitations in join movements in pa-

tients, especially of the hip, may interfere with the movement of the endoscopic instruments. Alternative positions for these instruments should be kept in mind.

One monitor suffices but we use always two monitors. They are placed to the right and to the left of the head of the patient. The video tower usually stands at the right side, and all cables come from that same side onto the operating table. There are usually seven different cables [camera, light, CO2, outside monopolar high frequency electrocoagulation (MHFE), inside monopolar HFE, suction, and irrigation].

28.3.3
Telescope

Irrespective of age, we always use a 6-mm cannula for a 5-mm 30° telescope.

28.3.4
Instruments

In larger children, classic 5-mm instruments are used. In smaller children we use 3.5-mm instruments of either 30 or 20 cm length, depending on the size of the child. For suturing, however, we always use a 6-mm cannula.

As a liver retractor, either an Allis type instrument with ratchet is inserted below the xiphoid process underneath the left lobe of the liver and grabbing the anterior hiatus underneath the liver. This instrument usually does not need any holding. Alternatively, a Dia-

Fig. 1.
Positioning of the patient, crew, and equipment

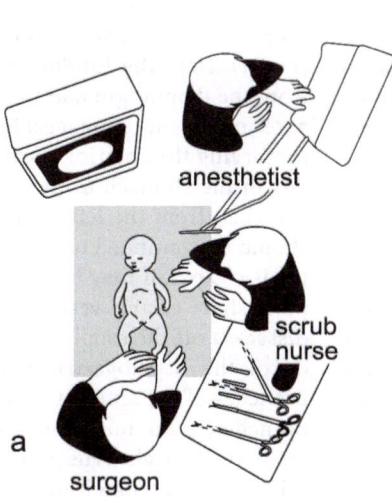

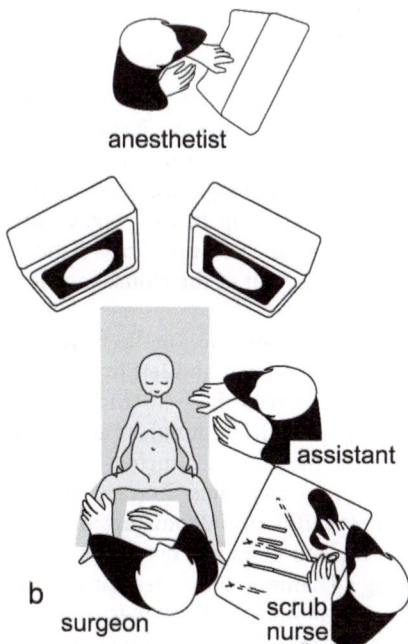

mond Flex retractor is inserted through a cannula, inserted below the right costal margin on the anterior axillary line. Such retractors are available in 5- and 3.5-mm sizes.

Once the distal esophagus has been mobilized, a vessel loop is passed around the esophagus and clipped together anteriorly with two 5-mm clips. We use a reusable clipping device for this purpose.

28.3.5
Suture Material

For the suturing we use 3_0 Ethibond interrupted sutures. The needle is straightened to fit in the 6-mm suturing cannula, and the length is cut to 10–15 cm.

28.3.6
Energy Source

MHFE usually suffices, but alternative energy sources such as ultrasonic energy can be used as well.

28.3.7
Pneumoperitoneum

The CO_2 pneumoperitoneum pressure is set at 8 mmHg and the flow at 5 L per min. It may be advantageous to increase pressure briefly up to 10 mmHg during the insertion of the secondary cannulae.

28.3.8
Cannulae

We insert five cannulae (Fig. 2). The first 6-mm cannula is inserted in an open way just below the inferior umbilical edge. If this position does not allow an adequate view of the hiatal region, a second 6-mm cannula can be inserted higher up in the epigastrium. The umbilical cannula can then be used for a Babcock for pulling on the anterior wall of the stomach or for introducing the sutures.

The two cannulae for the working instruments are placed in the right and left hypochondrium. The ideal angle in between these instruments is around 60°. The left hypochondrial cannula is always a 6-mm one and is used for dissection, suturing, and introduction of the vessel loop and clips. Retraction of the liver can be achieved either by introducing an Allis-type instrument into the abdomen just below the xiphoid process or by using a Diamond Flex retractor inserted subcostally on the right at the anterior axillary line. A last cannula is inserted pararectally at umbilical level for a Babcock to

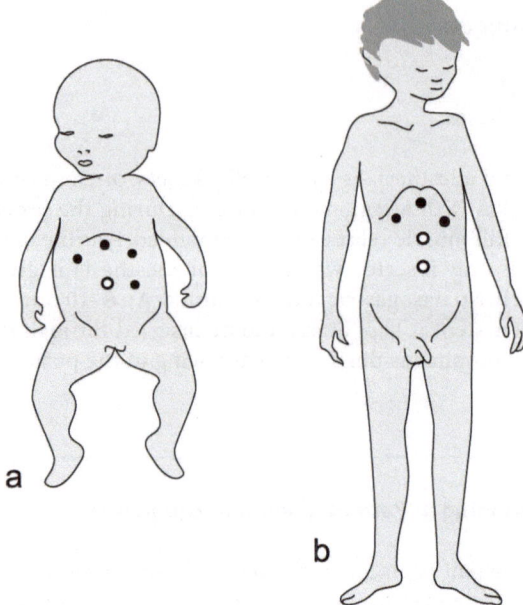

Fig. 2. Positioning of the cannulae

pull on the anterior wall of the stomach. This is only needed when the telescope has not been moved higher up in the epigastrium, in which case traction can be applied via the umbilical cannula.

28.3.9
The Procedure Itself

28.3.9.1
Hiatal Dissection and Closure

The procedure (Fig. 3) is started with the incision of the upper part of the hepatogastric ligament above the hepatic branches of the anterior vagal nerve, which are preserved. By this maneuver, the right crus is identified (Fig. 1). Next the fundus of the stomach is detached from the diaphragm and the left crus is identified. The anterior phrenoesophageal ligament is then transacted, preserving the anterior vagal nerve. By pulling the fundus of the stomach to the right, the esophagus can be detached from the left crus. The dissection on the left should be continued until the posterior part of the hiatus is cleared. It may be necessary to divide the uppermost short gastric vessels. The right crus can best be dissected off the esophagus by entering the pars flaccida of the hepatogastric ligament below the hepatic branches of the anterior vagal nerve. By elevating these branches, a thin but strong membrane is seen that covers both the right crus and the esophagus. By opening this membrane longitudinally, the groove between the

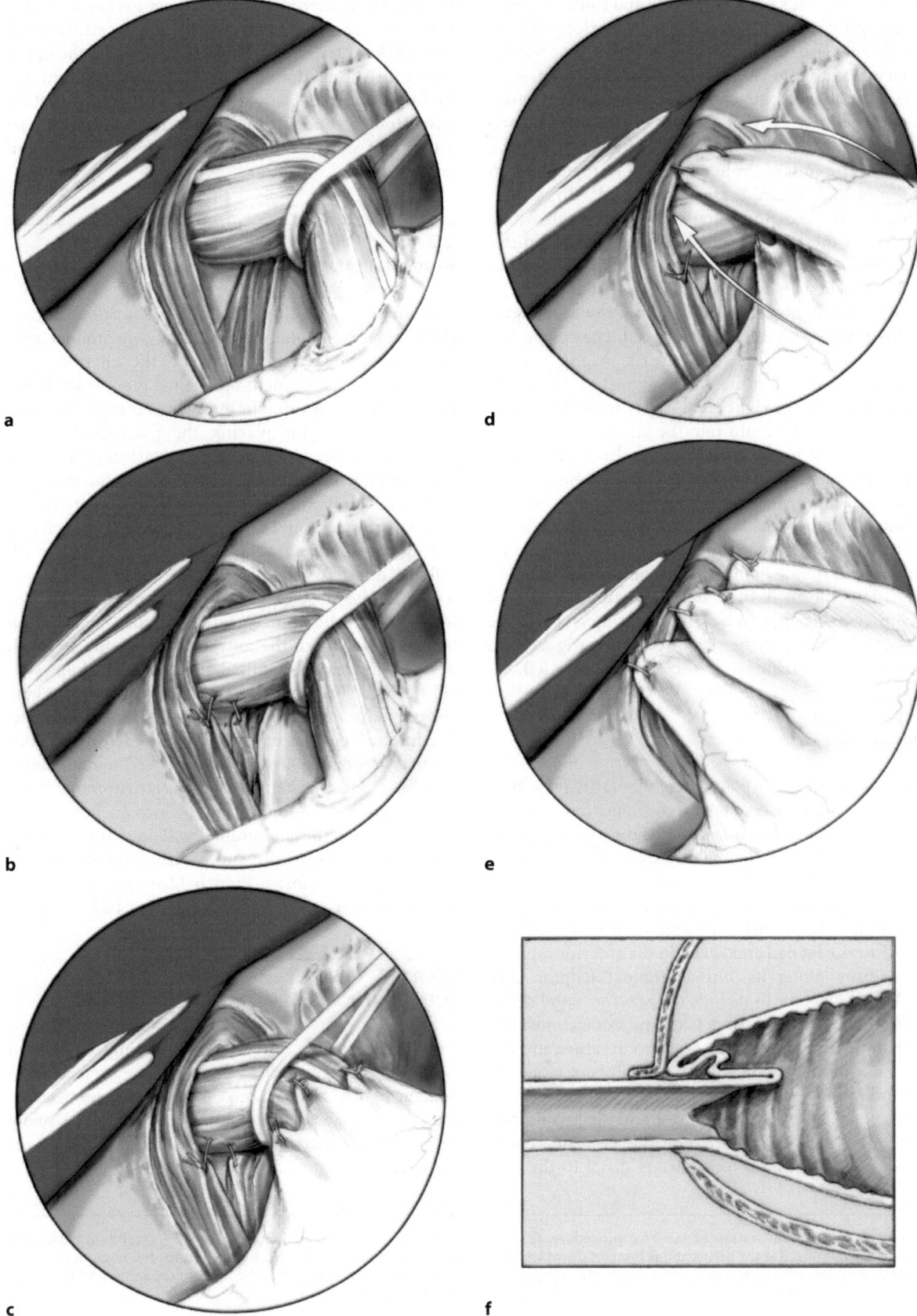

a

b

c

d

e

f

esophagus and crus becomes visible and can be dissected bluntly. By pushing the esophagus anteriorly, the area behind the esophagus opens up and the posterior vagal nerve comes into view. An instrument is now passed posterior to the nerve to enter the region above the fundus of the stomach. A vessel loop is inserted and passed behind the esophagus and above the hepatic vagal branches. The ends of the loop are clipped together with two 5-mm clips. The ends are now grasped with ratcheted forceps through the same cannula through which traction on the stomach has been exerted. The distal esophagus is now mobilized further until a sufficient part has reached an intraabdominal position.

The hiatus is now narrowed behind the esophagus. For that purpose a suture is introduced. The needle end is placed from the right behind the esophagus. The left crus is then taken, next the posterior part of the esophagus, and finally the right crus. We try to avoid including big bites of the crura into the stitches in order to prevent damage to the crura. Care is also taken not to include the posterior vagus in the stitch. Before intracorporeal tying, a stent is inserted through the esophagus into the stomach in order to prevent stenosis. In smaller children a stent diameter of 8 mm suffices, while in larger children a diameter of 10 mm is more appropriate. The suture is then tied. Sometimes a second stitch may be needed. In a case presenting a very large hiatus, the hiatus may be narrowed anteriorly as well. Alternatively, the hiatus may be closed from the left.

28.3.9.2
Fundoplication

For the fundoplication, two rows of three stitches will be placed. The stitching is started at the upper left. A bite of the stomach is taken just in front of the greater curvature a few centimeters below the esophagogastric junction. Next the left wall of the esophagus is taken about midway along the intraabdominal length. The next stitch is placed anteriorly on the stomach a few centimeters below the fat pad and again on the anterior esophagus halfway along its intraabdominal length. Care should be taken not to include the anterior vagal nerve in the stitch. The third stitch takes the stomach just anterior to the upper part of the lesser curvature and the right side of the esophagus again half-way along its intraabdominal length.

The vessel loop is now removed, and the second row of the three stitches is started on the left. The greater curvature is taken a few centimeters distal to the first

stitch and is anchored to the left upper part of the intraabdominal esophagus and the left crus. A second stitch anchors the anterior part of the stomach onto the upper part of the intraabdominal esophagus and the anterior rim of the hiatus. A last stitch takes the lesser curvature of the stomach and anchors it onto the uppermost part of the right side of the intraabdominal esophagus and the right crus.

28.3.10
Concomitant Gastrostomy

In children with feeding difficulties, as is often the case when they are mentally retarded, a concomitant gastrostomy may be required. As part of the anterior stomach wall has been brought up against the intraabdominal esophagus and diaphragm, less anterior stomach wall is available for placing the gastrostomy. Care should be taken not to insert the gastrostomy too low, as this may interfere with the gastric outlet, for example, causing intermittent balloon obstruction. Alternatively the gastrostomy should not be put into the stomach in a too-high position, as traction onto the anterior stomach wall may interfere with the fundoplication. The best way to identify the most appropriate place for the gastrostomy is to inflate the stomach with a gastroscope, and then to determine where the anterior wall of the stomach meets the anterior abdominal most easily. By doing so it will become clear that the optimal position for a gastrostomy after a Thal fundoplication is the upper epigastrium rather than midway along the left hypochondrium. We use a laparoscopic-controlled percutaneous technique for the placement of the gastrostomy catheter at the end of the fundoplication [6]. Two anchors are inserted through the abdominal wall into the stomach under both laparoscopic and gastroscopic control. In between both anchors a French 12 or 14 gastrostomy catheter is inserted with a Seldinger-type technique.

28.3.11
Postoperative Course

No nasogastric tube is left behind. Feedings are started the day after surgery. When these feeding are well tolerated, the patient is discharged. A urine catheter is left in situ for as long as epidural anesthesia is given. Usually the epidural catheter, as well as the urine catheter, is removed on the first postoperative day.

Fig. 3a–f. Schematic illustration of the Thal procedure. (**a**) The esophagus is mobilized at the hiatus and is brought down well below the diaphragm. (**b**) The hiatus is closed behind the esophagus, taking a bite of esophagus in the suture. (**c**) First row of three stitches of the fundoplication. The anterior gastric wall is sutured to the anterior esophagus halfway along its intraabdominal length. (**d**) The second row of three stitches sutures the anterior stomach to the upper part of the intraabdominal esophagus and to the adjacent diaphragm

28.4
Results

In the period 1993–2001, 149 patients underwent a laparoscopic antigastroesophageal reflux procedure [19]; 49% was mentally retarded. One hundred-forty of the patients underwent a laparoscopic Thal procedure (93%), the remaining nine a Nissen procedure. The median follow-up period was 4.5 years (range: 6 months to 9 years). Nineteen patients, all mentally retarded, died during the follow-up period. In only one patient was the cause of death related to the procedure. He developed multi-organ failure as a result of peritonitis due to incorrect use of the gastrostomy feeding tube. In 29 patients the results were less than optimal, and eight of these patients (5.7%) underwent a redo-operation. However, none of the patients with a follow-up of more than 5 years show any symptoms.

28.5
Discussion

The laparoscopic Thal procedure as described is a straightforward procedure and seems to work well [1, 19], not only in children but also in adults [22]. The effectiveness of an anterior fundoplication has also been proven experimentally [21]. Of interest is a recent publication reporting good results after a 90° anterior wrap [8]. The anterior fundoplication seems also to work well when applied in neurologically impaired children [10, 16]. Although the results of the anterior fundoplication in children after esophageal atresia repair are less good, the results are better than those of the Nissen fundoplication [11].

The technique of adding a gastrostomy has been described before [6]. Classically a gastrostomy is created in the left hypochondrium halfway between the costal margin and the umbilicus. As pointed out earlier in this chapter, the gastrostomy after an anterior fundoplication should be inserted higher up in the epigastrium. Otherwise the catheter may be too close to the gastric outlet, and the balloon of the gastrostomy may cause gastric outlet obstruction. In children who have had a prior percutaneous endoscopic gastrostomy, subsequent Thal fundoplication can be performed without much difficulty [18].

References

1. Ashcraft KW, Goodwin CD, Armoury RA (1978) Thal fundoplication: a simple and safe operative treatment for gastroesophageal reflux. J Pediatr Surg 13:643–647
2. Boix-Ochoa J, Rowe MI (1998) Gastroesophageal reflux, In: O'Neill JA Jr, Rowe MI, Grosfeld JL, Fonkalsrud EW, Coran AG (eds) Pediatric Surgery, Mosby-Year Book, St. Louis, pp 1007–1028
3. Bohmer CJ, Niezen-de Boer MC, Klinkenberg-Knol EC, Deville WL, Nadorp JH, Meuwissen SG (1999) The prevalence of gastroesophageal reflux disease in institutionalized intellectually disabled individuals. Am J Gastroenterol 94:804–810
4. Foglia RP (1997) Gastroesophageal reflux, In Oldham KT, Colombani PM, Foglia RP (eds) Surgery of Infants and Children, Lippincott-Raven, Philadelphia, pp 1035–1047
5. Gold BD, Freston JW (2002) Gastroesophageal reflux in children: pathogenesis, prevalence, diagnosis, and role of proton pump inhibitors in treatment. Paediatr Drugs 4:673–685
6. Hament JM, Bax NM, van der Zee DC, De Schryver JE, Nesselaar C (2001) Complications of percutaneous endoscopic gastrostomy with or without concomitant antireflux surgery in 96 children. J Pediatr Surg 36:1412–1415
7. Kimber C, Kiely EM, Spitz L (1998) The failure rate of surgery for gastro-oesophageal reflux. J Pediatr Surg 33:64–66
8. Krysztopik RJ, Jamieson GG, Devitt PG, Watson DI (2002) A further modification of fundoplication. 90 degrees anterior fundoplication. Surg Endosc 16:1446–1451
9. Pearl RH, Robie DK, Ein SH, Shanling B, Wesson DE, Superina R, Mctaggart K, Garcia VF, O´Connor FA, Filler RM (1990) Complications of gastroesophageal antireflux surgery in neurologically impaired versus neurological normal children. J Pediatr Surg 25:1169–1173
10. Ramachandran V, Ashcraft KW, Sharp RJ, Murphy PJ, Snyder CL, Gittes GK, Bickler SW (1996) Thal fundoplication in neurologically impaired children. J Pediatr Surg 31:819–822
11. Snyder CL, Ramachandran V, Kennedy AP, Gittes GK, Ashcraft KW, Holder TM (1997) Efficacy of partial wrap fundoplication for gastroesophageal reflux after repair of esophageal atresia. J Pediatr Surg 32:1089–1091
12. Sydorak RM, Albanese CT (2002) Laparoscopic antireflux procedures in children: evaluating the evidence. Semin Laparosc Surg 9:133–138
13. Tovar JA, Angulo JA, Gorostiaga L, Arana J (1991) Surgery for gastroesophageal reflux in children with normal pH studies. J Pediatr Surg 26:541–545
14. van der Zee DC, Rövekamp MH, Pull ter Gunne AJ, Bax NMA (1994) Surgical treatment for reflux esophagitis: Nissen versus Thal procedure. Pediatr Surg Int 9:334–227
15. van der Zee DC, Bax NMA (1995) Laparoscopic Thal fundoplication in severely scoliotic children. Surg Endosc 9:1197–1198
16. van der Zee DC, Bax NMA (1996) Laparoscopic Thal in mentally retarded children. Surg Endosc 10:659–661
17. van der Zee DC, Arends NJT, Bax NMA (1999) The value of 24-h Ph study in evaluating the results of laparoscopic antireflux surgery in children. Surg Endosc 13:918–21
18. van der Zee DC, Bax NM, Ure BM (2000) Laparoscopic secondary antireflux procedure after PEG placement in children. Percutaneous endoscopic gastrostomy. Surg Endosc 14:1105–1106
19. van der Zee DC, Bax NMA, Ure BM, Besselink MG, Pakvis DF (2002) Long-term results after laparoscopic Thal procedure in children. Semin Laparosc Surg 9:168–171
20. Watson DI, Jamieson GG (1999) Antireflux surgery in the laparoscopic era. Br J Surg 86 :571–572
21. Watson DI, Mathew G, Pike GK, Baigrie RJ, Jamieson GG (1998) Efficacy of anterior, posterior and total fundoplication in an experimental model. Br J Surg 85:1006–1009
22. Watson DI, Jamieson GG, Pike GK, Davies N, Richardson M, Devitt PG (1999) Prospective randomized double-blind trial between laparoscopic Nissen fundoplication and anterior partial fundoplication. Br J Surg 86:123–30
23. Wenner J, Nilsson G, Oberg S, Melin T, Larsson S, Johnsson F (2001) Short-term outcome after laparoscopic and open 360 degrees fundoplication. A prospective randomized trial. Surg Endosc 15:1124–1128

Chapter 29

Boix-Ochoa Procedure

29

Jose Boix Ochoa · Jesus Broto

Contents

29.1
Introduction

Although all existing techniques for the correction of GERD have the same aim, each surgeon has his or her own personal preference based on background and training [1, 2]. After reviewing some of the better-known techniques, such as Toupet, Nissen, and Thal, we will deal with a method specially applicable to pediatric patients: the Boix-Ochoa (BO) technique.

The open procedure [3] was described by Boix Ochoa in 1983. The basis of the philosophy that led to the development of this technique was the idea of restoring the anatomic mechanisms which, under physiological circumstances, prevent reflux [4]. The BO technique is fundamentally based on the physiological reconstruction of the cardiohiatal junction, seeking a normalization of the antireflux mechanisms and placing the organic structures as close as possible to their physiological location.

The fundamental aim of this procedure is to restore and maintain the length of the infradiaphragmatic segment of the esophagus. This is anchored to the margins of the diaphragmatic hiatus, with the goal of re-establishing the pressure barrier, while reconstructing an acute angle of His and unfolding the gastric fundus [5]. This enhances the mechanical closing of the esophagus in order to reinforce the lover esophageal sphincter (LES) [6].

The anterior wrap described by Boix Ochoa has the same success rate as that of the most commonly performed procedure, the 360° wrap described by Nissen, but also has the distinctive advantages of allowing most of the patients to burp and vomit, as well as causing a minimal incidence of serious "gas bloat" syndrome [7, 8].

29.2
Technical Details

To facilitate the approach to the distal esophagus, a pillow is placed under the patient's back at the level of the lower ribs, with a nasogastric tube already in place (Fig. 1).

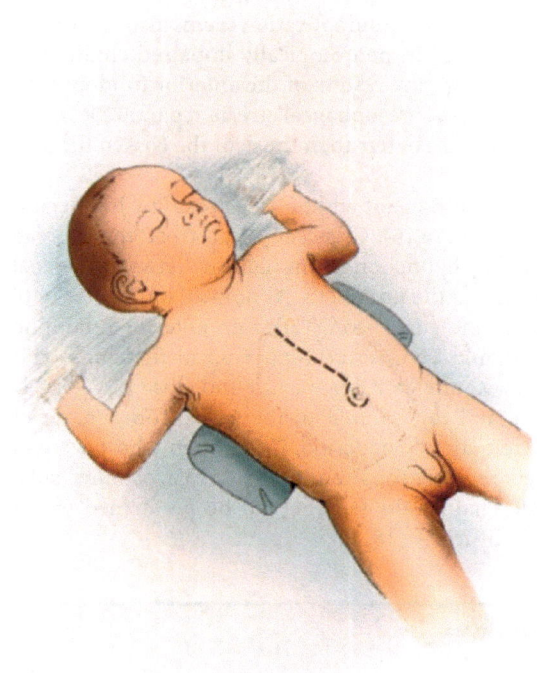

Fig. 1. (Hiatus 1) A pillow is placed under the patient at the level of the lower ribs

The hiatus area is approached through a supra-umbilical midline incision, ligating the umbilical vessels to ease the handling of the liver. This is retracted downwards, and the left triangular ligament which attaches the left liver lobe to the diaphragm is divided, paying special attention to not enlarge the dissection beyond the middle line in order to avoid injury to the suprahepatic veins.

Once the left lobe of the liver is free, it is turned downwards protected by a sponge and retracted to the right by the second assistant, who stands cranial to the surgeon. Then, in the right side of the stomach, the esophagohepatic ligament is divided, paying close attention to the potential existence of a left hepatic artery growing from the gastric artery, which must be preserved.

The distal esophagus is exposed by blunt dissection, allowing a dissector to be introduced behind it, permitting the passage of a vessel-loop, tape, or plastic sling to surround the esophagus, which is then used for downward traction. Stay sutures are placed on the right, left, and anterior arch of the pillars to retract them.

The distal intrathoracic esophagus is denuded by blunt dissection in a variable length of 3–6 cm depending on the infant's size, taking care to avoid injury to the pleural fold.

The hiatus should now be completely visible and the esophagus free and mobile (Fig. 2).

To maintain a fixed length of the infradiaphragmatic esophagus, three 2/0 non-absorbable U-sutures are passed pillar–esophagus–pillar to anchor it to hiatal margins, and tied while pushing the diaphragm cranially and pulling down the esophageal traction tape.

Once the esophagus is anchored to the hiatus, the posterior crossing of the pillars must be closed by applying two or three crural sutures, avoiding excessive tightening that can produce dysphagia or loosening that may lead to a parahiatal hernia (Fig. 3).

The greater curvature of the stomach must be dissected and mobilized so that the upper portion of the gastric fundus can be placed without any tension over the right pillar of the hiatus to create a new reinforced His angle. This step could require the division of the upper two short gastric vessels in order to obtain a tension-free gastric fundus covering the distal esophagus and right pillar (Fig. 4).

A nonabsorbable 0-suture is placed from the great curvature to the right crus/pillar, maintaining the tension on the tape that pulls down the esophagus in order to produce a more pronounced angle of His. A further three or four 2/0 nonabsorbable sutures are placed between the rim of mobilized gastric fundus and the right lateral margin of the intra-abdominal esophagus, consolidating the new His angle.

To maintain an open fundus, it must be unfolded upwards like an umbrella. To achieve this, three 2/0 non-

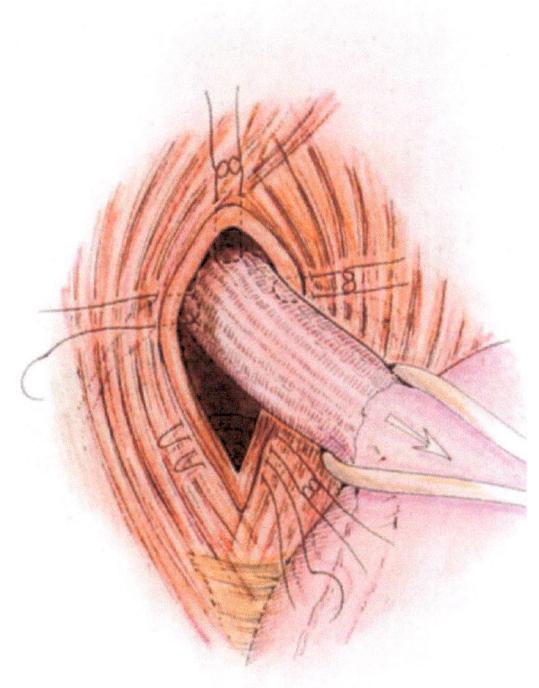

Fig. 2. (Hiatus 2) After the dissection, the esophagus should be free and mobile

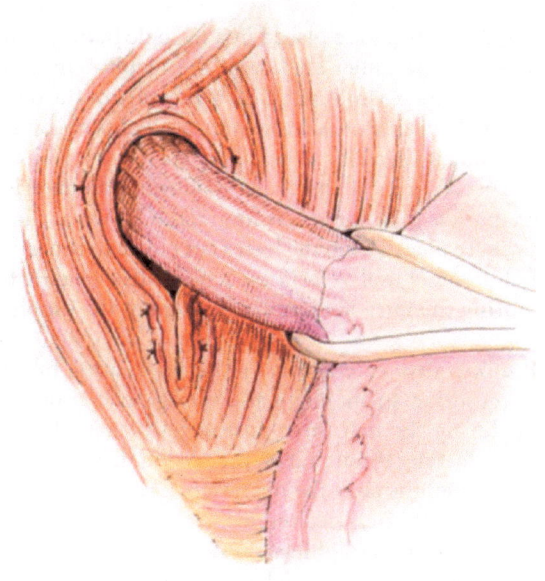

Fig. 3. (Hiatus 3) The esophagus is anchored to the hiatus with three nonresorbable sutures. The posterior crossing of the pillars must be closed with one or two sutures avoiding excessive tightening

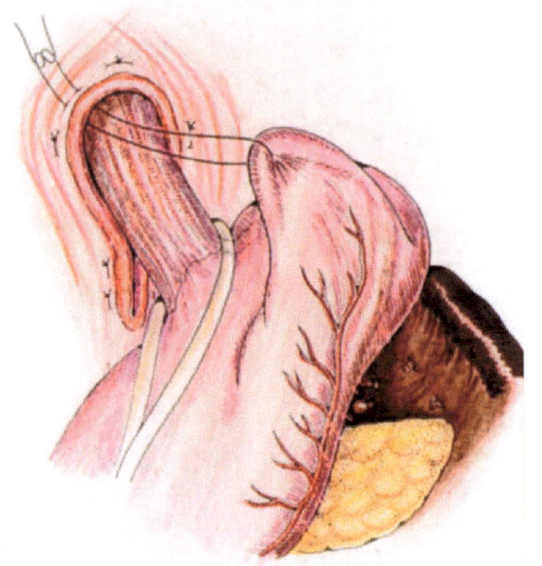

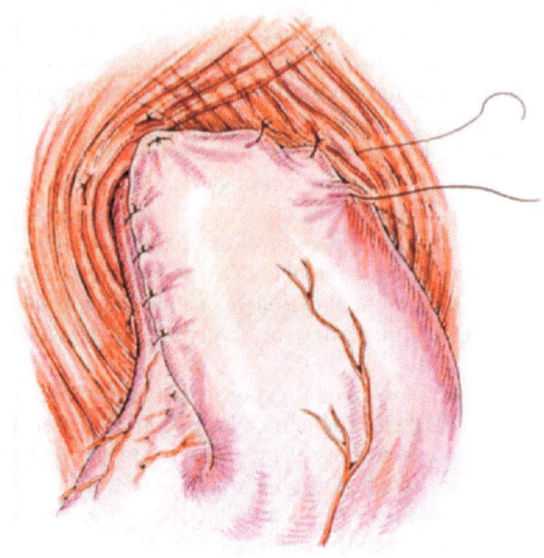

Fig. 4. (Hiatus 4) A fundus plap is performed in order to cover the distal esophagus and right pillar, consolidating the new His angle

Fig. 5. (Hiatus 5) Three nonresorbable sutures are placed in triangle between the fundus and the under surface of diaphragm

absorbable sutures are placed in a triangle between the fundus and the under surface of the diaphragm. This enables any increase in intragastric pressure of the open fundus to be transmitted against the wall of the esophagus, closing it (Fig. 5).

In special cases of shortened esophagus, an anterior Boerema-like gastropexy is recommended. Two or three sutures are placed from the lesser curvature to the anterior abdominal wall to facilitate tension-free healing by anchoring the intra-abdominal segment of the esophagus.

Postoperative care is most often uneventful, taking the precaution to maintain the nasogastric probe in place during the first three postoperative days, beginning the feeding through it on the second day.

Three months after the operation, a radiological assessment must be carried out to check the morphological aspect of the cardiohiatal crossroad and to evaluate whether the reflux has completely disappeared.

To complete the postoperative control, a 24-h pH study is performed at six-months postintervention.

References

1. Bettex M, Oesch I (1983) The hiatus hernia saga. Ups and downs in gastroesophageal reflux: past, present and future perspectives. J Pediatr Surg 18: 670–680
2. Boix Ochoa J (1986) Gastroesophageal reflux. In: Welch K et al., (eds) Pediatric Surgery, Mosby-Year Book, St. Louis
3. Boix Ochoa J, Casasa JM, Gil-Vernet JM (1983) Une chirurgie physiologique pour les anomalies du secteur cardiohiatal. Chir Pediatr 24: 117–120
4. Boix Ochoa J (1986) The physiologic approach to the management of gastric esophageal reflux. J Pediatr Surg 21: 1032–1039
5. Bardaji C, Boix-Ochoa J (1986) Contribution of the His angle to the gastroesophageal antireflux mechanism. Pediatr Surg Int 1: 172–174
6. Casasa JM, Boix-Ochoa J (1977) Surgical or conservative treatment in hiatal hernias in children: a new decisive parameter. Surgery 82: 573–575
7. Boix-Ochoa J, Casasa JM (1989)Surgical treatment of gastroesophageal reflux in children. Surg Annu 21: 97–118
8. Cohen Z, et al. (1999) Nissen fundoplication and Boix-Ochoa antireflux procedure: comparison between two surgical techniques in the treatment of gastroesophageal reflux in children. Eur J Pediatr Surg 9(5): 289–293

Chapter 30

Other Antireflux Procedures in Infants with GERD

30

Pedro Olivares · Antonio Leggio

Other surgical procedures have been used for the treatment of gastroesophageal reflux, and new endoscopic and laparoscopic techniques are still being proposed. Although seldom used these days, the operation proposed by Narbona enjoyed some popularity in the past in Europe. In this procedure, the liver round ligament is divided at its entrance into the parenchyme, passed around the distal intraabdominal esophagus, and sutured on itself to form a loop that tractions the incisura angularis downwards, thus lengthening the intraabdominal esophagus and sharpening the angle of His. Its technical simplicity made it suitable for laparoscopic approach [1–3]. There are no recent references about its use but, according to the existing clinical, manometric, and pH-metric evidence, it was effective in the treatment of reflux.

Another technique used in children is the gastropexy or anterior fixation of the stomach to the abdominal wall. It was performed as an isolated procedure or associated with other actions on either the crura or the angle of His. Although its rationale was sound and the clinical results were in general good, it seems that these were not maintained over time, with frequent recurrence of the symptoms and functional evidence of failure of the reconstructed barrier. The first references to this technique in children were by Vos and Boerema [4], who proposed it particularly for neurologically impaired children because the relatively high morbidity of regular fundoplication in them made a milder valve advisable (Fig. 1).

A 1983 study by De Laet and Spitz showed the clear advantages of Nissen fundoplication over gastropexy, both in terms of clinical results and postoperative morbidity, and after this publication, gastropexy lost some of its popularity [5]. Procedures used in adults such as Belsey Mark IV have not been used in children. This 270° transthoracic fundoplication does not seem well adapted to children, although its video-assisted performance has been occasionally proposed [6, 7].

Another interesting procedure adopted in children is the Lortat-Jacob operation. The aim of this procedure is to obtain a long abdominal esophageal segment of at least 3–4 cm and to restore the correct anatomy of the

cardiotuberosity region. The technique consists of reducing the width of the esophageal hiatus, securing the esophagus to diaphragmatic hiatus, recreating the His angle, and reestablishing the gastric fundus below the diaphragm (Fig. 2).

The prosthesis developed by Angelchik has not been applied in children, because of its allegedly frequent complications and reoperations. This crescent-shaped silastic prosthesis was easily inserted around the lower esophagus, but it was frequently dislodged and caused

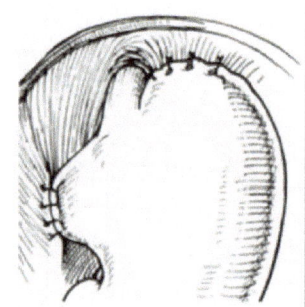

Fig. 1. Gastropexy according to Boerema's procedure

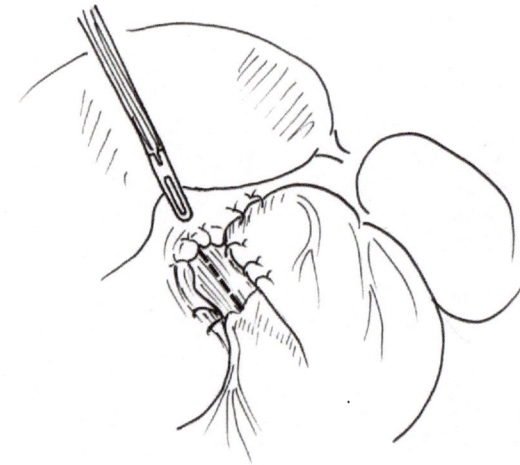

Fig. 2. Antireflux procedure according to Lortat-Jacob's technique

erosions of the wall, leading to up to 25% reoperations in some series. To our knowledge, it is not presently used in children [8–10].

Operations aiming at lengthening the intraabdominal esophagus and deepening the angle of His developed once suitable stapling instruments became available. Collis gastroplasty, in which the intraabdominal esophagus is lengthened by a double line of staples on the fundus parallel to the esophageal axis and starting at the angle of His and section of the gastric fundus along this line, has been performed several times, particularly in association with Belsey and Nissen antireflux procedures [11]. This operation is still used by some authors, particularly in older children. An uncut modification of the Collis technique was recently proposed, with apparently good results in the hands of its developers [12]. After the first descriptions of the endoscopic approach to the gastric chamber by Gauderer et al. [13] for creating a percutaneous gastrostomy, a combined endoscopic-laparoscopic approach was developed for plicating intragastrically the gastroesophageal junction using a laparoscopic endostapler. These procedures seem promising in the laboratory [14, 15]. The idea of performing an endoluminal plication is interesting because some postoperative problems such as dysphagia, stenosis, and valve failure could be controlled. Vagal or pleural lesions would be avoided, along with injury to other neighboring organs. However, these techniques have not become widespread, probably because of the current development of laparoscopic surgery for GER.

We are now witnessing the rapid development of more equipment and techniques for endoluminal or intraesophageal treatment of gastroesophageal reflux [16]. At least three such techniques have been developed. The first is the reinforcement of the intraesophageal barrier by plication with several stitches of the cardial area that would increase its thickness and improve the valve mechanism [17–19]. This procedure is spreading rapidly for the treatment of refluxing adults, but its application to children is limited due to problems with the size of the endoscopes required. Its development is based on the relatively easy insertion by intraesophageal route alone, its reversibility, its reduced cost, and the encouraging results observed in the short and midterms. It is contraindicated when a hiatal hernia or other associated anatomical anomalies are present. Severe esophagitis or columnar dysplasia (Barrett's esophagus) are other contraindications.

Another intraluminal technique proposed is the application of thermic energy (laser and radiofrequency) on the four quadrants of the distal esophagus. The device is easily located intraesophageally and consists of a balloon that, once positioned in the cardias under direct view, allows insertion of four electrodes that release thermic energy to the mucosa, submucosa, and muscle

layers of the esophagus, inducing burns and edema. The subsequent healing and scarring contribute to create an antireflux barrier that, according to the developers of the technique, would mature along the ensuing one or two years. Some comparisons between this procedure and long-term medication have been published [16, 19].

The third method is the implantation of a nondegradable, biocompatible polymer in several submucosal pouches at the lower esophageal or cardial levels [20–22]. This injectable fluid (Enteryx) is inspired by those currently used in the treatment of vesico-ureteral reflux, with good results in well selected cases. This alternative is easy and attractive and has been used by several groups with apparent good results [23]. Certainly other procedures are being developed. Reflux is frequent. The price of long-term or lifelong medication is high, and the demands of the adult and pediatric populations for new minimally invasive, endoluminal techniques able to provide a durable cure are growing.

References

1. Nathanson LK, Shimi S, Cuschieri A (1991) Laparoscopic ligamentum teres (round ligament) cardiopexy. Br J Surg 78: 947–951
2. Meyer C, De Manzini N, Rohr S, Thiry CL, Perraud V (1994) Traitement laparoscopique du reflux gastro-oesophagien. Cardiopexie par le ligament rond versus fundoplicature de type Nissen. Chirurgie 120:107–112
3. Narbona B, Olavarrieta L, Lloris JM, de Lera F, Calvo MA (1990) Le traitement du reflux gastro-oesophagien par pexie avec le ligament rond. A propos de 100 operés suivis entre 16 et 23 années. Chirurgie 116:201–210
4. Vos A, Boerema I (1971) Surgical treatment of gastroesophageal reflux in infants and children: Long-term results in 28 cases. J Pediatr Surg 6:101–111
5. De Laet M, Spitz L (1983) A comparison of Nissen fundoplication and Boerema gastropexy in the surgical treatment of gastro-oesophageal reflux in children. Br J Surg 70:125–127
6. Alexiou C, Salama FD, Beggs D, Brackenbury ET, Knowles KR (1999) Comparison of long-term results of total fundoplication gastroplasty and Belsey Mark IV antireflux operations in relation to the severity of oesophagitis. Eur J Cardiothorac Surg 15:320–326
7. Masclee AA, Horbach JM, Ledeboer M, Lamers CB, Gooszen HG (1998) Prospective study of the effect of the Belsey Mark IV fundoplication on reflux mechanisms. Scand J Gastroenterol 33:905–910
8. Bonavina L, DeMeester T, Mason R, Stein HJ, Feussner H, Evander A (1997) Mechanical effect of the Angelchik prosthesis on the competency of the gastric cardia: pathophysiologic implications and surgical perspectives. Dis Esophagus 10:115–118
9. Maxwell-Armstrong CA, Steele RJ, Amar SS, Evans D, Morris DL, Foster GE, Hardcastle JD (1997) Long-term results of the Angelchik prosthesis for gastro-oesophageal reflux. Br J Surg 84:862–864
10. Varshney S, Kelly JJ, Branagan G, Somers SS, Kelly JM (2002) Angelchik prosthesis revisited. World J Surg 26:129–133
11. Ritter MP, Peters JH, DeMeester TR, Gadenstatter M, Oberg S, Fein M, Hagen JA, Crookes PF, Bremner CG (1998) Treatment of advanced gastroesophageal reflux disease with Collis gastroplasty and Belsey partial fundoplication. Arch Surg 133: 523–528, discussion 8–9
12. Mutaf O, Abasiyanik A, Karaca I, Arikan A, Mir E (2003) Treatment of gastroesophageal reflux with a gastric tube cardioplasty. J Pediatr Surg 38:571–574

13. Gauderer MW, Ponsky JL, Izant RJ, Jr (1980) Gastrostomy without laparotomy: A percutaneous endoscopic technique. J Pediatr Surg 15:872–875
14. Mason RJ, Filipi CJ, DeMeester TR, Peters JH, Lund RJ, Flake AW, Hinder RA, Smyrk TC, Bremner CG, Thompson S (1997) A new intraluminal antigastroesophageal reflux procedure in baboons. Gastrointest Endosc 45:283–290
15. Jennings RW, Flake AW, Mussan G, Harrison MR, Adzick NS, Pellegrini CA (1992) A novel endoscopic transgastric fundoplication procedure for gastroesophageal reflux: An initial animal evaluation. J Laparoendosc Surg 2:207–213
16. Roy-Shapira A, Stein HJ, Scwartz D, Fich A, Sonnenschein E. (2002) Endoluminal methods of treating gastroesophageal reflux disease. Dis Esophagus 15:132–136
17. Swain CP, Mills TN (1986) An endoscopic sewing machine. Gastrointest Endosc 32:36–38
18. Swain CP, Brown GJ, Mills TN (1989) An endoscopic stapling device: The development of a new flexible endoscopically controlled device for placing multiple transmural staples in gastrointestinal tissue. Gastrointest Endosc 35:338–339
19. Galmiche JP, des Varannes SB (2003) Endoluminal therapies for gastro-oesophageal reflux disease. Lancet 361:1119–1121
20. Deviere J, Pastorelli A, Louis H, de Maertelaer V, Lehman G, Cicala M, Le Moine O, Silverman D, Costamagna G (2002) Endoscopic implantation of a biopolymer in the lower esophageal sphincter for gastroesophageal reflux: A pilot study. Gastrointest Endosc 55:335–341
21. Johnson DA, Ganz R, Aisenberg J, Cohen LB, Deviere J, Foley TR, Haber GB, Peters JH, Lehman GA (2003) Endoscopic, deep mural implantation of Enteryx for the treatment of GERD: 6-month follow-up of a multicenter trial. Am J Gastroenterol 98: 250–258
22. Mason RJ, Hughes M, Lehman GA, Chiao G, Deviere J, Silverman DE, DeMeester TR, Peters JH (2002) Endoscopic augmentation of the cardia with a biocompatible injectable polymer (Enteryx) in a porcine model. Surg Endosc 16: 386–391
23. Montinaro L, Paradies G, Leggio A (2002) The Lortat-Jacob operation by laparoscopic access to treat gastroesophageal reflux in pediatric patients. Surg Endosc 16 1438–1440

Chapter 31

Esophagogastric Dissociation   31

Adrian Bianchi

Contents

31.1
Introduction

Gastroesophageal reflux (GER) is a common condition affecting all age groups. It occurs in isolation but is also associated with other conditions such as hiatus hernia, esophageal atresia, and congenital diaphragmatic hernia, which themselves require surgery. GER is not infrequent in children suffering from mental subnormality. In infants and young children, the condition frequently follows a benign course and often resolves with growth and alteration in dietary habit. GER may however be persistent, leading to minor but controllable discomfort such as "intermittent heartburn," or it may be aggressive with serious consequences of esophagitis, such as significant gastrointestinal bleeding and esophageal obstruction from inflammatory or fibrous stenosis. Constant vomiting leads to failure to thrive physically, but there is often also a significant degree of emotional deprivation because of a reluctance to cuddle the child for fear of "vomiting and another mess."

In the otherwise normal child, GER commonly responds to a conservative "medical" approach involving dietary adjustments and reduction in gastric acid output. Failure of conservative management is an indication for surgery. The normally swallowing child is best managed by fundoplication, either through a conventional "open" abdominal approach or by the "minimally invasive" laparoscopic route, with the surgeon also able to convert to an open approach when relevant. Even in this group there is an appreciable incidence of recurrence of GER after fundoplication.

Mentally subnormal children and others with pharyngeal neuromuscular incoordination leading to swallowing difficulties and food aspiration are often nasogastrically tube-fed in order to maintain hydration and weight. As the child grows, the passage of a nasogastric tube becomes increasingly difficult for the child's caregivers, and such children are eventually referred to a surgeon for consideration of a feeding gastrostomy. In a study by Langer et al. [4], of 50 patients without demonstrable reflux, some 44% (22 patients) developed GER after insertion of a feeding gastrostomy alone, and 17 came to additional antireflux surgery. We disagree with those authors' conclusions and believe that serious consideration should be given to a "package" which includes a primary antireflux procedure and placement of a feeding gastrostomy.

GER in association with pharyngeal neuromuscular incoordination is of major concern. Swallowing difficulties are often exacerbated by a tendency for severe retching, and reflux and significant food aspiration into the trachea. Inadequate food intake and loss through vomiting lead to failure to thrive. Recurrent aspiration pneumonitis forces frequent, lengthy, and stressful hospitalization for debilitating "chest infections." In addition there is a constant need for replacement of the dislodged nasogastric feeding tube. Over time such "daily battles" detract severely from the quality of life of the child and his family. They seek permanent relief from these unending difficulties, which take up the major portion of their days and nights. It is often at this late stage that the surgeon is consulted, as a "last resort." Even in this group, surgical management may take the form of Open or Laparoscopic Fundoplication combined with a feeding gastrostomy. However some 7–35% of children will develop recurrent reflux some 2–5 years later, forcing unwelcome consideration of additional, more complex, and potentially hazardous surgery [5] with a much greater risk of esophageal injury, stricture formation, and possible esophageal replacement. The fragile subnormal child with established pharyngeal neuromuscular incoordination, compromised lungs, and failure to thrive physically and mentally can ill afford repeated and potentially catastrophic surgery. He asks for the least number of interventions towards an easier and more manageable feeding technique, and a guarantee of effective relief from the consequences of GER, with no risk of reflux recurrence or additional secondary surgery. Oesophagogastric dissociation (OGD) completely detaches the esophagus from the stomach, and is specifically designed as an alternative to fundoplication to eliminate the risk of recurrence of GER [1]. The esophagus is necessarily drained into an isoperistaltic and hence inherently antireflux, jejunal Roux loop and bowel continuity is established by end-to-side jejunojejunostomy. Access to the stomach is then only through the gastrostomy.

31.2
Investigations

By the time a child is referred to a surgeon, the primary diagnosis and the neurological status have already been well established. Clinical evidence of GER, failure to thrive, and "poor chest" are evident, as are the frustration and the necessary total commitment of the parents. Videofluoroscopic studies confirm incoordinate swallowing and may demonstrate aspiration, and contrast radiology shows reflux which can be further evaluated by lower esophageal pH monitoring. Detailed assessment of the respiratory tract is particularly relevant to anesthesia and a trouble-free postoperative course. It is often useful to determine esophageal pathology, e.g., stenosis, gastric motility, and pyloric function. Evidence of delayed gastric emptying may suggest consideration of a pyloroplasty.

31.3
Operative Technique

The abdomen is opened through a transverse left hypochondrial incision (Fig. 1). The left lobe of the liver is detached from the diaphragm and retracted medially to allow access to the esophagus and the esophageal hiatus. The lower esophagus is mobilized as for a fundoplication, visualizing and carefully preserving the vagus nerves, and is then transected at the gastroesophageal junction. The stomach is oversewn.

A 40-cm isoperistaltic jejunal loop is prepared in Roux-en-Y fashion on a liberal vascular pedicle, and is passed through the transverse mesocolon and behind the stomach to reach the esophagus at the lesser curve without torsion or tension on the blood supply. A wide esophago-jejunal anastomosis is performed, and a naso-jejunal tube appropriately positioned. Stomach-to-small bowel continuity is established by an end-to-side jejunojejunal anastomosis placed at least 40 cm below the esophageal anastomosis. A pyloroplasty is added in

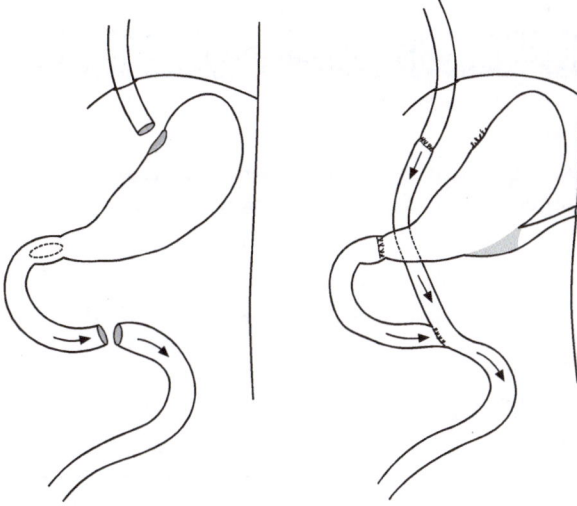

Fig. 1. Esophagogastric dissociation, fashioning of 40-cm isoperistaltic jejunal Roux loop, esophago-jejunal anastomosis, jejunojejunostomy, gastrostomy, and optional pyloroplasty

the event of possible injury to the vagus nerves, a history of severe retching, or delayed gastric emptying.

A tube or button gastrostomy is placed on the anterior surface of the stomach. Alternatively, a vascularized nonrefluxing gastric tube (Fig. 1) based on the right gastroepiploic vessels [2] is constructed from the greater curve of the stomach, and brought to the abdominal wall as an intermittently catheterizable feeding stoma. Antibiotics are given at surgery and postoperatively. The stomach is drained freely through an open gastrostomy until motility returns. Feeding is allowed in graded fashion, usually from the third postoperative day and once bowel function has returned. At this time and subsequently, oral food intake of any variety is also permissible to the child's tolerance and inclination.

31.4
Series

In our Unit, since inception of the technique, 32 children have undergone esophagogastric dissociation. The procedure was undertaken "primarily" (Group 1) as the single definitive antireflux operation in 13 children with severe permanent pharyngeal neuromuscular incoordination. There was no operative mortality. Morbidity was limited to a small left subphrenic collection requiring drainage in a young adult, and a small bowel hernia beneath the jejunal Roux loop requiring a laparotomy in a child.

Esophagogastric dissociation was used as a secondary "rescue" (Group 2) procedure on 10 occasions, of which nine were for recurrence of GER and one for esophageal obstruction after fundoplication. The proce-

Table 1. "Additional indications" for esophagogastric dissociation and outcome

Indication	N	Complications and outcome
Reflux to colon interposition	3	1: late death at 2 years post-EGD from adhesions and peritonitis; 2: thriving, no dumping, no reflux 2 years and 7 years post-EGD
Necrotic stomach from gas bloat after fundoplication	1	At 8 years: thriving, no dumping, no reflux
Bleeding gastric remnant after subtotal gastrectomy	1	Esophagojejunal dehiscence. At 2 years: thriving, no dumping, no reflux
Microgastria		
Long gap esophageal atresia	1	At 4 years: thriving, no dumping, no reflux
Congenital stenosis, lower third esophagus	1	Late death at 6 months post-EGD from small bowel hernia to chest
Congenital short esophagus		
L congenital diaph. hernia	1	Late death at 8 months post-EGD from chronic lung disease
Dysfunctional esophagus following tracheoesophageal cleft	1	At 2 years: thriving, no dumping, no reflux

dure is more complex since it is first necessary to undo any residual fundal wrap, with an increased risk of injury to the esophagus and the vagus nerves. In our series there was no morbidity or immediate mortality in this group. However, four children died a late death from their original condition.

As experience increased, esophagogastric dissociation was found useful in other circumstances (Table 1), and "additional indications" (Group 3) were developed.

In all three groups, early recovery was rapid with resumption of bowel activity and feeding within 3–5 days. Follow-up now spans a period of 6 months to 10 years. During this time there has not been any recurrence of reflux. Gastrostomy feeding has been much easier, but because of persistent and sometimes distressing retching, slower and smaller volume feeding has been necessary. Aspiration pneumonitis and hospitalization episodes were significantly reduced, and the children's overall health improved markedly. Quality of life for the child and the caregivers was also significantly better. In view of the parents' wish for minimal additional investigations, it has not been our standard practice to undertake in-depth postoperative studies unless clinically indicated. As such only one child had a barium study, and two other children had radioisotope milk scans through their gastrostomies because of a suspicion of reflux and food aspiration. At no time was it possible to demonstrate reflux of food placed in the stomach. Similarly, pH studies in these same children, with a probe placed at the esophagojejunal anastomosis, did not show any acid reflux. There was no clinical evidence of stenosis or strictures at the esophagojejunal anastomosis, with the children able to swallow saliva and food without difficulty. There were four late deaths in the "Rescue" OGD group, and three in those undergoing OGD for diverse reasons (Table 1), all occurring months or years after surgery and all unrelated to the operation.

31.5
Conclusions

The child with significant gastroesophageal reflux who has failed a medical conservative approach may benefit from surgery. For the normal child with normal swallowing reflexes, fundoplication remains the procedure of choice despite an inherent element of reflux recurrence. The child with pharyngeal neuromuscular incoordination, whether subnormal or otherwise and whether refluxing or otherwise, is plagued by serious swallowing and feeding difficulties, with recurrent food aspiration and pneumonitis. Oral feeding becomes an unpleasant "all-consuming occupation" such that the child becomes dependent on nasogastric feeds to maintain weight and hydration. In time the constant and repeated need to pass a nasogastric tube, particularly if followed by retching and profuse vomiting, creates difficulties for child and parents alike. It is often at this time that the surgeon is first involved with a request for a feeding gastrostomy or jejunostomy.

The management of children with pharyngeal neuromuscular incoordination and swallowing difficulties is best undertaken by a "specialist multidisciplinary team" with particular interest in this area. The surgeon should be an integral member of this "team," participating in assessment and management planning from the beginning and at all stages, to bring the potential benefits of surgery to the child and his family at an early and appropriate stage, and not "as a last resort and when all else fails." A prime consideration in the evaluation and management plan for such children and their families is good quality of life. Thus, should the swallowing difficulties and hence dependence on tube feeding be a long-term or permanent feature, it would be more logical to ease the feeding concerns and to protect the lungs from aspiration pneumonitis from an early stage. In such circumstances, OGD offers these children and their caregivers a much-improved long-term outlook and eliminates the potential risk of recurrence of GER inherent to fundoplication. Gatti et al. [3], in a nonrandomized prospective study, compared esophagogastric dissociation with fundoplication in neurologically impaired children. They assessed "effectiveness" 1 year later as measured by definitive resolution of GER, nutritional rehabilitation, and quality of life improvement for the child and the caregivers. They reported a "better and faster nutritional rehabilitation, testified by a more considerable increase in all anthropometric and biochemical parameters, except total protein." They observed a considerable reduction in respiratory infections after OGD, but not after conventional surgery. Relevantly, hospitalization was less frequent after a Nissen fundoplication and gastrostomy, but they noted "an extraordinary decrease with a significant improvement in quality of life" only after OGD. A caregiver questionnaire highlighted less frustration in caring for the child, with less time being taken up for the child's special needs. In Gatti et al.'s [3] series, postoperative complications occurred in both groups. Pertinently, there was no GER recurrence in the OGD group, but three patients presenting with wrap failure some months after fundoplication were successfully treated by a "rescue" OGD.

Our own series leads us to the conclusion that OGD indeed eliminates the risk of recurrence of reflux from the stomach or retrogradely from the isoperistaltic jejunal Roux loop. Furthermore, hospitalization episodes were markedly less with a much-reduced incidence of aspiration pneumonitis. The children's general health and well-being improved, and they demonstrated a steady weight gain and increased activity. Feeding was rendered much easier and more pleasant despite the persistent tendency to retch, which is also common to fundoplication. Our review of the caregivers' assertion of a major improvement in lifestyle after OGD is in agreement with that of Gatti et al. [3]. It is relevant to state that successful fundoplication is associated with similar findings, such that fundoplication is an excellent procedure in its own right. However it retains the not insignificant risk of GER recurrence and the potential need for additional complex surgery. These findings favor consideration of esophagogastric dissociation as the single most effective primary antireflux operation for this group of children. The additional operative time is minimal, and the necessary anastomoses are not particularly significant when placed in the context of the potential long-term advantages. Our series and that of

Gatti et al. [3] stresses the usefulness of OGD also as a secondary "rescue" procedure following failed fundoplication.

Experience with OGD has led us to develop "additional indications" (Table 1) with gratifying results in otherwise difficult situations. Thus OGD may also have a temporary role in acute circumstances, with planned reversal at a later date. In this context and perhaps most relevantly, we have found that following direct esophagojejunal anastomosis, the children were able to eat full normal meals orally without volume or quality limitation and particularly without "dumping." Furthermore, in the event of bowel obstruction, the Roux-en-Y esophagojejunal configuration carries the practical advantage of a safe "open chimney," rather than the "closed loop" inherent to effective fundoplication.

All things considered, the issue is not one of fundoplication versus esophagogastric dissociation, but rather of determining the best form of management for the child and family with a significant GER problem, particularly when long-term or permanent pharyngeal neuromuscular incoordination and swallowing difficulty exist. Such children should be offered the benefits of surgical as well as medical management at an early stage. This is best undertaken through the services of a dedicated specialist multidisciplinary team, which includes a "surgeon with a specific interest" immediately from the time of diagnosis. At the end of the day, it is a question of developing a tailored program that best meets the needs of the individual child and that is designed to give the best quality of life to that child and his family.

References

1. Bianchi A (1997) Total oesophagogastric dissociation: an alternative approach. J Pediatr Surg 32:1291–1294
2. Bianchi A, Pearse B (1997) The non-refluxing gastrostomy: an evaluation. Pediatri Surg Intl 12:494–496
3. Gatti C, Federici di Abriola G, Villa M, De Angelis P, Laviani R, La Sala E, Dall'Oglio L (2001) Esophagogastric dissociation versus fundoplication: which is best for severely neurologically impaired children? J Pediatr Surg 36:677–680
4. Langer JC, Wesson DE, Ein SH, Filler RM, Shandling B, Superina RA, Papa M (1988) Feeding gastrostomy in neurologically impaired children: is antireflux procedure necessary? J Pediatr Gastroenterol Nutr 7:837–841
5. Pearl RH, Robie DK, Ein SH, Shandling B, Wesson DE, Superina R, Mctaggart K, Garcia VF, O'Connor JA, Filler RM (1990) Complications of gastroesophageal antireflux surgery in neurologically impaired versus neurologically normal children. J Pediatr Surg 25:1169–1173

Chapter 32

Complications of Antireflux Surgery

32

Francois Becmeur · Isabelle Talon · Jurgen Schleef

Contents

32.1
Introduction

Gastroesophageal reflux (GER) is a common finding in children of all age groups. The treatment can be conservative and surgical. In the last decade, minimally invasive approaches became very popular, and the number of surgeons performing endosurgical procedures for GER is constantly rising. GER is a very complex pathology with different aspects influencing the course of the disease and also complications resulting from surgery. The indications for surgery are fairly well described and appear to be clear. However, every patient must of course be regarded as an individual, and the treatment should be adjusted according to individual patient-related symptoms and findings.

Every treatment in medicine is affected by a number of possible complications. These complications can be related to different aspects. Surgeons should be aware of complications, and meticulous analyses will not only help to detect the reason for a complication but also lead to correct handling and avoiding pitfalls and complications in the future.

Endoscopic gastroesophageal reflux surgery has a number of well-known and rare complications and side effects [2]. They can be divided in different groups. They can be specific to the procedure but also unspecific related to different aspects (Table 1). Concerning the time course, complications of surgery can be generally divided into four groups:

1. Intraoperative
2. Early postoperative
3. Mid-term
4. Long term

32.2
Unspecific Complications

This group of complications is very often neglected when complications of surgical procedures are analyzed and discussed. In many instances, however, especially mid-term and long-term problems might have their origin here. It is important to know that they are usually not related to the procedure and the surgical technique.

Table 1. Groups of complications related to GER surgery

Unspecific, related to:	Specific, related to:
Preoperative diagnostics	Access (endosurgical, open)
Bad nutritional status	Type of procedure (Nissen, Thal, Toupet, others)
Associated diseases (e.g., neurological impairment, seizures)	Associated interventions (gastrostomy, outlet procedures)
Indication for surgery in infants and toddlers	Surgical team
Social environment	

32.2.1
Pre-operative Diagnostics

The diagnostic approach to a patient with GER should include esophageal manometry, 24-h pH-metry, barium swallow, upper GI endoscopy, and a careful history regarding nutrition and nutritional habits. If these diagnostic steps are performed completely and meticulously, there will be rarely be an unexpected and unpleasant "surprise" after surgery.

Typical problems are motor problems of the esophagus. In some instances the peristalsis of the esophagus can be disturbed (e.g., children after esophageal atresia) or nonpropulsive. Manometry, barium swallow, or scintigraphic transit studies can detect this. In these cases a complete fundoplication (Nissen) might lead to severe swallow problems and will give in some cases the impression of a too-tight fundoplication with stenosis, in reality caused by the imbalance between the propulsive activity of the esophagus and the resistance created by the fundoplication. A further problem might be the upper GI transit. The barium swallow should demonstrate the complete upper GI passage with contrasting of the upper jejunum. Postoperative vomiting and stomach distension might have their origin in an upper GI stenosis, malposition, or connatal duodenal pathology. The pyloric region of the stomach should be carefully examined to rule out a functional stomach outlet problem. Severe inflammation of the mucosa of esophagus and stomach might mimic and cause peristalsis disturbances. In such a case with a verified esophagitis or gastritis, a conservative treatment with omeprazole and a repeated work-up are mandatory. It should be clear that every unclear examination or different diagnostic procedures giving non-concordant results must be repeated [6].

32.2.2
Bad Nutritional Status

It is well known that complications of surgery such as infection and wound healing are related to the nutritional status of the patient. Unfortunately, many patients with GER have a bad nutritional status; some because they vomit and retch constantly, others because they are mentally handicapped and not able to eat at all. Severe esophagitis might lead to painful swallowing and reduced nutritional intake. The sequels of these conditions are bad nutritional status and catabolism. In these cases, a pre-operative amelioration of the nutritional status by parenteral nutrition or even constant tube feeding (in some cases a jejunal tube might be necessary) will bring the patient to a better pre-op shape and reduce the risk of surgery and the number of complications related to catabolism [8, 15].

32.2.3
Associated Diseases

Many infants and children with GER have associated diseases [22]; some can be seen as a sequel of recurrent vomiting and aspiration, such as pulmonary obstruction or even asthma [16]. A thorough work-up should be made in these patients, since GER might be silent or undetected.

Allergic conditions or nutritional intolerance (celiac disease) might mimic or cause in some cases GER. The treatment or the adjustment of the nutrition should be the first step in all of these children. The symptoms of GER will usually disappear if the underlying condition is treated appropriately.

Neurological diseases affect a large group of pediatric patients with GER. In larger series, up to 70% of all operated infants and children are neurologically impaired [19, 22]. The complication and rate of recurrence of GER are higher in this group than in other patients. In severe cases with severe motility problems, retching, and cramps associated with the need for constant tube feeding, a jejunostomy tube for constant enteral nutritional support might be the better choice. A repeated work-up in such a patient can lead to the decision for GER surgery under better nutritional conditions, as mentioned above. Deviation procedures with Roux-Y esophago-jejunostomy should be reserved for a small number of disastrous situations.

32.2.4
Indications for GER Surgery in Babies and Toddlers

Gastroesophageal reflux is a common finding in children under 1 year of age. However, it is well known that with maturation of the muscle complex of the gastroesophageal junction, the changing of nutritional habits, and a more upright position, in most of these children GER will disappear. We would recommend being very conservative with GER surgery in this age group. In our institutions the patients are usually observed and treated conservatively, and a surgical intervention under 1 year of age needs a very thorough repeated work-up. Especially in this group of patients (under 1 year), other connatal conditions (partial duodenal obstruction, malposition of the stomach, pyloric hypertrophy) should be ruled out as a source of symptoms of GER. Nevertheless, babies with large hiatal hernia, status post-repair of esophageal atresia, short bowel syndrome, and respiratory problems related to GER must be regarded as candidates for GER surgery [3, 10].

32.2.5
Social Environment

As in many situations in medicine, the social environment can affect clinical findings and symptoms in children with GER disease. The nutritional habits in small infants should be evaluated carefully. In small children the regularity, number, and size of meals can affect symptoms of GER dramatically. Often symptoms disappear in this group of patients completely under hospital observation.

In patients with severe mental retardation, the follow-up and care must be observed carefully. Postoperative complications can occur due to poor care of the patient, irregular nutrition or unrecognized early symptoms.

A difficult situation can appear if a Munchausen syndrome by proxy (MSBP) is suspected. We had this experience with a young mother, provoking symptoms of GER in her child, influencing diagnostic results and visiting different physicians and hospitals. The diagnosis of MSBP was finally made because all symptoms persisted after surgery. If the diagnostic work-up in such a case is not clear and the information from the parents differs from findings gathered during stays in the hospital, and the conservative approach fails without any evident reason, an experienced family psychiatrist should be consulted to evaluate the interaction between members of the family and the child.

32.3
Specific Complications

This chapter deals with specific complications of endosurgical GER approaches in children and infants. These complications are regarded as conditions related to the surgical procedure itself. For better understanding and systematic reasons, complications are discussed in the order that they may appear chronologically.

32.4
Intraoperative Complications

Intraoperative pitfalls and complications are usually detected during the procedure and can be corrected in most instances. Nevertheless, they might result in an inappropriate result or cause further problems. The most dangerous condition is an unrecognized complication [18].

Intraoperative complications in GER surgery can be divided into two groups (Table 2). The first group includes complications related to the laparoscopic approach, and the second to the GER procedure.

32.4.1
Complications Related to the Laparoscopic Approach

32.4.1.1
Open Access

The discussion about the access to the abdominal cavity is as old as endosurgery. The blind access with the Veress needle or a trocar is associated with a number of severe complications reported in the literature. Many of them can be repaired immediately, but an unrecognized vessel or bowel injury can cause a disastrous situation. We strictly recommend the open access with introduction of the first trocar under vision. The position can be the umbilicus or even in adolescents above the umbilicus. This technique is basically without any complication [18].

32.4.1.2
Instrumentation and Trocar Position

The choice of instruments should be adjusted to the patient. Small infants and babies require atraumatic and small forceps and scissors. Liver lacerations with bleed-

Table 2. Intraoperative complications related to laparoscopic approach and GER procedure

Laparoscopic approach	GER procedure
Organ lesion by blind puncture	Bleeding
Liver laceration with retraction	Pneumothorax
Malposition of trocars	Mediastinal emphysema
Technical defects	Vagal lesion
Side effects of the pneumoperitoneum	Esophageal and stomach perforation
Surgeon and team	Splenic injury
	Hiatal rupture
	Torsion of the esophagus
	Hiatal stenosis

ing and hematoma usually result from traumatic retractors. In small children we often use a clamp introduced from the right abdomen to lift up the liver, grasping the diaphragm. The position of the trocars should be adjusted to the size of the patient, the position of the liver, and to the location of a pre-existing gastrostomy. In children with severe spine deformity, a completely atypical trocar position might be necessary. To avoid unrecognized organ injuries, introducing instruments following the rule "no handling without vision" should be respected [17].

For preparation, vessel occlusion, sealing, and cutting, a vast number of different devices are available. We recommend controlling the function before the procedure in every case. We have to be aware that uncontrolled coagulation (especially with monopolar cautery) might cause an unrecognized injury to bowel or organs [18].

32.4.1.3
The Pneumoperitoneum

A pneumoperitoneum is usually installed during endosurgical procedures. There are only a few reports about the use of abdominal wall lifts in children. The abdominal pressure is usually adjusted to the size and age of the patient and is usually not higher than 10 mmHg CO_2. In most cases this is well tolerated [10]. Nevertheless, there are a few cases with congenital heart disease or pulmonary disease, in which the pneumoperitoneum is not tolerated. We experienced in a small child (3 months) with status post-esophageal atresia a severely impaired ventilatory function, and a conversion was necessary.

32.4.1.4
The Surgeon and the Surgical Team

Endosurgery is becoming more and more common in pediatric surgery. Compared to conventional surgery, endosurgery requires different training and experience. GER surgery requires endoscopic suturing. The team at the OR table should be trained together and aware of the steps of the procedure. There is in all larger series a rate of complications and pitfalls which might be caused by the above-mentioned problems.

32.4.2
Complications Related to GER Procedures

The types of surgery being performed for GER have already been discussed extensively. The most popular and frequently used approaches are the Nissen technique (complete fundoplication), the Toupet, and the Thal hemifundoplication [11, 17, 20]. Many other modifica-

tions exist but play only a minor role in the surgical therapy of GER [12]. A number of intraoperative complications are reported (Table 2).

32.4.2.1
Bleeding

Bleeding is the most common complication. Bleeding occurred in larger series from diaphragmatic veins, from the short gastric vessels, and the retro- esophageal tissue [5]. In most instances bleeding can be controlled by clipping or coagulation. Local gastric necrosis and perforation are described as a sequelae of clipping and coagulation of short gastric vessels. If retroesophageal bleeding occurs, primary identification of the posterior vagus nerve should be achieved to avoid damage to the vagal tissue. In contrast, in cases of bleeding from the short gastric vessels, a conversion might become necessary, as reported even in the hands of an experienced surgeon.

32.4.2.2
Pneumothorax and Mediastinal Emphysema

In case of large sliding hiatal hernia or fixed hernia of the fundus into the thorax, a pneumothorax or mediastinal emphysema can occur. A pleural lesion can remain undetected. If a tension pneumothorax arises, immediate release should be achieved by placing of a thoracic drain. This incident does not require conversion, if ventilation is not impaired.

A pneumomediastinum might develop in case of extensive mediastinal preparation along the esophagus. If pulmonary function is not impaired, no further treatment is necessary. The CO_2 pressure should be reduced in these cases to as low as possible. CO_2 will be reabsorbed spontaneously.

32.4.2.3
Vagal Lesions

Injuries to the vagal nerve can lead to impairment of gastric and intestinal function. The anterior and posterior vagal nerves can be detected easily and should be preserved. A careful preparation of the gastroesophageal junction, avoiding uncontrolled cutting and coagulation, is mandatory. Grasping the stomach and traction on the stomach by traumatic forceps might injure the anterior vagus nerve on the anterior stomach surface. For traction on the stomach, a vessel loop or umbilical band around the distal esophagus are less traumatic. Injuries to the posterior vagal nerve and its branches can be avoided by meticulous preparation of the retroesophageal space. If a vagal lesion occurs, an impairment of the stomach emptying function and dumping syndrome-like symptoms might develop, which usually recover with time. If dysfunction persists, in rare cases an outlet procedure (pyloroplasty) must be performed.

32.4.2.4
Esophageal and Stomach Perforation

Perforation of the upper GI tract in GER surgery is rare. The distal esophagus is more commonly affected than the stomach. Perforation can occur, when the retroesophageal space is freed or a large hernia is present. If the margin of the posterior wall of esophagus and stomach are not clear, positioning of a gastroscope in the gastroesophageal junction might be helpful. The diaphanoscopy and the palpable instrument in the esophagus can be very helpful and clarify the situation. If a perforation occurs, it should be verified by the endoluminal application of methylene blue through a nasogastric tube. The perforation should be closed with sutures. The skills of the individual surgeon might decide to perform it laparoscopically or to convert and proceed open [4]. Positioning a drain in the area of the perforation might be recommended.

32.4.2.5
Splenic Injury

Laceration of the spleen can occur during the preparation of the left crura of the hiatus. Mostly these injuries are small and can be treated by simple compression, coagulation, or using fibrin glue. Tears to the splenic capsule during the preparation of short gastric vessels are more difficult to deal with. Good suction and good exposition are mandatory, and local monopolar coagulation should be avoided. If no blood control can be achieved by this means, in minor bleeding a sponge can be placed and left in place until the end of the procedure. Usually the bleeding will stop. If bleeding persists, conversion might become necessary.

32.4.2.6
Hiatal Rupture

In many children with GER, the hiatus is not normal and the tissue is fragile, and rupture of the fibers during preparation or performing of the hiatal adaptation can occur. In these cases using nonresorbable mesh can enforce the hiatus. This technique is well established in adults, but in children only a few reports exist. We have only one such experience, in a girl with a large hiatal hernia where a mesh was successful applied. Usually, positioning the sutures in a saw-toothed fashion can reconstruct the hiatus and adapt the crura.

32.4.2.7
Torsion of the Esophagus

As well in anterior as in posterior hemifundoplication, a torsion of the esophagus can occur. In a stomach with a small fundus, the fundoplication might result in a partial torsion of the distal esophagus. The fundus is not wrapped around the esophagus, but the stomach is torsioned and torquing of the distal esophagus occurs. Especially in anterior fundoplication this complication is difficult to recognize, since the distal esophagus is covered by the fundus anteriorly. We experienced this complication in a boy who needed to be reoperated. If the fundus appears to be small, a complete mobilization with dissection of the short gastric vessels is recommended. Especially in small infants after repair of esophageal atresia with a short distal esophagus, the fundus might be small. In one of these children we converted to open, since no traction-free fundoplication could be achieved.

32.4.2.8
Hiatal Stenosis

We believe that in every case of GER surgery, a posterior hiatoplasty should be performed. Many recurrences of GER with migrating of the wrap or posterior hernia in the literature are associated with an "untouched" posterior hiatus. Nevertheless, stenosis or strictures at the level of the gastroesophageal junction must be avoided. In open surgery, a finger should be placed between the posterior esophagus and the first hiatal suture having a large gastric tube inside. This distance can be overestimated in laparoscopic surgery. We use an open needle holder and calibrate the hiatoplasty, introducing the instrument behind the esophagus. The large gastric tube should be slid smoothly in and out of the stomach at the end of the procedure [14]. If the hiatoplasty is too narrow, postoperatively a fixed stenosis with vomiting and severe dysphagia can be seen. In one girl we performed a relaparoscopy and opened the anterior suture, of the hiatoplasty and symptoms disappeared.

32.4.2.9
Conversion

At the end of this chapter with intraoperative complications, a short comment on conversion to open surgery should be made. Conversion rates were of great interest in the early days of endosurgery. Currently, the conversion rate is of secondary importance. The conversion rate should stay under 15% in a routine procedure such as GER surgery in a surgical setting. The individual decision for a conversion depends on many different aspects, and must be respected. The primary rules for endosurgery should be safety and quality [22].

32.5
Postoperative Complications

As already mentioned, postoperative complications can be divided into three different categories. Those occurring early, immediately after surgery and generally during the hospital stay, others occurring weeks and months later after surgery, and long-term problems or complications after occurring several months after surgery. Each group has a typical pattern of sequels of GER endosurgery.

32.5.1
Early Postoperative Complications

Since these complications are seen during the early postoperative days, they are usually all related directly to the surgery. Again we can divide between unspecific (general) postoperative complications and specific complications.

Every surgical procedure has general potential complications. Most of them are well known and many are related to general risk factors of the patient [9]. Postoperative respiratory distress can be related to the duration of surgery and the cardiopulmonary situation of the patient. Postoperative fever due to atelectasis can be seen in many handicapped patients. Local wound problems are rare and of minor importance. But there are some important-, and sometimes life-threatening events-, every surgeon should be aware of.

32.5.1.1
Bleeding

Immediately postoperative bleeding is characterized by instability and distortion of circulation. If there is any doubt about an organ injury or laceration during the procedure, and the patient cannot be stabilized, a re-intervention should be performed. If the patient is stable and not endangered, diagnostic should be performed (x-ray, ultrasound, CT) to evaluate the situation. Usually minor postoperative bleeding can be handled conservatively.

32.5.1.2
Organ Perforation

As already mentioned, perforations of the intestinal tract might occur during endosurgical procedures and might not be recognized. Patients will present with signs of an acute abdominal distension and early sepsis. The symptom of "free abdominal air" as a typical sign of GI tract perforation after endosurgery is not helpful. Therefore, contrast studies of the upper GI tract should be performed to rule out the diagnosis of perforation. If a perforation is detected, it should be treated in a routine way. This can be done laparoscopically or open. In some instances, it can be very helpful to review the video recording of the initial procedure.

32.5.1.3
Omental Prolapse

The prolapse of parts of the omentum through a trocar incision is a fairly frequent complication occurring in the early postoperative period in small children. This occurs mostly in the umbilical incision. If it occurs, the wound must be reopened and closed by suturing the different layers, under general anesthesia. A surgeon should close all incisions at the fascia level to avoid this unpleasant complication [18].

32.5.1.4
Abdominal Distension

Postoperative abdominal distension is a typical problem after GER surgery. In to our experience this problem is less frequent after a laparoscopic intervention compared to open surgery. This can be related to less abdominal trauma and less postoperative bowel paralysis. If the patient suffers from distension, usually a nasogastric tube and rectal tube might be helpful. If a gastrostomy is in place, it can be opened to decompress the upper GI tract.

In a few cases, abdominal distension can be a sign of early bowel obstruction. A small incisional hernia at a trocar side can be the cause of an omental incarceration, leading to bowel obstruction and requiring surgery.

32.5.1.5
Dysphagia

Dysphagia after GER surgery is a very common problem. Early dysphagia can be detected in many patients and should be observed and treated by dietetic means. In only a few severe cases should early diagnostic by barium swallow studies be performed. If there is no sign of complete obstruction at the level of the hiatus, no primary intervention is necessary. If there are signs of complete obstruction, the videotape of the surgery should be reviewed. If the closure of the hiatus appears too tight, or if a torsion of the distal esophagus cannot be ruled out, a combined laparoscopic/gastroscopic intervention can be discussed. We detected in one patient a stenosis due to a stenotic hiatoplasty and in another patient a rotated distal esophagus. Both were corrected laparoscopically and the patients are free of symptoms.

32.5.2
Mid-Term Postoperative Complications

These problems occur weeks and months after the surgery. They can be persisting problems or symptoms arising after an uneventful postoperative course.

32.5.2.1
Dysphagia

Although dysphagia during the first days and weeks after surgery is common after GER surgery, persistent dysphagia over months is a severe and embarrassing problem for patients. Different causes can be named. Generally there is a strong relation between the problem and the type of procedure. We check all our pediatric patients with GER at 3 and 6 months after the operation by barium swallow and 24-h pH-metry. If one of these examinations is not normal, a manometry is performed.

Persisting dysphagia can be caused by a still narrow and stenotic closure of the hiatus. If this finding is present, we perform an endoscopy with repeated balloon dilatation [23]. This procedure was successful in our experience with two boys. If the esophagus shows a dilatation and no motility with a normal esophagogastric junction on barium swallow, the source of complaint might be the imbalance between the propulsive activity of the esophagus and the resistance created by the regular fundoplication. In these cases dietetic means will be successful on in the short-term. Pneumatic dilatation can be tried. However, we had two children who required finally a redo procedure; preferably a conversion from a Nissen to a hemifundoplication [1, 6].

Dysphagia occurring months after surgery can be the first symptom of a paraesophageal hernia, developing after surgery. These children suffer from a combination of recurrent reflux and partial obstruction by a paraesophageal hernia. In these cases a re-operation is necessary [21].

32.5.2.2
Recurrence of Reflux

A recurrence of GER months after surgery is often related to an operative error or pitfall. There are three typical reasons for early insufficiency after fundoplication. (1) The use of resorbable sutures for the fundoplication leads after several months to a complete rupture. (2) The "untouched hiatus". In these cases a posterior sliding of the wrap or the gastroesophageal junction above the diaphragm might be visible. (3) In severely handicapped children with progressive disease, the general motility disorders of the intestine can be the cause of recurrent reflux with an intact and functioning wrap. In these cases, alternatives such as jejunal tube feeding, medical therapy, and diversion operations should be discussed [4].

We would recommend in the latter group aa re-evaluation of the patient in cooperation with the pediatrician, because the prognosis, even with re-intervention, will be poor in most cases.

32.5.3
Long-Term Postoperative Complications

32.5.3.1
Bowel Obstruction

Late complications after surgery are usually related to adhesions and bowel obstruction. Laparoscopic antireflux surgery is less affected by bowel obstruction due to scar formation and adhesions, but there are cases with late acute bowel obstruction [7]. We experienced one case with an acute obstruction due to adhesion to a trocar side two years after initial surgery.

32.5.3.2
Trocar Hernia

Abdominal wall complications are frequent after open surgery. Endosurgical procedures are less affected by this problem, especially the problem of wound healing. Trocar hernias represent a typical problem after laparoscopic procedures. They can occur early, but usually appear months after the surgery. In many cases the hernia remains asymptomatic. However, many articles in the literature deal with this problem, and in nearly every larger series of pediatric and also adult patients, trocar hernias are described [13]. The diameter of the trocar used initially seems not to be important. Hernias are described after 10-mm, but also after 5- and 3-mm trocar insertion. In most cases, the fascia was not closed. It seems advisable to attempt a closure of the fascia even in very small trocar incisions to avoid later herniation. It remains to be determined whether the use of self-expanding trocars can minimize this problem.

32.5.3.3
Recurrence of GER

Recurrences of GER after antireflux surgery in the long term are present in every larger study. No technique can be described as superior to any other. We should consider that in severely handicapped children, the rate of recurrence is much higher than in normal children. If we diagnose a recurrent GER, a surgical redo should be discussed [4, 6]. Nevertheless in many patients a supportive medical treatment might be sufficient. In other cases a change in the strategy of nutrition can be proposed.

32.6
Complications Related to Feeding Ostomies

As was discussed earlier, in many cases simultaneous procedures are performed. A gastrostomy is the most frequently performed procedure during an operation for GER in children. In rare cases a simultaneous jejunostomy is performed. Gastrostomies are accompanied by a fairly high rate of complications. Especially in children with bad nutritional status and reduced immune response, wound healing problems with insufficiency and consecutive peritonitis are described [4, 5]. We prefer to perform first the gastrostomy (PEG), continue with enteral feeding, and perform the fundoplication later. The literature shows that the feasibility of a laparoscopic GER procedure is not impaired by a gastrostomy in place.

32.7
Conclusion

Surgery for gastroesophageal reflux in children is a complex entity. The extant literature provides encouraging data regarding the success rate and incidence of complications after open and laparoscopic surgery. Comparing the present studies, laparoscopic surgery seems to be favorable. Nevertheless, there is no prospective randomized study comparing open and laparoscopic surgery for GER in children. The present data show that in most institutions, the laparoscopic approach is the standard procedure.

The complications listed in this chapter show that there is a large number of pitfalls and unpleasant events and complications which can be avoided if systematic guidelines and a complete diagnostic approach to the problem of GER in children are followed. Thus, many of the complications can be avoided.

Severe intraoperative complications are usually related to inexperienced surgeons, or surgeons who are not trained in endoscopic procedures. Larger series demonstrate that the incidence of intraoperative catastrophes is related to the experience of the team. Adequate training and assistance of experienced colleagues can help to avoid a learning curve with a high rate of complications.

References

1. Ceriati E, Guarino N, Zaccara A, Marchetti P, la Sala E, Lucchetti I, Dall´Oglio, Rivosecchi M (1998) Gastroesophageal reflux in neurologically impaired children: partial or total fundoplication? Langenbecks Arch Surg 383:317–319
2. Esposito C, Ascione G, Garipoli V, De Bernardo G, Esposito G (1997) Complications of pediatric laparoscopic surgery. Surg Endosc 11:655–657
3. Esposito C, Montupet P, Reinberg O (2001) Laparoscopic surgery for gastroesophageal reflux disease during the first year of life. J Pediatr Surg 36:715–717
4. Esposito C, van der Zee DC, Settimi A, Doldo P, Staiano A, Bax NMA (2003) Risks and benefits of surgical management of gastroesophageal reflux in neurologically impaired children. Surg Endosc 17:708–710
5. Georgeson KE (1993) Laparoscopic gastrostomy and fundoplication. Paediatr Ann 92:675–677
6. Graziano K, Teitelbaum DH, McLean K, Hirschl RB, Coran AG, Geiger JD (2003) Recurrence after laparoscopic and open Nissen fundoplication. Surg Endosc 17:704–707
7. Holzinger F, Klaiber C (2002) Trokarhernien, eine seltene, potenziell gefährliche Komplikation nach laparoskopischen Eingriffen. Chirurg 73:899–904
8. Hüttl TP, Hohle M, Meyer G, Schildberg FW (2002) Antirefluxchirurgie in Deutschland. Chirurg 73:451–461
9. Iwanaka T, Arai M, Ito M, Kawashima H, Imaizumi S (2000) Laparoscopic surgery in neonates and infants weighting less than 5 kg. Pediatr Int 42:608–612
10. Mattioli G, Montobbio G, Pini Prato A, Repetto P, Carlini C, Gentilino V, Castagnetti M, Leggio S, Della Rocca M, Kotitsa Z, Jasonni V (2003) Anesthesiologic aspects of laparoscopic fundoplication for gastroesophageal reflux in children with chronic respiratory and gastroenterological symptoms. Surg Endosc 17:559–566
11. Meehan JJ, Georgeson KE (1996) Laparoscopic fundoplication in infants and children. Surg Endosc 10:1154–1157
12. Montinaro L, Paradies G, Leggio (2002) The Lortat-Jacob operation by laparoscopic access to treat gastroesophageal reflux in pediatric patients. Surg Endosc 16:1438–1440
13. Nakajiama K, Wasa M, Kawahara H, Hasegawa T, Soh H, Taniguchi E, Ohashi S, Okada A (1999) Revision laparoscopy for incarcerated hernia at a 5 mm trocar site following pediatric laparoscopic surgery. Surg Laparosc Endosc Percutan Tech 9:294–295
14. Ostlie DJ, Miller KA, Holcomb GW (2002) Effective Nissen fundoplication length and bougie diameter size in young children undergoing laparoscopic Nissen Fundoplication. J Pediatr Surg 37:1864–1666
15. Pessaux P, Arnaud JP, Ghavami B, Flament JB, Trebuchet G, Meyer C, Huten N, Tuech JJ, Champault G, Societe Francaise de Chirurgie Laparoscopique (2002) Morbidity of laparoscopic fundoplication for gastroesophageal reflux: a retrospective study about 1470 patients. Hepatogastroenterology 49:447–450
16. Powers CJ, Levitt MA, Tantoco J, Rossman J, Sarpel U, Brisseau G, Caty MG, Glick PL (2003) The respiratory advantage of laparoscopic Nissen fundoplication J Pediatr Surg 38:886–891
17. Rothenberg S (1998) Experience with 220 consecutive laparoscopic Nissen fundoplication in infants and children. J Pediatr Surg 33:274–278
18. Schleef J (2002) Endoskopische Chirurgie im Kindesalter – Spezielle Gefahren und ihre Vermeidung. Min Inv Chir 11:71–74
19. Schleef J, Deluggi S, Schaarschmidt K, Engels M, Willital GH (2000) Multi–institutional experience in laparoscopic surgery for gatsroesophageal reflux: a five–year experience with 30 children. J Laparoendosc Adv Surg Techn B 4:265–270
20. Schleef J, Steinau G, Willital GH (1994) Laparoskopische Hiatusrekonstruktion nach Thal im Kindesalter. Langenbecks Arch Chi Suppl Ii Verh Dtsch Ges Forsch Chir 577–579
21. Seelig MH, Hinder R, Klinger PJ (1999) Paraesophageal herniation as a complication following laparoscopic antireflux surgery. J Gastrointest Surg 3:95–99
22. Steyaert H, Al Mohaidly M, Lembo MA, Carfagna L, Tursini S, Valla JS (2003) Long-term outcome of laparoscopic Nissen and Toupet fundoplication in normal and neurologically impaired children. Surg Endosc 17:543–546
23. Yeming W, Somme S, Chenren S, Huiming J, Ming Z, Liu DC (2002) Balloon catheter dilatation in children with congenital and aquired esophageal anomalies. J Pediatr Surg 37:398–402

Chapter 33

Clinical Outcomes After Laparoscopic Antireflux Surgery

33

Craig T. Albanese · Mac Harmon · Keith Georgeson

Contents

33.1
Introduction

Laparoscopic surgery for gastroesophageal reflux disease (GERD) was first reported in adults in 1991 [10] and in children in 1993 [35]. The laparoscopic technique is rapidly becoming the "gold standard" despite the absence of outcomes from any randomized controlled trials comparing it to the open fundoplication in the pediatric population. However, many retrospective studies have been published and form the basis for this chapter (Table 1).

33.2
Technical Considerations

The single greatest advantage of the laparoscopic technique compared to open surgery is the visualization afforded by a telescope that magnifies, greatly illuminates and, when angled (e.g., 30°), extends the field of view. Additionally, with the use of gravity (e.g., the reversed Trendelenburg position) the bowel need not be manipulated, thus decreasing postoperative adhesions. This has been clearly noted in those children in whom an

Table 1. Select outcome measures after pediatric laparoscopic fundoplication using recent studies containing 25 or more patients

First author (year) [reference no.]	Number of patients (n)	Conversion rate (%)	Complication rate (%)	Rate of recurrent GERD (%)
Longis (1996) [36]	30	3.3	10	NA
Meehan (1996) [39]	160	7.5	7.4	1.4
Georgeson (1998) [22]	389	3.3	NA	5
Rothenberg (1998) [49]	220	1	Intraoperative 2.6 Postoperative 7.3	3.4
Dick (1999) [12]	50	8	8	6
Hopkins (1999) [28]	25	0	NA	NA
Esposito (2000) [17]	289	1.3	Intraoperative 5.1 Postoperative 3.4	2.1
Liu (2000) [34]	26	3.8	Intraoperative 3.8	NA
Allal (2001) [1]	142	2.1	Intraoperative 0.5 Postoperative 2	NA
Montupet (2001) [44]	284	NA	1	2
Iglesias (2001) [30]	104	1	11.5	2.9
Somme (2002) [53]	55	NA	0	2.6
Steyaert (2003)	53	3.8	0	6.6
Al-Mohaidaly (2003) [2]	45	NA	4.4	11.1

NA, not available, GERD, gastroesophageal reflux disease

upper abdominal reoperation has been performed. Instrumentation that is proportionately short (20-cm long) and small in diameter (3.5 mm) allows an ergonomically sound operation, with small skin incisions, for neonates as well as older children. The smaller and less conspicuous scars portend obvious cosmetic and possible psychological benefits to the child and parents. Laparoscopic robotic surgery has also been proven possible and may provide additional advantages in the future [4, 42, 25]. The summation of all of these technical advances allow laparoscopic fundoplication to be performed safely and effectively in the most difficult pediatric populations: children less than 5 kg [50], children with previous abdominal operations [34], children in the first year of life [18], and in disabled infants and children [29]. Should the primary operation fail for any reason, reoperation can be performed laparoscopically in many instances [23].

33.3
Learning Curve

The lack of size-appropriate instrumentation was a factor in the successful performance of antireflux procedures many years ago. Now, the learning curve is mainly a function of the ability to suture and tie knots intracorporeally in a small space. Four separate studies in children have noted this phenomenon in the laparoscopic treatment of GERD [17, 40, 1, 49]. In each, a learning curve of 25–50 cases was needed to achieve efficient operative times and led to decreased intraoperative complications. Operative time in each of these varied widely, but usually decreased on average from 100–200 min in the first group of procedures to 50–100 min after experience aggregated. In the latter cases, there was a reduced number of complications including conversions to open procedures, and costs decreased. What was responsible for this improvement was difficult to quantify. In many cases, technical facility with instrumentation, familiarity with the proper placement of trocars, optimized dissection, retraction, and knot-tying, and lastly the presence of a dedicated, minimal-access operating room team appeared to be vital components in this improvement.

33.4
Postoperative Analgesia Requirements

It is difficult to quantify and study the pain associated with the laparoscopic fundoplication in neonates, infants, and small children. In this population, administration of analgesics is usually based on subjective evaluation by a parent or nurse. Nevertheless, when studied prospectively in children, the total amount of morphine analgesia required was similar for both laparoscopic and open surgery [13]. However, the period for analgesia was significantly less in the laparoscopic group with the median length of opiate requirement being only one day [13]. In another study, oral or rectal analgesics were the only agents used in 89% of patients and treatment ceased within 48 h in 95% of patients [12]. As experience has accumulated, many interventions have been added to further diminish pain associated with the laparoscopic procedure. Pain from trocar sites has been reduced by preemptive application of long-acting local anesthetics during trocar placement, while peritoneal and diaphragmatic irritation has been decreased by subdiaphragmatic instillation of local anesthetics to diminish phrenic nerve irritation [51, 9]. In addition, pain from residual intra-abdominal gas can be minimized by its complete exsufflation from the peritoneal cavity and minimizing irrigation since carbon dioxide combines with water to make carbonic acid, which is a peritoneal irritant.

33.5
Physiologic Considerations

Theoretically, gas insufflation at 8–12 torr pressure with positioning in steep reverse Trendelenburg and concomitant carbon dioxide resorption may lead to impaired ventilation. However, hypo-oxygenation and hypercarbia with resultant acidosis due to cephalad diaphragmatic displacement and decreased lung volumes has not been significant and may be reversed by increasing minute ventilation 20–25% [12]. When studied postoperatively, laparoscopic fundoplication results in little to no physiologic alteration in respiration and as a large painful upper abdominal incision is not present, the approach translates to postoperative benefits [48]. There is little postoperative atelectasis and pneumonia, findings which may be linked to increased vital and total lung capacity [1]. Meehan reported a 1.8% rate of postoperative pneumonia in neurologically impaired children compared to a historical incidence of postoperative pneumonia after open surgery of 14–40% in a similar patient population [41].

Characteristics of the effect of laparoscopic fundoplication on lower esophageal sphincter (LES) have also been studied. Following fundoplication, a postprandial increase of basal LES pressure and significant residual LES pressure at the nadir of LES relaxation have been seen [32], a finding similar to that in studies following open procedures [31, 47].

33.6
Complications

Intraoperative complications during pediatric laparoscopic fundoplication occur in about 5% of cases [23]. Mortality is almost never reported and when present, is a complication of underlying disease. In a study of adults published in 1997, the rate of complications in one series of 2,453 patients demonstrated viscus perforation in 1%, transfusion in 1%, pneumothorax in 2%, splenectomy in 0.1%, and conversion to open procedures in 6% [46]. Reoperation was rarely necessary and was due to persistent bleeding, missed perforation, crural disruption, paraesophageal hernia, and gastric volvulus. Death occurred in 0.2% of cases. In children, intraoperative complications in large series are similarly infrequent [1, 22].

The majority of studies which compare complication rates between open and laparoscopic approaches show little difference, both in adults [8] and in children [15]. Nevertheless, some studies do show a trend toward increased complications in the open group (25% versus 14%; [26, 57]). In these studies, the greatest benefit of laparoscopic fundoplication appears to be in lowered rates of wound complication, which can occur in up to 20% of open procedures [14]. The mechanism behind this may be linked to a transient suppression of cell-mediated immunity in open procedures when compared to laparoscopic procedures, and the presence of a larger incision [43]. Other complications more likely to be seen with open procedures include adhesive bowel obstruction and postoperative pulmonary impairment. Estimated blood loss appears to be significantly reduced in laparoscopic procedures [14].

Intraoperative complications that are more common and/or more difficult to manage in laparoscopic procedures include bowel/vessel injury during trocar insertion, pneumothorax from diaphragmatic injury or pleural injury during mobilization of the distal esophagus, trocar site hernia, and bleeding. Many of these, if recognized, can be treated laparoscopically. Evidence suggests that the majority of complications in large series occur early in the experience of the surgeon (first 50 cases) and thereafter are significantly reduced [1].

Conversions from laparoscopic to open cases are infrequent and decrease as experience improves [29]. Rates vary from 0.9% [1, 16] to 7.5% [39] due to a combination of equipment problems, inadequate visualization, and dense adhesions. Some series have reported 0% conversion rates [28]. Overall, conversions to open procedures in children can be expected in 2% of cases [22]. Two-thirds are due to technical reasons and one-third to complications [7].

33.7
Hospital Stay, Feeding, and Activity

Perhaps the greatest benefit of laparoscopic fundoplication is seen in return of the patient to a normal level of function. In numerous studies, laparoscopic fundoplication is associated with a shorter length of stay in the hospital. This has been evaluated in two different ways: patients who go home following their operation are evaluated simply according to their length of stay, and those who have prolonged hospitalizations not related to their antireflux surgery are evaluated by time to full feeds. Using either of these methods, there has been a significant decrease in length of stay with the minimal access approach [1, 8]. Length of stay in children can be as low as 1–3 days in large series [22]. The significance of this is great, with considerable decrease in cost not only in terms of hospital charges but also the ability of parents to return to work and children to return to school and regular activities [3]. Several factors may be responsible for this, not the least of which is an earlier return of bowel function and decreased pain requiring less narcotic usage.

Over 50% of children undergoing minimal access procedures are feeding by postoperative day one and 85% by day two [39]. The patients are then kept on a soft diet for the first 7–10 days following surgery to avoid early complaints of dysphagia associated with postoperative edema. Patients undergoing concomitant gastrostomy placement are usually kept in the hospital a day longer because their feeds are not started until the first postoperative day.

33.8
Long-Term Outcome

Most long-term studies reporting results after laparoscopic fundoplication stem from the adult literature and describe satisfaction rates of 85–100% [5], a similar finding to the open approach [11, 27]. Failure rates for adults undergoing fundoplication, namely persistent or recurrent symptoms, are approximately 1% per year with both techniques.

In children, recurrence rates with open procedures are well known [33]. These are somewhat increased compared to the adult population since neurologically impaired children comprise a large percentage of operated patients and this group recurs more frequently. The largest experience to date, with over 7,400 cases, noted a recurrence rate of 7.1% [19]. When stratified, this rate was 5% in normal and 15% in neurologically impaired children. Higher rates of recurrence have also been seen in children with chronic lung disease [55], in children less than 3 months old [20], and in series with smaller numbers of patients [52, 37, 38]. In these latter studies, this number can be as high as 19% [6, 45, 21]. The failure rate with laparoscopy varies but can be as low as 2% [47] to 14% when physiologically studied [56]. The largest series in the pediatric literature demonstrate symptomatic recurrent reflux of 2–11.1% [23, 1, 49, 22, 24, 2, 53, 54, 36, 44, 30], a number lower than that of traditional open fundoplication.

References

1. Allal H, Captier G, Lopez M, et al (2001) Evaluation of 142 consecutive laparoscopic fundoplications in children: effects of the learning curve and technical choice. J Pediatr Surg 36: 921–926
2. Al-Mohaidaly M, Steyaert H, Valla JS (2003) Long term results of laparoscopic antireflux surgery in children. Saudi Med J 24: S29
3. Blucher D, Lobe TE (1994) Minimal access surgery in children: the state of the art. Int Surg 79:317–321
4. Cadiere GB, Himpens J, Vertruyen M, et al (2001) Evaluation of telesurgical (robotic) Nissen fundoplication. Surg Endosc 15: 918–923
5. Campos GM, Peters JH, DeMeester TR, et al (1999) Multivariate analysis of factors predicting outcome after laparoscopic Nissen fundoplication. J Gastrointest Surg 3:292–300
6. Caniano DA, Ginn-Pease ME, King DR (1990) The failed antireflux procedure: analysis of risk factors and morbidity. J Pediatr Surg 25:1022–1026
7. Chen MK, Schropp KP, Lobe TE (1996) Complications of minimal-access surgery in children. J Pediatr Surg 31:1161–1165
8. Collins JB, III, Georgeson KE, Vicente Y, et al (1995) Comparison of open and laparoscopic gastrostomy and fundoplication in 120 patients. J Pediatr Surg 30:1065–1071
9. Cunniffe MG, McAnena OJ, Dar MA, et al (1998) A prospective randomized trial of intraoperative bupivacaine irrigation for management of shoulder-tip pain following laparoscopy. Am J Surg 176:258–261
10. Dallemagne B, Weerts JM, Jehaes C, et al (1991) Laparoscopic Nissen fundoplication: preliminary report. Surg Laparosc Endosc 1:138–143
11. DeMeester TR, Bonavina L, Albertucci M (1986) Nissen fundoplication for gastroesophageal reflux disease. Evaluation of primary repair in 100 consecutive patients. Ann Surg 204: 9–20
12. Dick AC, Potts SR (1999) Laparoscopic fundoplication in children–an audit of fifty cases. Eur J Pediatr Surg 9:286–288
13. Dick AC, Coulter P, Hainsworth AM, et al (1998) A comparative study of the analgesia requirements following laparoscopic and open fundoplication in children. J Laparoendosc Adv Surg Tech A 8:425–429
14. Eshraghi N, Farahmand M, Soot SJ, et al (1998) Comparison of outcomes of open versus laparoscopic Nissen fundoplication performed in a single practice. Am J Surg 175:371–374
15. Esposito C, Garipoli V, De Pasquale M, et al (1997a) Laparoscopic versus traditional fundoplication in the treatment of children with refractory gastro-oesophageal reflux. Ital J Gastroenterol Hepatol 29:399–402
16. Esposito C, Ascione G, Garipoli V, et al (1997b) Complications of pediatric laparoscopic surgery. Surg Endosc 11:655–657
17. Esposito C, Montupet P, Amici G, et al (2000) Complications of laparoscopic antireflux surgery in childhood. Surg Endosc 14: 622–624
18. Esposito C, Montupet P, Reinberg O (2001) Laparoscopic surgery for gastroesophageal reflux disease during the first year of life. J Pediatr Surg 36:715–717
19. Fonkalsrud EW, Ashcraft KW, Coran AG, et al (1998) Surgical treatment of gastroesophageal reflux in children: a combined hospital study of 7467 patients. Pediatrics 101:419–422
20. Fonkalsrud EW, Bustorff-Silva J, Perez CA, et al (1999) Antireflux surgery in children under 3 months of age. J Pediatr Surg 34:527–531
21. Fung KP, Seagram G, Pasieka J, et al (1990) Investigation and outcome of 121 infants and children requiring Nissen fundoplication for the management of gastroesophageal reflux. Clin Invest Med 13:237–246
22. Georgeson KE (1998) Laparoscopic fundoplication and gastrostomy. Semin Laparosc Surg 5:25–30
23. Graziano K, Teitelbaum DH, McLean K, et al (2003a) Recurrence after laparoscopic and open Nissen fundoplication. A comparison of the mechanisms of failure. Surg Endosc 17: 704–707
24. Graziano K, Teitelbaum DH, McLean K, et al (2003b) Recurrence after laparoscopic and open Nissen fundoplication. Surg Endosc 17:704–707
25. Gutt CN, Markus B, Kim ZG, et al (2002) Early experiences of robotic surgery in children. Surg Endosc 16:1083–1086
26. Heikkinen TJ, Haukipuro K, Koivukangas P, et al (1999) Comparison of costs between laparoscopic and open Nissen fundoplication: a prospective randomized study with a 3-month followup. J Am Coll Surg 188:368–376
27. Heikkinen TJ, Haukipuro K, Bringman S, et al (2000) Comparison of laparoscopic and open Nissen fundoplication 2 years after operation. A prospective randomized trial. Surg Endosc 14:1019–1023
28. Hopkins MA, Stringel G (1999) Laparoscopic Nissen fundoplication in children: a single surgeon's experience. JSLS 3:261–266
29. Humphrey GM, Najmaldin AS (1996) Laparoscopic Nissen fundoplication in disabled infants and children. J Pediatr Surg 31:596–599
30. Iglesias JL, Kogut K, Owings E, et al (2001) Safety and efficacy of laparoscopic Nissen fundoplication in early infancy. Ped Endosurg Innov Tech 5:379–384
31. Kawahara H, Imura K, Yagi M, et al (1998) Mechanisms underlying the antireflux effect of Nissen fundoplication in children. J Pediatr Surg 33:1618–1622
32. Kawahara H, Imura K, Nakajima K, et al (2000) Motor function of the esophagus and the lower esophageal sphincter in children who undergo laparoscopic Nissen fundoplication. J Pediatr Surg 35:1666–1671
33. Kimber C, Kiely EM, Spitz L (1998) The failure rate of surgery for gastro-oesophageal reflux. J Pediatr Surg 33:64–66
34. Liu DC, Flattmann GJ, Karam MT, et al (2000) Laparoscopic fundoplication in children with previous abdominal surgery. J Pediatr Surg 35:334–337
35. Lobe TE, Schropp KP, Lunsford K (1993) Laparoscopic Nissen fundoplication in childhood. J Pediatr Surg 28:358–361
36. Longis B, Grousseau D, Alain JL, et al (1996) Laparoscopic fundoplication in children: our first 30 cases. J Laparoendosc Surg 1:S21–S29
37. Martinez DA, Ginn-Pease ME, Caniano DA (1992a) Recognition of recurrent gastroesophageal reflux following antireflux surgery in the neurologically disabled child: high index of suspicion and definitive evaluation. J Pediatr Surg 27: 983–990
38. Martinez DA, Ginn-Pease ME, Caniano DA (1992b) Sequelae of antireflux surgery in profoundly disabled children. J Pediatr Surg 27:267–273
39. Meehan JJ, Georgeson KE (1996) Laparoscopic fundoplication in infants and children. Surg Endosc 10:1154–1157
40. Meehan JJ, Georgeson KE (1997a) The learning curve associated with laparoscopic antireflux surgery in infants and children. J Pediatr Surg 32:426–429
41. Meehan JJ, Georgeson KE (1997b) Laparoscopic fundoplication yields low postoperative pulmonary complications in neurologically impaired children. Ped Endosurg Innov Tech 1: 11–14
42. Meininger DD, Byhahn C, Heller K, et al (2001) Totally endoscopic Nissen fundoplication with a robotic system in a child. Surg Endosc 15:1360
43. Mendoza-Sagaon M, Hanly EJ, Talamini MA, et al (2000) Comparison of the stress response after laparoscopic and open cholecystectomy. Surg Endosc 14:1136–1141

44. Montupet P, Mendoza-Sagaon M, De Dreuzy O, et al (2001) Laparoscopic Toupet fundoplication in children. Ped Endosurg Innov Tech 5:305–308
45. Pearl RH, Robie DK, Ein SH, et al (1990) Complications of gastroesophageal antireflux surgery in neurologically impaired versus neurologically normal children. J Pediatr Surg 25:1169–1173
46. Perdikis G, Hinder RA, Lund RJ, et al (1997) Laparoscopic Nissen fundoplication: where do we stand? Surg Laparosc Endosc 7:17–21
47. Peters JH, Heimbucher J, Kauer WK, et al (1995) Clinical and physiologic comparison of laparoscopic and open Nissen fundoplication. J Am Coll Surg 180:385–393
48. Powers CJ, Levitt MA, Tantoco J, et al (2003) The respiratory advantage of laparoscopic Nissen fundoplication. J Pediatr Surg 38:886–891
49. Rothenberg SS (1998) Experience with 220 consecutive laparoscopic Nissen fundoplications in infants and children. J Pediatr Surg 33:274–278
50. Rothenberg SS, Chang J (1997) Experience with advanced endosurgical procedures in neonates and infants. Ped Endosurg Innov Tech 1:107–110
51. Rowney DA, Aldridge LM (2000) Laparoscopic fundoplication in children: anaesthetic experience of 51 cases. Paediatr Anaesth 10:291–296
52. Smith CD, Othersen HB, Jr, Gogan NJ, et al (1992) Nissen fundoplication in children with profound neurologic disability. High risks and unmet goals. Ann Surg 215:654–659
53. Somme S, Rodriguez JA, Kirsch DG, Liu DC (2002) Laparoscopic vs open fundoplication in infants. Surg Endosc 16:54–56
54. Steyaert H, Al Mohaidaly M, Lembo MA, et al (2003) Long-term outcome of laparoscopic Nissen and Toupet fundoplication in normal and neurologically impaired children. Surg Endosc 17:543–546
55. Taylor LA, Weiner T, Lacey SR, et al (1994) Chronic lung disease is the leading risk factor correlating with the failure (wrap disruption) of antireflux procedures in children. J Pediatr Surg 29:161–166
56. Tovar JA, Olivares P, Diaz M, et al (1998) Functional results of laparoscopic fundoplication in children. J Pediatr Gastroenterol Nutr 26:429–431
57. Viljakka MT, Luostarinen ME, Isolauri JO: Complications of open and laparoscopic antireflux surgery (1997) 32-year audit at a teaching hospital. J Am Coll Surg 185:446–450

Chapter 34

Redo Surgery in Cases of Recurrent GER

34

Ciro Esposito · Hossein Allal · Philippe Montupet

Contents

34.1
Introduction

Gastroesophageal fundoplication can actually be considered one of the most common operations performed by pediatric surgeons on infants and children [5, 15].

In about 3–7% of cases, the laparoscopic technique can be adopted to treat patients in whom antireflux surgery has failed [1, 18]. Laparoscopic redo operations after unsuccessful antireflux procedure are rarely reported in children, whereas there is a wealth of such reports on adults series [2, 9, 10, 16, 20, 23, 25].

After an unsuccessful antireflux procedure, careful preoperative evaluation, planning and preparation are necessary to achieve optimal outcome [10]. Surgical interventions need to be tailored to the specifics of each patient, above all in case of neurologically impaired children [10]. Our aim focus here is to describe the feasibility of laparoscopic revision surgery following previous open and laparoscopic antireflux operations in children.

34.2
Mechanisms Responsible for the Failure of a Fundoplication

There are several reasons for which a fundoplication may fail. The first is the development of a recurrent GER; the second is the onset of severe postoperative symptoms, such as dysphagia, pain, retching, or dumping syndrome; and the third is the slipping of the wrap, usually upwards into the thorax. The patient with a slipped fundoplication may be asymptomatic or may present with dysphagia, pain, retching, or recurrent reflux. The diagnosis is usually made on the basis of the clinical history and radiological findings.

Failure of the fundoplication may occur either for technical errors in the performance of the operation or because of patient-related risk factors, which should nevertheless be investigated before surgery, with careful patient selection.

Technical errors are extremely rare events, since fundoplications are considered elective surgery and must therefore be performed only in centers with sound experience in the treatment of gastroesophageal reflux.

In contrast, two important reasons for failure may be represented by the wrong indication for surgery, and the presence of neurological impairments in the patient. Concerning the first aspect, it is important for the surgeon to always perform a complete pre-operative evaluation and to study all the aspects of the patient's GER before performing a fundoplication.

In any case, a major problem is the management of neurologically impaired children (NIC) affected by GER, because these patients have a high incidence of complications after fundoplication, and the issue of which is the best treatment to adopt in these cases is still matter of debate. For this reason, a redo surgery in a neurologically impaired child may be very challenging and extremely difficult for a pediatric surgeon.

34.3
Preoperative Evaluation

A complete preoperative evaluation represents an essential step in patients who have experienced unsuccessful antireflux surgery. A careful evaluation of the dysfunction requiring correction, of the reason for the previous failure, and the therapeutic strategies adopted during the first operation (e.g. closure of the crura, fixation of the valve) is fundamental. The operating notes from the previous operation should be reviewed.

Radiological studies are an invaluable guide to the anatomy and provide a road map for the other investigations. The surgeon must accurately evaluate the anatomic lesion, its etiology, and functional consequences.

Our team's procedure is to control preoperatively all the aspects of GERD by means of 24-h pH-metry, manometry, and endoscopy. In NIC patients, it is especially important to verify gastric emptying, either by ultrasonography or scintigraphy. As a matter of fact, the choice of the type of fundoplication may depend on the results of these exams, as may the decision of whether to add a feeding gastrostomy or eventually a feeding jejunostomy.

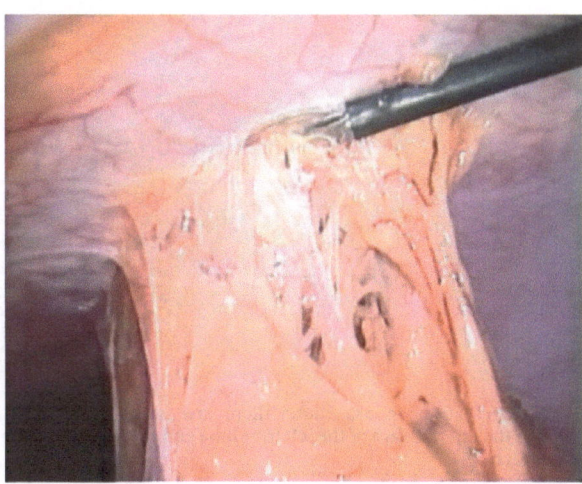

Fig. 1. The first step of the redo procedure consists of lysis of the adhesions, which are particularly strong after a first open operation

34.4
Operative Strategy

The operating strategy to adopt in a patient who has had a previous antireflux surgery should be carefully planned preoperatively. On the basis of preoperative evaluation, the surgeon must have clearly in mind the technique to adopt. In case of dysphagia following the previous antireflux procedure, it may be preferable to perform a less tight procedure, such as the 270° fundoplication according to Toupet.

Pre-operative planning is extremely important in NIC. In fact, after a failed antireflux procedure in NIC, some surgeons prefer to always add a feeding gastrostomy or jejunostomy to the fundoplication; others prefer to perform an esophagogastric disconnection in cases of several recurrences of GER after several surgical procedures [24].

34.5
Surgical Technique in Cases of Redo Surgery

Four or five trocars may be used to perform a redo antireflux surgery. The first step of the operation consists in the lysis of the adhesions, which are particularly strong after open procedures (Fig. 1). Thereafter, the old antireflux mechanism is dismounted, the anatomic structures identified, and a new fundoplication performed.

The type of fundoplication is generally decided by the surgeon on the basis of preoperative exams and the patient's neurological status. Our team prefers to perform a 270° wrap according to Toupet or a 360° fundoplication according to Nissen. In all of our patients, we performed a posterior closure of the crura with one or two stitches of nonresorbable suture. The valve wall is always fixed at the end of procedure to the right crura with one or two stitches to stabilize the wrap.

Redo procedures are successfully completed laparoscopically in about 70–80% of cases. In about 20% of cas-

es of recurrence of GER after open surgery, it is necessary to convert to open surgery as a consequence of a difficult dissection of the anatomic planes.

Operating time is longer compared to a first operation for GER, and ranges, in our experience, between 70 and 150 min (median 95 min).

The hospitalization is similar to the first operation for GER.

34.6
Discussion

Reports of failure of an antireflux procedure, possibly caused by recurrent GERD or migration of the valve into the thorax, have been rarely reported in pediatric literature.

The laparoscopic approach may be used successfully to treat patients in whom antireflux operations have failed. Good results have been achieved in adults despite the technical difficulty of the procedure [4, 6, 21, 22]. We believe that it is extremely important to have an overview of this problem, on the basis of our experience and on a review of the literature. First of all, it is important to underline that it is completely different to operate on children who have undergone unsuccessful open surgery, compared to laparoscopic fundoplication [8, 16].

Indeed, patients operated in open surgery the first time present at laparoscopic redo surgery a large number of adhesions between the epiploon and the abdominal wall scar, as well as between the internal face of the left liver lobe and the anterior part of stomach (Fig. 2). Therefore, in case of recurrence after open surgery, the first part of redo laparoscopic procedure consists in the lysis of the adhesions: this is generally simple at the be-

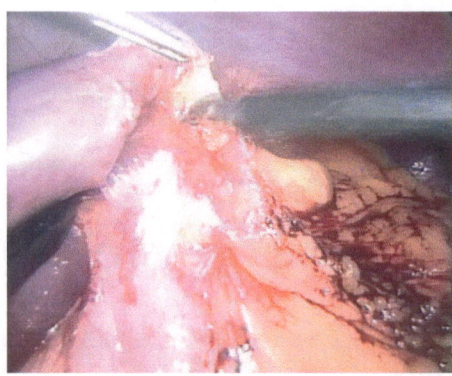

Fig. 2. After an open procedure, there are several adhesions between the internal face of the left liver lobe and the anterior part of stomach

ginning but may become extremely difficult when trying to identify a correct dissection plane between the liver and the stomach [12, 13, 17]. In contrast, the esophagogastric junction is approached quite simply in laparoscopy .

The second problem depends on the type of fundoplication performed the first time: in Thal's procedure, for instance, the posterior part of the esophagus is free from adhesions because it is not involved in the first procedure. In cases of Toupet's or Nissen's approaches, the dissection of the two crura and the posterior wall of the esophagus may also be difficult during redo surgery.

The third difficulty may depend on the cause of the recurrence. In cases of valve disruption, it is not difficult to create a new valve and fix it stably at the end of the procedure [6, 7]. Even in case of recurrent reflux, it is sufficient to have a longer endoabdominal esophageal portion and change the type of fundoplication if necessary, although in most cases a 360° fundoplication according to Nissen may be needed [7].

In case of thorax migration of the valve, the redo procedure may be difficult; to reduce the possibility of iatrogenic complications, a conversion to open surgery may be advisable. Patients who experience valve migration often suffer from neurological impairment that leads to abnormal movements of the diaphragm and esophagus, and this, in turn, produces a great work load on the fundoplication [14, 16]. The operation in these cases consists of reducing the migration, bringing the crura closer and redoing the fundoplication, preferably according to Nissen. Contrarily to adults, prostheses to close the crura are not adopted in children after reducing the valve migration [11, 19].

The key factors to a successful redo procedure are closing the crura, creating a solid valve, and fixing it to the right crura at the end of the procedure. To reduce the incidence of complications, a blunt and delicate dissection is performed at the beginning of the redo proce-

dure to exactly identify the anatomic structures, and a correct dissection plane.

In NIC, it is necessary to choose whether the best strategy would be to perform a new fundoplication or, alternatively whether it may be useful to perform an antireflux procedure together with a feeding jejunostomy, to avoid the delayed gastric emptying that is so common in this type of patient.

In conclusion, laparoscopic reoperative antireflux surgery is feasible if performed by skilled laparoscopic surgeons. Reoperation is likely to be more difficult following failure of an open procedure than a laparoscopic one.

References

1. Croce E, Azzola M, Russo R, Golia M, Olmi S (1997) Laparoscopic re-operation from gastro-oesophageal reflux. Hepatogastroenterology 44(15):912–917
2. Curet MJ, Josloff RK, Schoeb O, Zucker KA (1999) Laparoscopic reoperation for failed antireflux procedures. Arch Surg 134(5):559–563
3. Domini R (1972) Chirurgia delle Ernie Diaframmatiche e del reflusso gastroesofageo. Piccin, Padova
4. Esposito C (2003) Fundoplication: certainly a friend for children if the indication for surgery is correct. J Pediatr Gastr Nutr 7:545–546
5. Esposito C, Becmeur F, Centonze A, Settimi A, Amici G, Montupet P (2002) Laparoscopic reoperation following unsuccessful antireflux surgery in childhood. Semin Laparosc Surg 3:179–182
6. Esposito C., Montupet P, Amici G, Desruelle P (2000) Complications of laparoscopic antireflux surgery in childhood. Surg Endosc 14(7):658–660
7. Esposito C, Van Der Zee DC, Settimi A, Doldo P, Staiano A, Bax NM (2003) Risks and benefits of surgical management of gastroesophageal reflux in neurologically impaired children. Surg Endosc 17:708–710
8. Edye MB, Canin-Endres J, Gattorno F, Salky BA (1998) Durability of laparoscopic repair of paraesophageal hernia. Ann Surg 228(4):528–535
9. Floch NR, Hinder RA, Klingler PJ, Branton SA, Seelig MH, Bammer T, Filipi CJ (1999) Is laparoscopic reoperation for failed antireflux surgery feasible? Arch Surg 134(7):733–737
10. Fonkalsrud EW, Ashcraft KW, Coran AG, Ellis DG, Grosfeld JL, Tunell WP, Weber TR (1998) Surgical treatment of gastroesophageal reflux in children: a combined hospital study of 7467 patients. Pediatrics 101(3 Pt 1):419–422
11. Fontaumard E, Espalieu P, Boulez J (1995) Results of the celioscopic treatment of gastroesophageal reflux according to Nissen-Rossetti. Apropos of 94 cases. Ann Chir 49(6):507–512
12. Frantzides CT, Carlson MA (1997) Laparoscopic redo Nissen fundoplication. J Laparoendosc Adv Surg Tech A 7(4):235–239
13. Langer JC (2003) The failed fundoplication. Semin Pediatr Surg 12(2):110–117
14. Lillehei CW, Shamberger RC (2003) Reoperative esophageal surgery. Semin Pediatr Surg 12(2):100–106
15. Liu DC, Flattmann GJ, Karam MT, Siegrist BI, Loe WA, Hill CB (2000) Laparoscopic fundoplication in children with previous abdominal surgery. J Pediatr Surg 35(2):334–337
16. O'Reilly MJ, Mullins S, Reddick EJ (1997) Laparoscopic management of failed antireflux surgery. Surg Laparosc Endosc 7(2):90–93
17. Pointner R, Bammer T, Then P, Kamolz T (1999) Laparoscopic refundoplications after failed antireflux surgery. Am J Surg 178(6):541–544
18. Simpson B, Ricketts RR, Parker PM (1998) Prosthetic patch stabilization of crural repair in antireflux surgery in children. Am Surg 64(1):67–69; discussion 69–70

19. Stirling MC, Orringer MB (1986) Surgical treatment after the failed antireflux operation. J Thorac Cardiovasc Surg 92(4): 667–672
20. Szwerc MF, Wiechmann RJ, Maley RH, Santucci TS, Macherey RS, Landreneau RJ (1999) Reoperative laparoscopic antireflux surgery. Surgery 126(4):723–728; discussion 728–729
21. Turnage RH, Oldham KT, Coran AG, Blane CE (1989) Late results of fundoplication for gastroesophageal reflux in infants and children. Surgery 105(4):457–464
22. van der Zee DC, Arends NJ, Bax NM (1999) The value of 24-h pH study in evaluating the results of laparoscopiantireflux surgery in children. Surg Endosc 13(9):918–921
23. van der Zee DC, Bax NM, Ure BM (2000) Laparoscopic refundoplication in children. Surg Endosc 14(12):1103–1104
24. van der Zee DC, Bax NM, Ure BM (2000) Laparoscopic secondary antireflux procedure after PEG placement in children. Surg Endosc 14(12):1105–1106
25. Watson DI, Jamieson GG, Game PA, Williams RS, Devitt PG (1999) Laparoscopic reoperation following failed antireflux surgery. Br J Surg 86(1):98–101

Chapter 35

The Management of GER in Neurologically Impaired Patients

35

Thom E. Lobe · Tarun Kumar

Contents

35.1
Introduction

The optimal management today for GER in neurologically impaired (NI) children is a subject of great controversy, and there is no conformity of thought. Several authors have studied the role of gastrostomy tube placement in NI children, stressing facilitation of care and family satisfaction [1]. Others extensively evaluated the need for an antireflux procedure in these patients [2, 3].

Neurological impairment is defined as an abnormality of the central nervous system, manifest during the developmental period, that results in lifelong disability in any of the physical, cognitive, sensory, speech and language, or neuropsychological functions [4]. The incidence of neurological impairment ranges from 6 to 20 per 1,000 with a slight male preponderance [4]; 0.3% of the general population have severe neurological impairment [4, 5] and 0.1% need continuous care [6]. The vast majority of causes of neurological impairment remain unknown and among the known ones, prenatal genetic disorders represent the majority (40–60%) [6].

35.2
The Problem

Recent reports indicate that the number of NI children is constantly increasing due to advances in medical care for premature babies [6]. These children commonly have feeding and nutritional problems leading to malnutrition [1]. This can have serious consequences leading to potentially irreversible impairment of physical and brain growth, with further developmental delay in the critical period for brain maturation. It may also undermine their immune response and respiratory muscle strength, and result in recurrent pulmonary infections [7, 8]. The nutritional problem is complicated because NI children often demonstrate abnormal feeding behavior with poor sucking ability, improper jaw-lip and tongue control, inability to maintain head posture during feeds, and incoordination of oropharyngeal and tongue reflexes with defective swallowing. All these factors result in making oral feeding an unpleasant and sometimes dangerous experience for both the child and caregiver [9] and can consume many hours daily [10]. Feeding often results in choking, coughing, retching, and gagging, and puts the child at risk of aspiration [1]. This in turn predisposes the child to a wide spectrum of airway and pulmonary problems including recurrent pneumonias, bronchitis, asthma exacerbation, and wheezing and apnea and bradycardia [9]. Other issues that contribute to difficulty and refusal to eat include gastrointestinal dysmotility and delayed gastric emptying due to a presumed autonomic neuropathy [1], constipation due to immobility, ventilation dependency due to severe brain damage or associated anomalies, and gastroesophageal reflux disease. The end result is a nutritionally depleted child with failure to thrive.

35.3
Gastroesophageal Reflux Disease (GERD)

Gastroesophageal reflux is a common problem in these patients, ranging in incidence ranging between 15% and

75% [11, 12]. Predisposing factors include a higher incidence of hiatal hernia, adoption of a prolonged supine position, increased intraabdominal pressure due to spasticity, scoliosis, seizures, or respiratory distress and coughing from aspiration [13]. The use of sedatives and relaxants to relieve spasticity further compromises the lower esophageal sphincter mechanism and promotes reflux [14]. Ventilator-dependent NI children subjected to positive airway pressure have a weaker lower esophageal sphincter barrier due to decreased length of intraabdominal esophagus and constant increase of intragastric pressure. This results in a higher incidence of GERD [14].

Recent studies using electrogastrography suggest that vomiting in children with central nervous system disease involving the brainstem nuclei may result from widespread activation of the emetic reflex, and differentiate it from GERD proper [15]. Infants with a hyperactive emetic reflex usually have a prodromal phase and forceful vomiting associated with retching and gagging.

Neurologically impaired patients with GERD can present in a array of ways. The most frequently seen is vomiting, usually effortless, in the supine and upright position and even during sleep [14]. Pulmonary complications also are common and include chronic lung disease, recurrent pneumonias and bronchitis, asthma and wheezing, stridor, apnea and bradycardia, cyanosis, hypoxemia, and sometimes sudden infant death syndrome [14]. In neonates, GERD often complicates respiratory distress syndrome and ventilator management. Reflux esophagitis causes pain that makes the child refuse to eat and can lead to stricture formation with dysphagia and later development of Barrett's changes in adolescence. Severe dental caries, hoarseness of voice, recurrent ear infections, subglottic stenosis, and anemia occur frequently [14].

35.4
The Solution

The many factors that lead to malnutrition and failure to thrive with difficulty of oral feeding in the neurologically impaired child dictate the need for alternative measures to improve nutrition. A temporary alternative is tube feeding (nasogastric or nasojejunal). Insertion of these tubes is unpleasant for the child and caregiver and may even hinder resumption of oral feeding later, as these children often associate feeding with the noxious experience of tube insertion [1]. When it becomes apparent that tube feeding will be necessary for longer than 6–8 weeks, a permanent feeding tube such as a gastrostomy should be considered [1].

35.5
Gastrostomy Tubes

The most common indications for gastrostomy tube placement in these patients include dysphagia, failure to thrive, aspiration, vomiting, ventilator dependence, and intolerance of prolonged tube feeding. Most studies show improvement of nutritional status after gastrostomy placement including weight gain, decreased coughing and choking, and improved patient's well-being and caregivers' satisfaction [1]. Vomiting improved in those who had an additional fundoplication, while the rate of pulmonary infection, pain, and epilepsy were not affected despite easier administration of medicine. It seems that gastrostomy feeding, even after an antireflux procedure, does not reduce the incidence of aspiration in these children, many of whom cannot swallow their own saliva [1]. Complications have been described in up to 28% of patients [15].

Fashioning of a gastrostomy to provide enteral nutrition was first suggested by Egeberg in 1837 [16], although it was not until 1876 that a patient survived the attempt [17]. The most commonly accepted method of gastrostomy placement in children remained the Stamm's gastrostomy technique for years. The next major advance in gastrostomy placement occurred in 1979, when percutaneous endoscopic gastrostomy was introduced by Ponsky [18]. Since then, several modifications of the basic technique have been suggested [19]. Percutaneous nonendoscopic (fluoroscopic) techniques for creation of a gastrostomy were first described by Prewshaw in 1981 and have also undergone minor modifications [20]. With increasing interest in minimally invasive surgery in the 1990's, it is not surprising that attempts at laparoscopic gastrostomy insertion were made, the first report in the literature appearing in 1991 [21].

Another major evolution in gastrostomy placement was the introduction of the low-profile devices (buttons) in the late 1980's by Gaurder et al. [22]. Buttons prove far superior to latex or even silicon tubes, as they sit securely at skin level, creating less torque at the insertion site and hence fewer wound problems, better cosmetic appearance, and less accidental dislodgement or distal migration [20].

Laparoscopic button placement also became feasible as a simple and safe technique of gastrostomy insertion that can be combined with a fundoplication. Several modifications have been devised to ensure the simplest technique and the best results [22, 23].

Although conventional open insertion of a gastrostomy is always safe and associated with few complications, it has the disadvantage and morbidity of an open procedure, especially in the nutritionally compromised [22]. The minimally invasive percutaneous procedure and the fluoroscopic gastrostomy are appealing options, but they are relatively contraindicated in the presence of uncontrolled ascites, coagulopathy, a large hiatus hernia, gastric wall pathology, presence of gastroesophageal reflux, and previous abdominal surgery [22, 24]. They also are absolutely contraindicated when it is not possible to pass an endoscope or nasogastric tube into the stomach. Failure of insertion is still reported in up to 24% of cases [25]. In addition, these techniques do not allow optimal control of the site of the gastrostomy on the gastric or abdominal walls, and can even result in a higher incidence of visceral injury [22]. Furthermore, lack of fixation of the stomach to the abdominal wall can result in separation of the stomach from the abdominal wall, air embolization, or even peritonitis if premature attempts at tube replacement are made [26]. Other problems common to either open or percutaneous gastrostomy tubes that can be minimized by using a laparoscopic primary button include leakage, excessive granulation, skin irritation, wound infection or dehiscence, and device migration or malfunction [18, 26].

Laparoscopy, however, is not without its problems. It requires the availability of special and expensive equipment and may take longer than percutaneous placement [22]. Major complications, namely, injury to viscera and major vessels and gas embolization, occur in up to 0.2% of cases [27]. These, and the problems of CO_2 pneumoperitoneum, can be minimized by the routine use of open laparoscopy [28], appropriate instrumentation, monitoring, and an understanding of safe laparoscopic practice [22].

35.6
The Need for an Antireflux Procedure

Although long-term follow-up studies show the efficacy of a gastrostomy alone, one of the most significant complications after its placement is the development of GERD [29, 30]. The reported incidence of GERD with gastrostomy placement in neurologically impaired children ranges from 14% to 91% [31, 32]. Even with the percutaneous approach in neurologically impaired patients, GERD occurs 25% of the time [33]. Twenty years ago it was routine practice to perform a protective wrap along with gastrostomy placement [14], even in the absence of documented GERD.

This attitude has changed, however, over the past decade to reserving a wrap for those who have preoperative evidence of GERD. There are several reasons for this change. The advent of percutaneous techniques, which only require sedation, makes the addition of a wrap (a procedure requiring general anesthesia) seem like a safer or at least more appealing option. There is increasing evidence from several centers that gastrosto-

mies do not consistently promote GERD [34], thus reducing the performance of concomitant antireflux procedures in those centers to between 4% and 14% [34]. The results of studies on proton pump inhibitors in children demonstrates their high efficacy in controlling reflux, even after surgery [2], and the increasing recognition of significant morbidity associated with antireflux surgery in neurologically impaired patients also caused surgeons to reconsider the addition of a wrap in NI children undergoing gastrostomy placement.

With NI children comprising the majority of those undergoing wraps [13], there are high failure rates and significant morbidity and mortality [34]. The failure rate and complications vary between 12% and 59%, and the mortality is as high as 40.6% [1]. One study reports twice the complication rate, three times the morbidity rate, and four times the re-operation rate for NI children undergoing wraps compared with neurologically normal children, over a mean follow-up of only 1.6 years [35]. In another study, more than 30% of NI patients had major complications or died within 30 days of surgery. Within a mean follow-up of 3.5 years, 25% have documented operative failure and, overall, there is return of one or more preoperative symptoms of GERD in 71% [36]. Although the operative mortality for wraps ranges from 1% to 3% for both normal and NI candidates [12], there is increased late mortality for NI children related to co-existing abnormalities and intraabdominal complications, notably adhesive bowel obstruction and paraesophageal hernia [34].

The most frequent complication in NI children is recurrence of GERD symptoms due to paraesophageal herniation or disruption of the wrap [34]. Predictors of recurrence include severe neurological impairment, hypertonic cerebral palsy, esophageal dysmotility and delayed gastric emptying [2], preoperative evidence of severe reflux with esophagitis [33], and persistent postoperative retching [13]. The technique chosen does not appear to affect the rate of recurrence [35]. Objective evidence of recurrent reflux after fundoplication ranges from 6% to 36% [34], often is difficult to elucidate, and its detection requires a high index of suspicion with repeated testing over time using multiple modalities [34]. Initial management of recurrent reflux should be medical, and the need for redo surgery is only 5–15% [34].

Another distressing problem is postoperative retching with or without recurrent vomiting [13]. This occurs mainly in those having a hyperactive emetic reflex as reported by Richards et al. [13], and may explain the high failure rate of wraps in NI children who were misdiagnosed with GERD. These patients should not undergo antireflux procedures (ARP) as it may even worsen the symptoms. They are better served by measures to suppress the emetic reflex, e.g. antiemetics and modulators of gastric vagal afferents (tricyclic antidepressants), and continuous drip feeds. If these measures fail, jejunostomy feeding or even esophagogastric dissociation may be required as "a once and for all effective procedure" [36].

Other complications include the gas-bloat syndrome, particularly with complete wraps, and the dumping syndrome that may present with hypoglycemia and unresponsiveness.

An additional compounding factor is the high prevalence of delayed gastric emptying and gastrointestinal dysmotility that have been postulated by some to increase the failure rate of antireflux surgery, posing more stress on the wrap. Some authors thus have recommended the addition of a gastric emptying procedure (pyloroplasty, pyloromyotomy, or anteroplasty) at the time of the wrap to avoid failure [37]. Others recommend a partial wrap to allow for belching and vomiting [38]. However, no general consensus regarding the need for an emptying procedure has been reached. Studies show the inaccuracy of preoperative gastric scans in predicting postoperative gastric emptying and failure of gastric emptying to improve after emptying procedures in most cases [39].

The current recommendations from most authors are that: A wrap should be performed only in those with documented moderate to severe reflux, proven by contrast studies, endoscopy or 24-h pH monitoring, although the latter has been unreliable in NI patients, with a sensitivity of 38.5% and specificity of 71.4% [40]. Patients with mild GERD can be offered a trial of gastrostomy alone with close follow-up to monitor for secondary GERD. If this occurs, an attempt can be made to control symptoms medically with a change to continuous feeds [34]. Secondary GERD in these patients sometimes is a temporary event accompanying an intercurrent infection or inadequate seizure control, and medical management may be sufficient [34]. If GERD persists, as evidenced by upper gastrointestinal radiographs, a wrap is needed. An attempt also should be made to clinically identify those patients with a hyperactive emetic reflex in whom a wrap probably should be avoided.

Several different types of operations have been devised to fulfill these goals. The most widely accepted one is the fundoplication originally described by Nissen and Rosetti [41]. Although modifications have been adopted, it remains the gold standard for the treatment of reflux, especially in patients with severe GERD fed by gastrostomy. It is effective with more than 92% of patients having long-term resolution of their symptoms [14].

A Thal anterior fundoplication [3] is preferred by some surgeons in NI children and those with esophageal dysmotility, because they maintain the ability to burp or vomit. Results are comparable to a Nissen fundoplication with less operative time and hospital stay, but a higher incidence of recurrent GERD [42]. The Toupet partial fundoplication [43] also is recommended in patients with abnormal esophageal motility or manometry to reduce the incidence of postoperative dysphagia [14]. However, in a recent study comparing laparoscopic Toupet with laparoscopic Nissen fundoplication, there was a higher incidence of dysphagia, epigastric pain, and early recurrence with the Toupet procedure [44].

Other procedures include the Boix-Ochoa procedure, Borema gastropexy, Collis gastroplasty, and Belsey-Mark IV procedure; all have been used in adults with few applications in children [14]. Finally, wraps can be performed safely in premature infants, those less than 10 kg [45] and in those less than 3 months old [46].

Nissen fundoplication relieves emesis in 76–100% of children [14]. Pulmonary symptoms either are cured or relieved in 66–96% of patients, weight gain is achieved in 38–100% of patients with failure to thrive and asthmatic symptoms, and esophagitis resolves in a high proportion of patients [14]. In one study, 90% of those with isolated GERD improved, compared to 64% of those with associated anomalies [14]. Complications are more common and outcome less favorable in NI children. Complications of the procedure, but not particularly prevalent in NI patients, are rare operative complications (pneumothorax, splenic injury, or bowel perforation) [14], gastric volvulus [47], delayed gastric necrosis, and wound infection (<2%) [14].

35.7
Surgical Management of GERD

The main indication for surgery is persistent symptomatic esophagitis despite adequate medical treatment [39]. For children with severe complications of reflux such as aspiration, failure to thrive, esophagitis, or stricture, antireflux surgery can be performed shortly after the diagnosis is established [14].

The major objectives of operative repair are to increase the high-pressure zone in the lower esophagus, to accentuate the angle of His, and to increase the length of the abdominal esophagus [14].

35.8
Laparoscopic Nissen Fundoplication (LNF)

Minimally invasive surgery in children has revolutionized the management of many conditions. The first GERD cured by laparoscopy in an adult was reported in 1991 by Dallemagne et al. [37]. Georgeson and Lobe et al. published their first experiences in children in 1992 [40, 48]. Since then, the procedure gained popularity as the procedure of choice for severe, symptomatic GERD. With its short postoperative stay, decreased postoperative pain, and complete relief of most reflux symptoms, the frequency of laparoscopic wraps is increasing [39].

All wraps can be performed with the laparoscope with results comparable to those of their respective open techniques. A study comparing laparoscopic Nissen, Rosetti, and Toupet procedures in adults found no differences with regard to conversion rate, morbidity, and reintervention rate. With the Toupet procedure, however, the operative time and the postoperative complaints were greater than those reported in the Nissen group [49]. A gastric emptying procedure can always be added laparoscopically in those who need it.

Results of laparoscopic Nissen wraps are comparable to those of open Nissen fundoplications, including the higher incidence of complications and late mortality in NI children. The procedure effectively reduces heartburn and regurgitation in 91–95% of patients, and oral feeding is rendered asymptomatic in 71.7% of patients [45]. While the laparoscopic wrap can be performed safely in small infants less than 10 kg and younger than 1 year of age [46], it is reported by some to be less effective in controlling cough and dysphagia [49].

Laparoscopic fundoplication is associated with an intraoperative complication rate of 0–8.3% and a postoperative complication rate of 0.07–6.1%, even in a study population where 75.4% of patients were NI [45, 50]. Recurrence of GERD is reported in 3.2–20% [39, 45, 46], the conversion rate varied between 0.9% and 8% [46, 51], and redo surgery was required in 3.6–11.1% [39, 45]. All the aforementioned problems closely resemble those reported in studies on open Nissen procedures [14]. Despite the fact that no study evaluating the incidence of postoperative complications in children with neurological impairment after laparoscopic wraps is available, collective data indicate that there is a higher complication and failure rate in these children. In one study, 78% of children who required redo surgery had neurological impairment [52]. Persistent dysphagia, gas bloating, and distressing retching and gagging are also more prevalent in these children [45], making careful evaluation necessary prior to surgery.

Despite these problems, a laparoscopic wrap has several advantages over the open technique. The procedure appears to be associated with fewer complications such as adhesive intestinal obstruction, wound complications, and postoperative pulmonary complications [53]. Moreover, there appears to be a shorter hospitalization and an earlier return to enteral alimentation and unrestricted activities [53]. Restoration of postoperative feeding is possible on the day of surgery in most studies [45, 51], and the postoperative stay ranges between 1.2 and 15 days, with the majority of reports in the 3- to 4-day range [39]. When the cost-effectiveness of the laparoscopic procedure is evaluated, the hospital savings is $5,391 [54]. Postoperative pain is reported to be less after laparoscopy, although one study cites that while the total amount of morphine analgesia is similar for the laparoscopic and open procedures, the period for which analgesia is required is significantly less in the laparoscopic group [44]. Cosmetic benefits are argued by some authors [14], and there is high family satisfaction with the small port wounds [53]. In NI children, laparoscopy is reported to decrease morbidity compared with laparotomy [45].

The main disadvantage of laparoscopy is the operative time, which ranges between "a little over an hour" [55] and 221 min [56]. Lengthy procedures were reported at the beginning of the learning curve from many centers, but these generally trend towards shorter times. Some investigators also report that significant early dysphagia is more common in patients who have undergone laparoscopy, but this usually resolves with time [45].

35.9
Which Approach is Better?

To evaluate the efficacy and outcome of gastrostomy in NI children, we reviewed the records of 130 NI patients who had gastrostomies placed either laparoscopically (n=56) or open (n=74) between January 1999 and October 2001.

Data collected included demographic data (age, sex, race, and weigh), admission diagnosis, reason for gastrostomy placement, operative data (procedure description, operative time, additional procedures, and type of tube placed) postoperative course (time to 1st feed and postoperative stay), early complications (operative complications, conversion to open in cases of laparoscopic procedures, early postoperative problems, e.g. fever, atelectasis, or ileus; mortality), late complications (feeding problems, e.g. dysphagia, intolerance of oral feeds or high gastrostomy residuals; device complications, e.g. tube breakage, dislodgement, clogging, or migration; site complications, e.g. granulation, infection, bleeding, leakage or persistent fistula; and development of GERD symptoms), analgesic requirements (Acetaminophen, Morphine Sulphate, Codene or Fentanyl), and follow-up data (re-admissions, emergency visits, and surgery related to gastrostomy tubes as well as clinic visits and frequency of tube changes).

All patients were evaluated with a modified barium swallow to identify swallowing dysfunction or aspiration, in addition to an upper gastrointestinal tract contrast radiograph or milk scan to identify associated GERD. The contrast study was always done as the initial investigation to identify GERD and to evaluate the anatomy before surgery. Milk scans were done whenever the results of the contrast study were equivocal in high-risk symptomatic patients, despite failure of the study to demonstrate reflux. It was also used to detect delayed gastric emptying and dysmotility.

An attempt was always made to maximize the nutritional status (as expressed by weight gain and improvement of prealbumin levels) of these patients before surgery, either through tube feeds or the parenteral route. In patients with aspiration pneumonia or other infectious issues, treatment with a course of antibiotics was always considered. Those with GERD had a trial of medical treatment for at least 2–4 weeks prior to surgery.

Open gastrostomies were placed using the standard Stamm gastrostomy technique through a midline incision. Latex tubes usually were used in these cases and were exteriorized through a separate stab incision in the left upper quadrant. Occasionally, in latex-sensitive patients and in those whose family requested placement of a low-profile device, a primary button was placed. Latex tubes usually were changed to a button in the clinic after an average of 2 months. Laparoscopic gastrostomies were placed after institution of CO_2 pneumoperitoneum (using the open or closed technique) using a two-port technique. A low-profile, gastrostomy replacement button of appropriate size was inserted using the Seldinger technique through the left upper quadrant trocar site and secured with two "U" stitches, and was connected to a right-angled drainage catheter. Open Nissen fundoplications were performed through a midline abdominal incision with division of the short gastric vessels to assure a loose 360° wrap. The crura were always approximated. The gastrostomy was placed along the greater curvature of the stomach, midway between the wrap and the pylorus, at the end of the procedure. The laparoscopic wraps were performed using a five-port technique after institution of CO_2 pneumoperitoneum. The loose 360° wrap and the primary button were constructed as described above. We evaluated the patients in four groups: Group I ($n=12$) was composed of those who had laparoscopic gastrostomy placement alone (or combined with other minor procedures), Group II ($n=44$) was the patients who had open gastrostomy placement alone (or combined with other minor procedures), Group III ($n=44$) was those who had laparoscopic gastrostomy with Nissen fundoplication, and Group IV ($n=30$) was those who had open gastrostomy with Nissen fundoplication. Data were statistically verified using Student's t-test for unequal variances. Institutional Review Board approval was obtained.

35.10
Results

The children consisted of 47 females (36.2%) and 83 males (63.8%); their mean age was 3.64 years (range 10 days to 17.7 years) and their weight averaged between 1.2 kg and 63.4 kg (mean 12.8 kg).

Neurological impairment was ascribed to a variety of conditions, namely, genetic disorders (e.g. Down's syndrome, Cornellia De Lange) ($n=32$), traumatic head injury ($n=8$), encephalitis (infectious and noninfectious) ($n=8$), neoplasia ($n=8$), vascular accidents ($n=14$), anoxic brain injury ($n=11$), seizure disorder ($n=13$), hydro- or microcephaly ($n=9$), and cerebral palsy ($n=24$).

The indication for gastrostomy tube placement included aspiration ($n=24$), failure to thrive ($n=49$), ventilator dependence ($n=14$), oropharyngeal dysphagia ($n=20$), and GERD ($n=23$). GERD was found in 74 of our patients (56.9%), and these patients were offered a Nissen fundoplication together with the gastrostomy, either open ($n=30$) or laparoscopic ($n=44$). Only 15 of these patients (20%) had silent GERD detected either by the upper gastrointestinal contrast study or the milk scan.

The groups all showed similar characteristics with regards to age, weight, cause of mental impairment, and the reason for placement of the gastrostomy. These characteristics are shown in Tables 1–3.

The average operative times for Groups I and II were similar. The average time for Group III was 117.4 min versus 79.7 min for Group IV ($p<0.05$). There were no significant differences in the performance of additional

Table 1. Patient characteristics

Group	I	II	III	IV
n	12	44	44	30
Weight (kg)	23.5	14	6.6	7.2
Age (Y)	7.18	3.7	1.7	2

Table 2. Causes of neurological impairment

Group	I	II	III	IV	n
Genetic disorder	5	8	11	8	32
Cerebral palsy	3	5	12	4	24
Hemorrhage	0	4	5	5	14
Seizures	0	5	4	4	13
Anoxic brain injury	0	3	7	1	11
Hydro or Microcephaly	0	7	0	2	9
Trauma	3	4	0	1	8
Encephalitis	0	1	3	4	8
Neoplasia	1	6	1	0	8
Others	0	1	1	1	3

Table 3. Reasons for gastrostomy placement

Group	I	II	III	IV
Aspiration	3	12	7	2
FTT	2	18	19	10
Vent dependence	3	6	2	3
Dysphagia	4	8	3	5
GERD	0	0	13	10

procedures between groups, and the postoperative course is shown in Table 4. Analgesic requirements were no different between groups.

Complications (Table 5) appeared to be fewer with laparoscopy 25% (Group I) vs. 41% (Group II) and 45% (Group III) vs. 53% (Group IV); however, these differences were not significant.

Follow-up showed less long-term morbidity and fewer complications with the laparoscopic gastrostomy compared to the open one (Table 5). Re-operation was only required in the open gastrostomy group for an ARP in two patients (one laparoscopic) and twice for revision of the gastrostomy. Emergency department visits for Groups III and IV patients were due to recurrent respiratory problems (three in Group III, two in Group IV), feeding problems (three in each group) or cardiopulmonary arrest (one in Group III, three in Group IV). Re-operation in the ARP groups consisted of one redo laparoscopic Nissen (Group III), revision of the gastrostomy sites (two in each group), and repair of a bowel perforation by the gastrostomy (one in each group).

Table 4. Operative data and postoperative course

	I	II	p	III	IV	p
Op time (min)	66.3	44.5	ns	117.4	79.7	0.00003
Other procedure	66	43	ns	16	33	ns
Postop stay (days)	11.2	13.1	0.7	8.4	17.9	0.4
Time to feed (days)	1.1	2.1	0.005	1.6	1.7	0.9

ns, not significant

Table 5. Mean percent complications and follow-up data

Group	I	II	p	III	IV	p
Total complications	25	41	ns	45	53	ns
Operative complications	0	0	ns	2.3	0	ns
Other early complications	8	11	ns	11	16	ns
Conversion	0	0	0	0	0	0
Early postoperative death	0	0	ns	2	0	ns
Device complication	0	4.5	0	16	13	ns
Site complication	0	23	0.0001	20	30	ns
Feeding problems	0	11	0.02	11	10	ns
GERD	8	4.5	ns	7	0	ns
Recurrent respiratory problems	16	9	ns	6.8	6.7	ns
Re-admissions	0	11.4	0.04	16	13	ns
Additional surgery	0	10	0.04	9	10	ns
Emergency department	0	22.7	0.002	25	33	ns
GT change	8	27.3	0.04	22.7	47	ns

ns, not significant

35.11
Discussion

This study was conducted in an attempt to define the best procedure for placement of a gastrostomy in NI children with or without a fundoplication. All our patients with GERD had a course of medical treatment, including the use of proton pump inhibitors, before surgery, in an attempt to avoid a wrap with its added morbidity [34]. The overall complication rate (both early and late) in this series, regardless of the procedure, was 41% over the 2-year period with only one operative mortality (0.7%). Operative complications and early postoperative complications (within 30 days of surgery) occurred in only 13% of our patients. These results compare favorably with the high morbidity reported with gastrostomy alone or with a wrap (12–56%) and with a mortality of up to 40% [1, 36]. Results of our study demonstrate a significant benefit to laparoscopic gastrostomy over the open technique, with no added morbidity or mortality. We found earlier resumption of feeding, fewer feeding problems and dysphagia, fewer gastrostomy site complications, fewer hospital admissions, no re-operation for gastrostomy problems, fewer emergency department visits, and fewer gastrostomy changes. These results suggest the superiority of the technique. New-onset GERD after gastrostomy placement occurred in only three patients (6.25%) (one in the laparoscopic group and two in the open group) and required surgery in two (the open gastrostomy patients). This figure is much lower than other reports [1, 31, 32].

When a wrap was added to the gastrostomy, this added morbidity. Overall complications occurred in 49% of those who had an additional fundoplication, compared to 33% in the gastrostomy-alone groups. Early operative and postoperative complications occurred in 15% of the fundoplication groups, compared to 11% with gastrostomy alone. This confirms the conclusions of other studies that the addition of a wrap at the time of gastrostomy placement is associated with more complications in the neurologically impaired and should not be done routinely as a prophylactic procedure [34]. When comparing laparoscopic and open techniques, there are no statistically significant differences except that the operative time is longer in the laparoscopic group (average 117.4 min). These results are in accordance with the literature [14, 45, 53].

Our low intraoperative complication rate (2.3%) was similar to those of other reports (0–8.3%) [45, 50, 51], despite the fact that the other studies were not conducted solely on NI patients. Neurological impairment may explain the higher incidence of perioperative complications (11%) compared to other studies (0.07–6.1%) [45, 51]. The postoperative stay in the laparoscopic group was slightly longer than that cited elsewhere (3–4 days)

[45, 57] due to the complexity of the patients' medical conditions. The re-institution of enteral feeds at an average of 1.1 days was similar to other reports [45, 51].

In conclusion, it appears that laparoscopic placement of a low-profile gastrostomy in NI children is a safe, simple, and well tolerated and should be the procedure of choice for enteral feeding in those who do not have evidence of moderate to severe reflux. All NI children should be studied before surgery to identify those who have moderate to severe reflux. A course of medical treatment, preferably with proton pump inhibitors, always should be tried first in those with GERD to obviate the need for a wrap. In patients who need a wrap, laparoscopy is a good option and has results comparable to those of the open technique, with apparently fewer complications and shorter hospital stays.

References

1. Tawfik R, Dickson A, Clarke M, et al (1997) Caregivers' perceptions following gastrostomy in severely disabled children with feeding problems. Dev Med Child Neurol 39:746–751
2. Gunasekaran TS, Hassall E (1993) Efficacy and safety of omeprazole for severe gastroesophageal reflux in children. J Pediatr 124:148–154
3. Thal AP (1968) A unified approach to surgical problems of the esophagogastric junction. Ann Surg 168:542–546
4. Kinsbourne M, Graffin W (2000) Disorders of mental development. In: Menkes J, Sarnat H (eds) Child neurology, 6th edn. Lippincott, Williams & Wilkins, Philadelphia, pp 1155–1212
5. Hagberg B, Kyllirman M (1983) Epidemiology of mental retardation–a Swedish survey. Brain Dev 5:441
6. Swaiman K (1994) Mental retardation. In: Swaiman K (ed.) Pediatric neurology principles and practice, 2nd edn. Mosby Year Book, St. Louis, pp 133–146
7. Patrick J, Boland M, Stoski D, Murray GE (1986) Rapid correction of wasting in children with cerebral palsy. Dev Med Child Neurol 28:734–739
8. Ballabriga A (1990) Malnutrition and the central nervous system. In: Suskind RM (ed) The malnourished child. Nestle Nutrition Workshop Series. Vevey Raven Press, New York, pp 177–195
9. Gisel EG, Patrick J (1988) Identification of children unable to maintain a normal nutritional state. Lancet I 283–286
10. Johnson CB, Deitz JC (1985) Time use of mothers with preschool children: a pilot study. Am J Occup Ther 39:578–583
11. Rice H, Seashore JH, Touloukian RJ (1991) Evaluation of Nissen fundoplication in neurologically impaired children. J Pediatr Surg 26:697–701
12. Spitz L, Roth K, Kiely EM, et al (1993) Operation for Gastroesophageal reflux associated with severe mental retardation. Arch Dis Child 68:347–351
13. Halpern LM, Jolley SG, Johnson DG (1991) Gastroesophageal reflux: a significant association with central nervous system disease in children. J Pediatr Surg 26:171–173
14. Fonkalsrud EW, Ament ME (1996) Gastroesophageal reflux. Childhood. Curr Probl Surg 33:1–70
15. Marin OE, Glassman MS, Schoen BT, Caplan DB (1994) Safety and efficacy of percutaneous endoscopic gastrostomy in children. Am J Gastroenterol 89:357–361
16. Cunha F (1946) Gastrostomy: its inception and evolution. Am J Surg 72:610–634
17. Gauderer MW, Stellato TA (1986) Gastostomies: evolution, techniques and complications. Curr Probl Surg 23:657–719
18. Gauderer MWL, Ponsky JL, Izant RJ (1980) Gastrostomy without laparotomy: a percutaneous technique. J Perdiatr Surg 15:872–875
19. Stroedel WE, Lemmer J, Eckhauser F, et al (1983) Early experience with endoscopic percutaneous gastrostomy. Arch Surg 118:449–453
20. Gaurderer MWL, Olsen MM, Stellato TA, et al (1988) Feeding gastrostomy button: experience and recommendations. J Pediatr Surg 23:24–28
21. Gray R, St Louis EL, Grosman H (1987) Percutaneous gastrostomy and gastro-jejunostomy. Br J Radiol 60:1067–1070
22. Humphrey GM, Najmaldin A (1997) Laparoscopic gastrostomy in children. Pediatr Surg Int 12:501–504
23. Rothenberg SS, Bealer JF, Chang JH (1999) Primary laparoscopic placement of gastrostomy buttons for feeding tubes. Surg Endosc 13:995–997
24. Miller PE, Kummer BA, Kotler P, Tiszenkel HI (1995) Percutaneous endoscopic gastrostomy; a safe method for obtaining enteral access. J Surg Res 58:1–5
25. Larson DE, Burton DD, Schroeder KW, DiMagno EP (1987) Percutaneous endoscopic gastrostomy: indications, success, complications and mortality in 314 consecutive patients. Gastroenterology 93:48–52
26. Von Sonnenburg E, Wittich GR, Cabrera OA (1986) Percutaneous gastrostomy and gastroenterostomy; 2 clinical experiences. AJR 146:581–586
27. Chamberlain G, Carron-Brown J (1978) Report of the working party of the confidential inquiry into gynecological laparoscopy. Royal College of Obstetricians and Gynecologists, London, pp 116–117
28. Humphrey GME, Najmaldin A (1994) Modification of the Hasson technique in paediatric laparoscopy. Br J Surg 81:1319
29. Mollitt DL, Golladay ES, Seibert JJ (1985) Symptomatic gastroesophageal reflux following gastrostomy in neurologically impaired patients. Pediatrics 75:1124–1126
30. Grunow JE, al-Hafidh A, Tunell WP (1989) Gastroesophageal reflux following percutaneous endoscopic gastrostomy in children. J Pediatr Surg 24:42–44
31. Turnage RH, Oldham KT, Coran AG, et al (1989) Late results of fundoplication for gastroesophageal reflux in infants and children. Surgery 105:457–463
32. Winkelstein A (1935) Peptic esophagitis; a new clinical entity. J Am Med Assoc 104:906–910
33. Marin OE, Glassman MS, Schoen BT, Caplan DB (1994) Safety and efficacy of percutaneous endoscopic gastrostomy in children. Am J Gastroenterol 89:357–361
34. Sullivan PB (1999) Gastrostomy feeding in the disabled child: when is an antireflux procedure required? Arch Dis Child 81:463–464
35. Pearl RH, Robie DK, Ein SH (1990) Complications of gastroesophageal antireflux surgery in neurologically impaired versus neurologically normal children. J Pediatr Surg 25:1169–1173
36. Martinez DA, Ginn-Pease ME, Caniano DA (1992) Sequelae of antireflux surgery in profoundly disabled children. J Pediatr Surg 27:267–273
37. Georgeson KE (1993) Laparoscopic gastrostomy and fundoplication. Pediatr Ann 92:675–677
38. Dallemagne B, Weets JM, Jehaes C, et al (1991) Laparoscopic Nissen fundoplication. Preliminary report. Surg Laparosc Endosc 1:138–143
39. Esposito C, Montupet P, Reinberg O (2001) Laparoscopic surgery for gastroesophageal reflux disease during the first year of life. J Pediatr Surg 36:715–717
40. Heine RG, Reddihough DS, Catto-Smith AG (1995) Gastroesophageal reflux and feeding problems after gastrostomy in children with severe neurological impairment. Dev Med Child Neurol 37:320–329
41. Nissen R, Rosetti M (1959) Die behandlung von hiatus hernie und reflux oesophagitis mit gastropexie und fundoplication. George Thieme Verlag, Stuttgart
42. Tuggle DW, Tunell WP, Hoelzer DJ, et al (1988) The efficacy of Thal fundoplication in the treatment of gastroesophageal reflux: the influence of central nervous system impairment. J Pediatr Surg 23:638–640
43. Toupet A (1963) La technique d'oesophago-gastroplastie avec phreno-gastropexie appliqué dans la cure radicale des hernies

hiatales et comme complement de l'operation de Heller dans les cardiospasmes>Mem Acad Chir 89:394–399

44. Dick AC, Coulter P, Hainsworth AM, Boston VE, Potts SR (1998) A comparative study of the analgesia requirements following laparoscopic and open fundoplication in children. J Laparoendosc Adv Surg Tech A 8:425–429

45. Allal H, Captier G, Lopez M, Forgues D, Galifer R (2001) Evaluation of 142 consecutive laparoscopic fundoplications in children: effects of the learning curve and technical choice. J Pediatr Surg 36:921–926

46. Fonkalsrud EW, Bustorff-Silva J, Perez CA, et al (1999) Antireflux surgery in children under 3 months of age. J Pediatr Surg 34:527–531

47. Fung KP, Rubin S, Scott RB (1990) Gastric volvulus complicating Nissen fundoplication. J Pediatr Surg 25:1242–1243

48. Lobe TE, Schropp KP, Lunsford K (1993) Laparoscopic Nissen fundoplication in childhood. J Pediatr Surg 28:358–361

49. Hui TT, Fass SM, Giurgiu DI, Iida A, Takagi S, Phillips EH (2000) Gastroesophageal disease and nausea: does fundoplication help or hurt? Arch Surg 135:545–549

50. Pessaux P, Arnaud JP, Ghavami B, et al (2000) Laparoscopic antireflux surgery: comparative study of Nissen, Nissen-Rosetti, and Toupet fundoplication. Societe francaise de chirurgie laparoscopique. Surg Endosc 14:1024–1027

51. Meehan J, Georgeson KE (1997) The learning curve associated with laparoscopic antireflux surgery in infants and children. J Pediatr Surg 32:426–429

52. Dalla Vecchia LK, Grosfeld JL, West KW, et al (1997) Re-operation after Nissen fundoplication in children with gastroesophageal reflux: experience with 130 patients. Ann Surg 226:315–321

53. Lobe TE (1993) Laparoscopic fundoplication. Semin Pediatr Surg 3:1978–1981

54. Luks FI, Logan J, Breuer CK, Kurkchubasche AG, et al (1999) Cost-effectiveness of laparoscopy in children. Arch Pediatr Adolesc Med 153:965–968

55. Georgeson KE (1998) Laparoscopic fundoplication and gastrostomy. Semin Laparosc Surg 5:25–30

56. Hopkins MA, Stringel G (1999) Laparoscopic Nissen fundoplication in children: a single surgeon's experience. JSLS 3:261–266

57. Wadie GM, Lobe TE (2002) GERD in neurologically impaired children, the role of the gastrostomy tube. Semin Lap Surg 9:180–189

Chapter 36

Results and Follow-up Antireflux Surgery in Neurologically Impaired Children

36

Ashwin Pimpalwar · Azad Najmaldin

Contents

36.1
Introduction

Gastroesophageal reflux (GER) is a common and relatively benign condition in children. Most patients recover during the first few years of life. In older children, however, GER is less likely to resolve spontaneously. Neurologically impaired (NI) children have an increased incidence of GER. The exact etiology is not clear. Opinions suggest that the high incidence of GER in NI children is multifactorial in origin, including central nervous system factors, esophageal dysmotility [1], impaired lower esophageal pressure [2], increased intraabdominal pressure, from spasticity, kyphoscoliosis, frequent seizures, and frequent chest infections [3], delayed gastric emptying [4], and probably positional effects from the time spent in bed or wheelchair [5].

In NI children, the symptoms and signs of GER are difficult to interpret, and delayed diagnosis is common. Difficulty with feeds and swallowing, retching, vomiting, signs of discomfort, and failure to thrive are common features for both advanced GER and neurological disease. Compared with neurologically normal (NN) children, NI children have an increased incidence of GER-related complications. Esophagitis is seen in 66–100% of NI [6, 7], hiatus hernia in 51% [5], and respiratory problems requiring hospitalization 35–85% [5–7]. Barrett's changes and esophageal stricture are also common [9–11]. In general, diagnostic studies in this group of patients are the same as for the NN children. However, modifications may be required, depending on the circumstances, severity of symptoms, and whether

there are signs of complications. Assessment of swallowing, esophageal motility, manometry, and gastric emptying are important diagnostic and prognostic measures in NI children.

Medical treatment remains the therapy of choice for as long as the patients remain asymptomatic and free of complications. However, cost is becoming an increasingly important consideration, and long-term therapy may prove more expensive than surgery. Surgical treatment is indicated for children in whom medical therapy fails or complications develop. In general, surgery is safe and effective. Several antireflux procedures exist, namely Nissen's fundoplication, Thal procedure, Hill's repair, Toupet procedure, and Belsey repair. Although there is no convincing evidence to suggest that one procedure is superior to others, the Nissen's fundoplication, despite its drawbacks, remains the most commonly performed procedure for children [12].

Children with neurological impairment constitute a large proportion of the patients who require surgery for GER [12]. Conventional open antireflux procedures in such patients are known to be associated with significant mortality and morbidity [13, 14]. Up to 46% may suffer from recurrent reflux, wrap dysfunction, or stomach herniation into the chest, and the incidence of reoperation is high [12–15]. Despite the relatively high complication rates associated with conventional open surgery 70–85% of patients' family and care givers are satisfied with the results of surgery, making antireflux surgery a worthwhile exercise in NI children who are resistant to conservative medical therapy [12–16].

Laparoscopic Nissen fundoplication was first performed in adults by Dallemagne et al. [17] in 1991. Sporadic reports and short series from pediatric centers soon followed [18–21].

More recent published large series indicate that postoperative analgesia requirements, time to feed, hospital stay, and return to normal activities are shorter in children with laparoscopic antireflux surgery compared to open techniques; the complication rates are similar or lower in laparoscopy patients; and short- and intermediate-term results appear comparable [22–28]. Although the published data are flawed by the absence of controlled randomized studies, and consequently historical and retrospective data have been used for comparison, laparoscopic antireflux surgery in children is fast becoming, as in adult practice, the technique of choice in the surgical management of GER.

Given the complex presentation of NI children with GER and the fact that co-existent illness and complications which are common in these children may contribute to the symptoms and progress of GER, any pre- and postoperative assessment is bound to be difficult to conduct and evaluate.

36.2
Results and Follow-up in Antireflux Surgery

Neurological status is the major predictive factor of success or failure of antireflux surgery in children. Dedinsky et al. [19] reported the results of 429 open technique Nissen's fundoplications in children, 297 of whom were NI. This group accounted for all four of the postoperative deaths, 24 of 28 wrap herniations into chest, and most of the re-operations. Pearl et al. [14] reported 234 children who had open technique antireflux surgery (81 NN, 153 NI). The failure rate was 28% in NI and 6% NN; mortality 9% NI and 1% NN, and NI underwent re-operation four times more frequently than NN children.

In 1995, we first reported the feasibility, safety, and success of laparoscopic Nissen fundoplication with or without gastrostomy in a group of 15 NI children [30]. Bufo et al. [30] reported a comparative study of 212 children who had either laparoscopic or open Nissen fundoplication (67% NI children proportionately distributed between the two groups). There was no statistically significant difference in the early complication rates between the two groups, but significantly lower late complication rates were detected in the laparoscopy group. Early and late complication rates after laparoscopic procedures were 41% in NI and 17% NN, and 13% in NI and 0% NN, respectively.

As for open surgery, data on functional assessment following laparoscopic antireflux surgery, especially in NI children, is scarce. Van der Zee et al. [31] reported 15 NI children who had laparoscopic Thal fundoplication (13 had feeding gastrostomy). All of their patients underwent postoperative pH studies. Two children showed silent reflux, but none had symptomatic reflux. Tovar et al. [32] reported 20 postoperative pH studies in 27 children (11 NI) who had laparoscopic Nissen. The reflux index decreased from $20.2\pm20\%$ to normal in all but four children, who were later found to have wrap disruption, and two of these were NI. However, both of these functional studies involved short-term follow-up. Conversion to an open procedure during laparoscopic fundoplication has been reported in 0% to 8% of children [23, 25, 32, 33]. Learning curve, appropriate instru-

mentation and assistance, previous surgery, skilled anesthesia, and unusual anatomy are the major predictive factors of success or failure with laparoscopy, especially in NI patients. In our unit including 54 NI children, so far the nonpredicted conversion rates for laparoscopic Nissen fundoplication is 0% NN (unpublished data) and 2% NI (one child with perforated esophagus) [34]. In addition, we have had two (3.5%) further NI children who had a predicted conversion (one small child with major neurological impairment, Fallott's tetralogy, and hepatomegaly; another because of faulty camera and lack of adequate assistance). Like previous authors [35] we have found that previous abdominal surgery, minor or major (15% in our series) is not a contraindication for laparoscopic antireflux surgery.

In NI children, postoperative pain is difficult to assess and evaluate. In a comparative analysis of the analgesia requirements of 20 laparoscopic versus 20 open fundoplication procedures, Dick et al. [26] reported that the total amount of morphine analgesia required was similar for the two groups. However, the period for which analgesia was required was significantly less in the laparoscopic group, yet the requirement for morphine during the first 24 h was greater in the laparoscopic group. We routinely provide either epidural or morphine IV infusion for all laparoscopic fundoplication in both NI and NN children for the first 12–18 h. This is followed by regular nonsteroidal analgesia orally, rectally, or via the gastrostomy for a further 1 or 2 days.

It has been suggested that delayed gastric emptying contributes significantly to the high incidence of GER in NI children, as does operative failure [4, 36, 37]. However, the issue of concomitant pyloroplasty at the time of fundoplication remains controversial. Sampson et al. [38] reported 61 combined laparoscopic fundoplication and pyloroplasty in patients who had GER associated with delayed gastric emptying. Four patients (7%) had to be converted to an open procedure for technical reasons, while the remaining 57 recovered uneventfully with clinical resolution of both reflux and delayed gastric emptying. On the other hand, Maxon et al. [39] reported a series of 40 NI children with delayed gastric emptying. Nineteen (48%) of them did not receive a drainage procedure. There was no difference in the incidence of recurrent symptoms, re-admissions, or re-operations between these groups. However, those who had a drainage procedure developed significantly higher pos-operative complication rates. Others have reported similar experiences [40, 41]. In our series of 54 NI patients, six had delayed gastric emptying on contrast radiology, none received a drainage procedure, yet all improved initially following laparoscopic Nissen fundoplication with gastrostomy.

During the follow-up (3 months–8.5 years), only two children have shown recurrent and/or persistent symptoms. It would, however, seem reasonable to suggest that pyloroplasty should be considered as a secondary procedure for those who become or remain symptomatic after fundoplication and who demonstrate convincing signs of delayed gastric emptying on investigations.

Peri-operative death and complications have occurred with both conventionally and laparoscopically performed fundoplications, with the incidence rates being higher in NI compared to NN children [13, 14, 20, 42]. Van de Zee et al. [43] reported 53 laparoscopic Thal procedures (28 NI) over a 35-month period. There were no deaths but two re-operations, one for major bleeding and the other for a tight wrap. Montupet et al. [44] reported 125 laparoscopic Toupet's fundoplications from three centers over a 5-year period. There were no deaths; however, their re-operation rate was 4% (three pneumothorax, one bleeding, and one sutured NGT). Meehan and Georgeson [23] reported one (0.7%) death and 11 (7.4%) complications in a series of 160 Nissen fundoplication. Esposito et al. [24] reported 289 Nissen and Toupet laparoscopic fundoplications for three different centers over a 6-year period. They had no deaths; however, there were 6% major perioperative complications (six pneumothorax, three perforated esophagus, two perforated stomach, one pericardial perforation, five hernia epiploica). Those authors concluded that their results for the laparoscopic technique are better than or comparable to traditional open fundoplication. In a series of 54 NI Children, we had one perforated esophagus (2%), but no other laparoscopic complications or early re-operation and no deaths.

Recurrent symptoms/reflux affect 10–19% of NI children treated conventionally [12–14, 42, 45–48]. Similar figures have been quoted for laparoscopic procedures [23, 24, 43]. Our results appear to be similar (16%). Re-operation for recurrent symptoms, disrupted fundoplication, and herniation into the chest affect 6–19% of the NI children treated conventionally [12–14, 29, 42]. Information about intermediate- and long-term outcomes of laparoscopic fundoplication in NI children are not available. Rothenberg reported 3% re-operation in a series of 220 infants and children (12% NI) over a 4-year period for Nissen fundoplication [25], Van Der Zee and Bax 4% in 100 (mixture of NI and NN) over a 6-year period for the Thal procedure [49], and Esposito et al. [24] 0.7% in 289 children (no mention of NI) who had Nissen and Toupet procedures (51% and 49%, respectively). These figures and our experience of 1 in 54 (2%) re-operation for a symptomatic recurrent hiatus hernia appear to be well within the lines of previously reported studies on laparoscopic fundoplication in general, and much better than previously mentioned figures for open surgery.

Postoperative intestinal obstruction, which is not a neurological status-specific complication, has been reported in 2.6–6.5% of children treated conventionally

[12, 14, 17]. In our experience, there has been no incidence of intestinal obstruction. Others have shown similar observations [23–25, 43, 44].

36.3
Personal Experience

Although conventional open fundoplication with or without gastrostomy is commonly performed in children, its application in NI children can be a major challenge and is associated with significant mortality and morbidity [12, 13].

Fixed limb contracture and kyphoscoliosis that may displace the internal organs severely restricts access to the operating field. The minimal invasive and remote manipulative nature of laparoscopy on the other hand allows for easier access, better visualization, and reduced trauma of surgery. There is no absolute contraindication for laparoscopic antireflux surgery in NI children. The limitations are essentially related to the experience of the surgeon and availability of instruments. Failure due to anesthetic difficulties is exceedingly rare [22–27]. However, awareness of the differences in access and risks between NI and NN children is important. Maximum surgical ability and safety are achieved if the following are considered carefully before each laparoscopic cannula is inserted: the size of the child; severity of limb, chest, and spine deformity; shape of the subphrenic space (use of pre-operative x-ray and/or contrast GI studies); and presence of a palpable liver, spleen, or aorta. At surgery, displaced anatomical landmarks are assessed and caution is advised during manipulation and dissection.

Between 1993 and 2001, 54 NI children underwent laparoscopic Nissen's fundoplication (NF), all performed by one surgeon. The patient weight was 2.7–42 kg. Hiatus hernia was present in 26%, delayed gastric emptying on contrast study was 11%, and abdominal scar from previous surgery was 15%. Forty-seven patients had concomitant insertion of gastrostomy. The average operating time for fundoplication was 2.2 h (range 1.05–3 h). The procedure was converted to an open procedure in three patients (two predicted – major cardiac problem and camera fault, one nonpredicted – perforation of esophagus). There was no bleeding, or anesthetic or operative complications. For the majority of patients the hospital stay ranged from 3–7 days (depending on whether the patient had a gastrostomy or not). Nine patients stayed longer for social reasons. One child developed food bolus obstruction three days after operation. During follow-up (median 5.8 years, range 0.3–8.6 years), most patients had improved clinically, but 17% (nine children) had persistent or recurrent retching, chest infection, or vomiting. Contrast and pH study or endoscopy in the latter group showed minor reflux in three patients and recurrent hiatus hernia in one patient. So far, only one child has required re-operation. Six have died from their background conditions.

36.4
Summary

Children with neurological impairment account for a large proportion of the patients who suffer from GER. Although in NI children GER is unlikely to resolve spontaneously, conservative measures remain the therapy of choice in such patients and surgical treatment (antireflux procedure) is indicated for children in whom medical therapy fails or complications develop. These children have a high incidence of GER complications. This and the fact that NI patients are difficult to assess make the outcome of antireflux surgery in NI children difficult to measure. Several antireflux procedures exist, and none appear superior to others. Conventional open antireflux procedures are associated with significant mortality and morbidity. In spite of this, the majority of patients' family and caregivers are satisfied with the results of surgery, making antireflux procedures a worthwhile exercise in NI children who are resistant to conservative therapy. Laparoscopic approach is becoming increasingly popular. Compared with historical data for the open technique, laparoscopic antireflux procedures in NI children have lower mortality and morbidity rates but similar intermediate and long-term results.

References

1. Cucchiara S, Staiano A, Di Lorenzo C, D'Ambrosio R, Andreotti MR, Prato M, De Filippo P, Auricchio S (1986) Esophageal motor abnormalities in children with gastroesophageal reflux and peptic esophagitis. J Pediatr 108(6):907–910
2. Vane DW, Shiffler M, Grosfeld JL, Hall P, Angelides A, Weber TR, Fitzgerald JF (1982) Reduced lower esophageal sphincter (LES) pressure after acute and chronic brain injury. J Pediatr Surg 17(6):960–964
3. Kassen NY, Groen JJ, Fraenkel M (1965) Spinal deformities and oesophageal hiatus hernia. Lancet 1:887–889
4. Hillemeier AC, Grill BB, McCallum R, Gryboski J (1983) Esophageal and gastric motor abnormalities in gastroesophageal reflux during infancy. Gastroenterology 84(4):741–746
5. Guttman FM (1972) On the incidence of hiatal hernia in infants. Pediatrics 50(2):325–328
6. Byrne WJ, Campbell M, Ashcraft E, et al. (1983) A diagnostic approach to vomiting in severely retarded patients. Am J Dis Child 137:259–262
7. Bohmer CJM, Niezen-de Boer MC, Klinkenberg-Knol EC, et al. (1997) Gastroesophageal reflux disease in intellectually disabled individuals: leads for diagnosis and the effect of omeprazole therapy. Am J Gastroenterol 92:1475–1479
8. Spitz L (1982) Surgical treatment of gastroesophageal reflux in severely mentally retarded children. J R Soc Med 75:525–529
9. Vane DW, Harmel RP Jr, King DR, et al. (1985) The effectiveness of Nissen fundoplication in neurologically impaired children with gastroesophageal reflux. Surgery 98:662–666
10. Wilkinson ID, Dudgeon DL, Sondheimer JM (1981) A comparison of medical and surgical treatment of gastroesophageal reflux in severely retarded children. J Pediatr 99:202–205

11. Roberts IM, Curtis RL, Madara JL (1986) Gastroesophageal reflux and Barrett's esophagus in developmentally disabled patients. Am J Gastroenterol 81:519–523
12. Fonkalsrud EW, Ashcraft KW, Coran AG, Ellis DG, Grosfeld JL, Tunell WP, Weber TR (1998) Surgical treatment of gastroesophageal reflux in children: a combined hospital study of 7467 patients. Pediatrics 101(3 Pt 1):419–422
13. Spitz L, Roth K, Kiely EM, et al (1993) Operation for gastroesophageal reflux associated with severe mental retardation. Arch Dis Child 68:347–351
14. Pearl RH, Robie DK, Ein SH, et al (1990) Complications of gastro-esophageal antireflux surgery in neurologically impaired versus neurologically normal children. J Pediatr Surg 25:1169–1173
15. Martinez DA, Ginn-Pease ME, Caniano DA (1992) Sequellae of antireflux surgery in profoundly disabled children. J Pediatr Surg 27:267–273
16. O'Neill JK, O'Neill PJ, Goth-Owens T, et al (1996) Care-giver evaluation of anti-gastroesophageal reflux procedures in neurologically impaired children: What is the real-life outcome? J Pediatr Surg 31:375–380
17. Dallemagne B, Weerts JM, Jehaes C, Markiewicz S, Lombard R (1991) Laparoscopic Nissen fundoplication: preliminary report. Surg Laparosc Endosc 1(3):138–143
18. Georgeson KE (1993) Laparoscopic surgery for gastroesophageal reflux in 15 infants and children. Presented at the 8th International Paediatric Congress, Berlin, Germany
19. Lobe TE, Schropp KP, Lunsford K (1993) Laparoscopic Nissen fundoplication in childhood. J Pediatr Surg 28:358–361
20. Schier F, Waldschmidt J (1994) Laparoscopic fundoplication in a child. Eur J Pediatr Surg 4(6):338–340
21. Humphrey GM, Najmaldin AS (1995) Laparoscopic Nissen fundoplication in disabled infants and children. Presented at the 42nd Annual International Congress of the British Association of Paediatric Surgeons Sheffield, England, July, 1996
22. Humphrey GM, Najmaldin AS (1996) Laparoscopic Nissen fundoplication in disabled infants and children. J Pediatr Surg 31(4):596–599
23. Meehan JJ, Georgeson KE (1996) Laparoscopic fundoplication in infants and children. Surg Endosc 10(12):1154–1157
24. Esposito C, Montupet P, Amici G, Desruelle P (2000) Complications of laparoscopic antireflux surgery in childhood. Surg Endosc 14(7):622–624
25. Rothenberg SS (1998) Experience with 220 consecutive laparoscopic Nissen fundoplications in infants and children. J Pediatr Surg 33(2):274–278
26. Dick AC, Coulter P, Hainsworth AM, Boston VE, Potts SR (1998) A comparative study of the analgesia requirements following laparoscopic and open fundoplication in children. J Laparoendosc Adv Surg Tech 8:425–429
27. Rowney DA, Aldridge LM (2000) Laparoscopic fundoplication in children: anaesthetic experience of 51 cases. Paediatr Anaesth 10(3):291–296
28. Allal H. Captier G, Lopez M (2001) Evaluation of 142 consecutive laparoscopic fundoplications in children: effects of the learning curve and technical choice. J Pediatr Surg 36(6):921–926
29. Dedinsky GK, Vane DW, Black T, Turner MK, West KW, Grosfeld JL (1987) Complications and reoperation after Nissen fundoplication in childhood. Am J Surg 153(2):177–183
30. Bufo AI, Chen MK, Lobe TE, et al (1997) Laparoscopic fundoplication in children: a superior technique. Pediatr Endosurg Innovative Tech 1:71–76
31. Van der Zee DC, Bax NM (1996) Laparoscopic Thal fundoplication in mentally retarded children. Surg Endosc 10(6):659–661
32. Tovar JA, Olivares P, Diaz M, Pace RA, Prieto G, Molina M (1998) Functional results of laparoscopic fundoplication in children. J Pediatr Gastroenterol Nutr 26(4):429–431
33. Dick AC, Potts SR (1999) Laparoscopic fundoplication in children–an audit of fifty cases. Eur J Pediatr Surg 9(5):286–288
34. Pimpalwar A, Najmaldin A (2002) Results of laparoscopic antireflux procedures in neurologically impaired children. Semin Laparosc Surg 9(3):190–196

35. Liu DC, Flattmann GJ, Karam MT, Siegrist BI, Loe WA Jr, Hill CB (2000) Laparoscopic fundoplication in children with previous abdominal surgery. J Pediatr Surg 35(2):334–337
36. Fonkalsrud EW, Ament ME (1996) Gastroesophageal reflux in childhood. Curr Probl Surg 33:10–70
37. Papaila IG, Wilmot D, Grosfeld JL, et al (1989) Increased incidence of delayed gastric emptying in children with gastroesophageal reflux. Arch Surg 124:933–936
38. Sampson LK, Georgeson KE, Royal SA (1998) Laparoscopic gastric antroplasty in children with delayed gastric emptying and gastroesophageal reflux. J Pediatr Surg 33(2):282–285
39. Maxson RT, Harp S, Jackson RI, et al (1994) Delayed gastric emptying in neurologically impaired children with gastroesophageal reflux: The role of pyloroplasty. J Pediatr Surg 29:726–729
40. Campbell JR, Gilchrist BF, Harrison MW (1989) Pyloroplasty in association with Nissen fundoplication in children with neurologic disorders. J Pediatr Surg 24:375–377
41. Brown RA, Wynchank S, Rode H, et al (1997) Is a gastric drainage procedure necessary at the time of antireflux surgery? J Pediatr Gastroenterol Nutr 25:377–380
42. Rice H, Seashore JH, Touloukian RJ (1991) Evaluation of Nissen fundoplication in neurologically impaired children. J Pediatr Surg 26(6):697–701
43. Van der Zee DC, Bax NMA (1999) Laparoscopic Thal fundoplication in infants and children. In: Bax NM et al (eds) Endoscopic surgery in children. Springer, Berlin Heidelberg New York, pp 174–183
44. Montupet P, Cargill G, Valla JS (1999) Laparascopic Toupet fundoplication. In: Bax NM et al (eds) Endoscopic surgery in children. Springer, Berlin Heidelberg New York, pp 184–190
45. Fung KP, Seagram G, Pasieka J, Trevenen C, Machida H, Scott B (1990) Investigation and outcome of 121 infants and children requiring Nissen fundoplication for the management of gastroesophageal reflux. Clin Invest Med 13(5):237–246
46. Wheatley MJ, Wesley JR, Tkach DM, Coran AG (1991) Long-term follow-up of brain-damaged children requiring feeding gastrostomy: should an antireflux procedure always be performed? J Pediatr Surg 26(3):301–304; discussion 304–305
47. Martinez DA, Ginn-Pease ME, Caniano DA (1992) Sequelae of antireflux surgery in profoundly disabled children. J Pediatr Surg 27(2):267–271; discussion 271–273
48. Chang JHT, Coln CD, Stricland AD, et al (1987) Surgical management of gastroesophageal reflux in severely mentally retarded children. J Ment Defic Res 31:1–7
49. Van der Zee DC, Bax NM, Ure BM (2000) Laparoscopic refundoplication in children. Surg Endosc 14(12):1103–1104

Subject Index